I0064570

Endocrinology and Metabolism

Endocrinology and Metabolism

Edited by **Joy Foster**

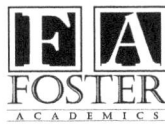

FOSTER
ACADEMICS

New Jersey

Published by Foster Academics,
61 Van Reypen Street,
Jersey City, NJ 07306, USA
www.fosteracademics.com

Endocrinology and Metabolism
Edited by Joy Foster

© 2016 Foster Academics

International Standard Book Number: 978-1-63242-467-9 (Hardback)

This book contains information obtained from authentic and highly regarded sources. Copyright for all individual chapters remain with the respective authors as indicated. All chapters are published with permission under the Creative Commons Attribution License or equivalent. A wide variety of references are listed. Permission and sources are indicated; for detailed attributions, please refer to the permissions page and list of contributors. Reasonable efforts have been made to publish reliable data and information, but the authors, editors and publisher cannot assume any responsibility for the validity of all materials or the consequences of their use.

The publisher's policy is to use permanent paper from mills that operate a sustainable forestry policy. Furthermore, the publisher ensures that the text paper and cover boards used have met acceptable environmental accreditation standards.

Trademark Notice: Registered trademark of products or corporate names are used only for explanation and identification without intent to infringe.

Printed in the United States of America.

Contents

Preface

Endocrinology is the branch of medicine that deals with the endocrine system. This system consists of various glands present in all parts of the body. It focuses on all the functions and behavioral activities performed by hormones such as sleep digestion, mood, excretion, stress, reproduction, lactation, movement, etc. Metabolism is the set of life-sustaining activities occurring within the cells of the living organisms. It is a sub-field of endocrinology. This book includes some of the vital pieces of work being conducted across the world, on various topics related to endocrinology and metabolism. It aims to shed light on some of the unexplored aspects related to these fields. Those in search of information to further their knowledge will be greatly assisted by it. This text will serve as a valuable source of reference for endocrinologists, academicians and students.

This book is a result of research of several months to collate the most relevant data in the field.

When I was approached with the idea of this book and the proposal to edit it, I was overwhelmed. It gave me an opportunity to reach out to all those who share a common interest with me in this field. I had 3 main parameters for editing this text:

1. Accuracy – The data and information provided in this book should be up-to-date and valuable to the readers.
2. Structure – The data must be presented in a structured format for easy understanding and better grasping of the readers.
3. Universal Approach – This book not only targets students but also experts and innovators in the field, thus my aim was to present topics which are of use to all.

Thus, it took me a couple of months to finish the editing of this book.

I would like to make a special mention of my publisher who considered me worthy of this opportunity and also supported me throughout the editing process. I would also like to thank the editing team at the back-end who extended their help whenever required.

Editor

The Effects of Amino Acid Nutritional Deficiency on the Expression of Protein Metabolism-Related Genes in the Mammary Gland and Muscle Tissues of Lactating Mice

Xueyan Lin*, Miaomiao Wu*, Guimei Liu, Yun Wang, Qiuling Hou, Kerong Shi, Zhonghua Wang#

College of Animal Science and Technology, Shandong Agricultural University, Tai'an, China
Email: linxueyan@sdau.edu.cn, #zhwang@sdau.edu.cn

Abstract

The mammary gland tissue exhibits a series of responses that are different from those of muscle and other peripheral tissues under amino acid deficiency. So, this present study was designed to investigate the effects of amino acid nutritional deficiency on the expression of protein metabolism-related genes in the mammary gland and muscle tissues of lactating mice. A total of 60 postpartum, lactating Kunming white mice were selected and randomly divided into 5 groups; each group contained 12 mice. Group A was the control group. The mice in group A were maintained on a normal diet after the initiation of lactation. Group B (starved) was given normal saline via intragastric administration. Group C (energy) was given glucose solution via intragastric administration. Groups D and E received a sodium caseinate solution via intragastric administration, which provided 0.5 g protein/d and 1.5 g protein/d, respectively. The results showed the following. 1) When the mice were exposed to nutritional stress caused by dietary amino acid deficiency, the β-casein mRNA expression level was increased in the mammary gland tissue. The increase in β-casein expression was the most significant in the energy-supplemented group, followed by the starved group ($P < 0.01$). In addition, the expression level of myosin heavy chain 2A (MHC2a) mRNA was markedly reduced in the muscle tissue ($P < 0.05$). 2) Different dietary treatments significantly affected the mRNA expression of ubiquitin system enzymes such as PolyUbC, $E2_{14k}$ and C2 ($P < 0.01$). The expression levels of the enzymes were upregulated. 3) The blood level of insulin-like growth factor 1 (IGF-1) was significantly decreased in the treatment groups ($P < 0.01$). 4) The phosphorylation level of the p70S6 kinase (p70S6K) was markedly enhanced in the mammary gland tissues collected from the treatment groups ($P < 0.05$). 5) The phosphorylation level of

---

*The authors have equal contribution to this article.
#Corresponding author.

p70S6K was elevated in the muscle tissues collected from the treatment groups. However, the magnitude of the increase was far smaller compared to that in the mammary gland tissues.

Keywords

Amino Acid Nutritional Deficiency, Mammary Gland Tissue, Muscle Tissue, Protein Metabolism

---

1. Introduction

Under amino acid deficiency, mammary gland tissue exhibits a series of responses that are different from those of muscle and other peripheral tissues. The rate of amino acid uptake from the blood by the mammary gland tissue increases to meet the needs of milk protein synthesis. In contrast, muscle and other tissues degrade proteins and release the deposited amino acids into the blood circulation. Therefore, lactation takes precedence over maintenance metabolism in amino acid and nutrient distribution in the body.

The reasons behind the different responses of mammary gland and muscle tissues are not yet clear. However, some or all of the following aspects may be involved. 1) The types of proteins synthesized by mammary gland and muscle tissues are different. Mammary epithelial cells synthesize exocrine proteins, which are secreted into the extracellular space soon after being synthesized and then are no longer under the cells' control. Muscle cells synthesize their own structural proteins, which are deposited in the cells and can be degraded. 2) The responses of mammary gland and muscle tissues to changes in humoral signals are different. Amino acid deficiency induces changes in the concentrations of amino acids and related hormones in body fluids. The mechanisms of signal reception or sensitivities to the signals are different between mammary gland tissue and muscle tissue, resulting in differences in metabolism. 3) The metabolic regulatory mechanisms are different between the cells of mammary gland and muscle tissues. Both mammary epithelial cells and muscle cells are highly differentiated, but the natures of the cell types are very different. Therefore, differences may exist between the metabolic regulatory mechanisms of the cell types, leading to different responses of the two types of tissues to amino acid deficiency (Bauman *et al.*, 2000; Vernon *et al.*, 1998) [1] [2]. This study was designed to investigate the effects of amino acid nutritional deficiency on the expression of protein metabolism-related genes in the mammary gland and muscle tissues of lactating mice.

2. Materials and Methods

2.1. Experimental Materials

Clean grade Kunming white mice were purchased from Shandong Taibang Biological Products Co. Ltd., Taian City, China. Trizol reagent was purchased from Invitrogen (Carlsbad, CA, USA). The reverse transcription kit (Code: DRR037A) and real time polymerase chain reaction (PCR) kit (Code: DRR420A) were purchased from TaKaRa Co., Ltd. The primers were purchased from TaKaRa Bio., Inc. The mammalian target of rapamycin (mTOR) antibody (rabbit), phospho-mTOR (P-mTOR) antibody (rabbit), p70S6 kinase (p70S6k) antibody (rabbit), phospho-p70S6k (P-p70S6k) antibody (rabbit), eukaryotic translation initiation factor 4E-binding protein 1 (4EBP1) antibody (rabbit) and phosphor-4EBP1 (P-4EBP1) antibody (rabbit) were all purchased from Cell Signaling Technology, Inc. The cationic amino acid transporter 1 (CAT1) antibody (rabbit) and ASC amino-acid transporter 2 (ASCT2) antibody (rabbit) were purchased from Abcam plc.

2.2. Experimental Design

A total of 55 male and 110 female Kunming white mice were selected for the present study. The male and female mice were similar in age (measured in days) and body size. The male mice were housed singly while the female mice were housed together (3 female mice per cage) until the mice reached breeding age (male mice at approximately 10 weeks of age and the females at approximately 8 weeks of age). Healthy and active mice were selected and bred at a male-female mating ratio of 1:2. Upon confirmation of breeding success (approximately two weeks after mating), the male mice were removed. The female mice with confirmed pregnancies were housed singly until they gave birth. Starting on the first day of lactation, the female mice were subjected to 1 of the 5 different types of treatment described below. Each treatment group contained 12 mice.

Group 1 (control) was fed the normal diet after the initiation of lactation. Group 2 (starved) was given intragastric administrations of 0.5 mL of normal saline at 7:00 and 19:00 on the first day of lactation and at 7:00 the following day (a total of 3 times). Group 3 (energy) received intragastric administrations of glucose solution (1.1 g/mL) at 7:00, 11:00, 15:00, 19:00 and 23:00 on the first day of lactation and at 7:00, 11:00 and 15:00 the next day (a total of 8 times). The amount of energy provided by the glucose solution was 94.325 KJ/d, which met the energy needs of the mice. Group 4 (low Pro.) received intragastric administrations of sodium caseinate solution (0.55 g/ml) at 7:00 on the first day of lactation and at 7:00 the next day (a total of 2 times). The treatment provided 0.5 g of protein per day, which was insufficient for the protein needs of the mice. Group 5 (high Pro.) received intragastric administrations of sodium caseinate solution (0.55 g/mL) at 7:00, 14:00 and 21:00 on the first day of lactation and at 7:00 and 14:00 the next day (a total of 5 times), which provided a total of 1.5 g protein per day. The mice in all of the treatment groups were fasted but allowed free access to drinking water. The mice were sacrificed at 36 h after the first intragastric administration (shandong agriculture university animal care and use committee approved this experiment).

2.3. Sample Collection and Measurement Methods

2.3.1. Collection and Examination of Blood Samples
The mice in all of the treatment groups were caused death by cervical dislocation. Blood samples were collected from the mice, allowed to settle for approximately 30 min at 4°C and then centrifuged at 5000 rpm for 20 min at 4°C. The supernatants were collected, transferred to labeled centrifuge tubes, and stored at −80°C. The biochemical indices of the blood samples were examined for blood glucose, insulin, insulin-like growth factor 1 (IGF-1), growth hormone (GH) and prolactin (PRL). The hormone indices in the blood samples were analyzed by radioimmunoassay. The blood glucose levels were determined using an automatic biochemistry analyzer.

2.3.2. Collection and Examination of the Tissue Samples
After the blood samples were collected from the mice, a ventral midline skin incision was made, and mouse mammary gland tissue in the inguinal region was collected using forceps. In addition, skin was stripped from the hind limbs of the mice, and muscle tissue was collected. The tissue samples were placed into numbered 1.5 mL centrifuge tubes and quickly stored at −80°C. The mRNA expression level of β-casein in the mammary gland tissue as well as those of α-actin, myosin heavy chain I (MHC I), MHC IIα, MHC IId/x, C2, 14-kDa ubiquitin-conjugating enzyme (E2$_{14k}$) and polyubiquitin-C (PolyUbC) in the muscle tissue were determined. The phosphorylation levels of mTOR, p70S6k and 4EBP1 and the protein expression levels of ASCT2 and CAT1 were measured in both types of tissues.

2.3.3. Determination of the Levels of mRNA Expression in Mammary Gland and Muscle Tissues
In the experiments, glyceraldehyde 3-phosphate dehydrogenase (GAPDH) was utilized as an internal reference. Total RNA was extracted from mammary gland tissue and muscle tissue using the Trizol method. After the quality of the extracted RNA was verified, reverse transcription was conducted in an improved 20 μL reaction system using the PrimeScriptTMRT reagent kit (Perfect Real Time) purchased from TaKaRa Co., Ltd. (Code: DRR037A). The steps of the reverse transcription reaction were as follows: 37°C, 15 min; and 85°C, 5 sec, 1 cycle.

Fluorescence-based quantitative real-time PCR was performed using the SYBR Green I dye and the SYBR Premix Ex TaqTM (Perfect Real Time) kit purchased from Takara Biotechnology (Dalian) Co., Ltd. (Code: DRR420A). The PCR reaction was conducted on the Applied Biosystems® 7500 Real-Time PCR Instrument (USA). The total volume of the reaction was 20 μL. The sequences of the primers utilized in the PCR reactions are summarized in **Table 1**.

2.3.4. Determination of the Levels of Protein Expression in Mammary Gland and Muscle Tissues
Proteins were extracted from various tissue samples, and the concentrations of total protein were measured. The amount of protein to be loaded was calculated. Based on the calculated results, corresponding amounts of sample loading buffer and lysis buffer were added to the protein samples. The protein samples were then boiled in a denaturing instrument for 5 min and analyzed by sodium dodecyl sulfate polyacrylamide gel electrophoresis (SDS-PAGE) and western blot.

Table 1. Primer sequences for each gene.

Gene	Primers	Primer sequences (5' → 3')	Product size
GAPDH	Forward	AAGGTGGTGAAGCAGGCAT	244 bp
	Reverse	GGTCCAGGGTTTCTTACTCCT	
β-casein	Forward	TCACTCCAGCATCCAGTCACA	126 bp
	Reverse	GGCCCAAGAGATGGCACCA	
α-actin	Forward	GTGAGATTGTGCGCGACATC	156 bp
	Reverse	GGCAACGGAAACGCTCATT	
MHC I	Forward	ACAACCCCTACGATTATGCGT	100 bp
	Reverse	ACGTCAAAGGCACTATCCGTG	
MHC IIα	Forward	CGACAACTCGTCTCGCTTTG	187 bp
	Reverse	CATTTCGATCAGTTCTGGCTTCT	
MHCIId/x	Forward	CACCAGGCTGCTTTAGAGGAA	207 bp
	Reverse	CCTGCTCCTAATCTCAGCATCC	
PolyUbC	Forward	GGCATGCAGATCTTTGTGAA	265 bp
	Reverse	TCTTGCCTGTCAGGGTCTTC	
E2$_{14k}$	Forward	CAGAAGGGACACCCTTTGAA	306 bp
	Reverse	CAATGGCCGAAACTCTCTTC	
C2	Forward	CTTTATGCGCCAGGAGTGTT	301 bp
	Reverse	TTCATCCAAATTGCACTCCA	

2.4. Data Processing and Statistical Analysis

The experimental data were organized using Excel and subjected to univariate analysis of variance (ANOVA) using the SAS 9.0 software. P values less than 0.05 were considered statistically significant while p values less than 0.01 were considered to be statistically highly significant. All results obtained by statistical analysis were expressed using the mean and standard error.

3. Results

3.1. Effects of Different Dietary Treatments on mRNA Expression Levels in Mammary Gland and Muscle Tissues

As shown in **Table 2**, nutritional stress induced by diets deficient in amino acids significantly affected the expression of β-casein and MHC2α ($P < 0.01$, $P < 0.05$). The expression level of β-casein mRNA was enhanced in mammary gland tissues collected from the treatment groups. The most significant increase in β-casein mRNA expression was observed in mice supplied with only energy, followed by mice in the starved group ($P < 0.01$). β-casein mRNA expression was also elevated in the rest of the treatment groups. However, the differences were not statistically significant. The experimental treatments did not significantly affect the expression of α-actin mRNA in muscle tissue. However, a clear decreasing trend was detected, and the starved group exhibited the largest decrease in α-actin mRNA expression. In addition, the expression level of MHC2α mRNA was significantly reduced in the treatment groups ($P < 0.05$). There were no significant differences in MHC2α mRNA expression between the treatment groups.

3.2. Effects of Different Dietary Treatments on mRNA Expression of the Factors of the Ubiquitin System in Muscle Tissue

It can be observed from **Table 3** that different dietary treatments significantly affected the mRNA expression of

Table 2. Effect of treatment on the mRNA expression of different genes in mammary and muscle tissue.

	A	B	C	D	E	SEM	P
β-casein	150.04^{b}	230.36^{a}	257.85^{a}	156.92^{b}	165.86^{b}	18.16	<0.01
α-actin	1.53^{a}	1.11^{b}	1.33^{ab}	1.29^{ab}	1.40^{ab}	0.11	0.22
MHCI	0.05	0.03	0.04	0.04	0.04	0.01	0.38
MHC2α	0.19^{a}	0.13^{b}	0.13^{b}	0.13^{b}	0.13^{b}	0.01	0.03
MHC2d/X	0.24	0.21	0.30	0.29	0.32	0.03	0.22

Note: The experimental data are expressed using the mean and standard error of measurement (SEM). Different letters in superscript following the values in the same row of the table ((a), (b), (c)) indicate statistically significant differences ($P < 0.05$).

Table 3. mRNA level of UPP system genes in muscle tissue.

	A	B	C	D	E	SEM	P
PolyUbC	0.42^{c}	0.51^{bc}	0.62^{b}	0.59^{b}	0.76^{a}	0.04	<0.01
E2$_{14k}$	0.16^{b}	0.15^{b}	0.25^{a}	0.14^{b}	0.21^{ab}	0.02	<0.01
C2	0.02^{c}	0.04^{bc}	0.12^{a}	0.04^{bc}	0.06^{b}	0.01	<0.01

Note: The experimental data are expressed using the mean and SEM. Different letters in superscript following the values in the same row of the table ((a), (b), (c)) indicate statistically significant differences ($P < 0.05$).

the proteins in the ubiquitin system, including PolyUbC, E2$_{14k}$ and C2 ($P < 0.01$). Although significant differences existed between some of the treatment groups, the expression levels of PolyUbC, E2$_{14k}$ and C2 were all upregulated. Compared with mice from the starved group, the expression levels of E2$_{14k}$ and C2 mRNAs were highest in mice supplied with energy.

3.3. Effects of Different Dietary Treatments on the Levels of Hormones and Glucose in the Blood

Table 4 demonstrates that the blood level of IGF-1 was markedly decreased in the treatment groups in comparison with the normal control group ($P < 0.01$). However, the differences between the treatment groups were not statistically significant. The prolactin (PRL) content was decreased in the starved group but was elevated in the other treatment groups. Again, the differences between the treatment groups were not statistically significant.

3.4. Effects of Different Dietary Treatments on the Expression Levels of Factors of the mTOR Pathway and Amino Acid Carrier Proteins in Mammary Gland Tissue

Table 5 showed that the dietary treatments significantly affected the phosphorylation level of p70S6K in the casein synthesis pathway ($P < 0.05$). The phosphorylation level of p70S6K was elevated in all treatment groups. The magnitude of increase was more significant in starved mice and in mice supplied with only energy. The expression level of the Lys/Arg carrier protein CAT1 was increased in the mammary gland tissues collected from the treatment groups ($P < 0.05$). Compared with mice supplied with protein, the magnitude of increase was slightly smaller in the starved mice and in mice supplied with energy. The expression level of the Met carrier protein ASCT2 tended to be decreased. In addition, the phosphorylation levels of mTOR and 4EBP1 were enhanced in the treatment groups. However, the differences were not statistically significant.

3.5. Effects of Different Dietary Treatments on the Expression Levels of Factors of the mTOR Pathway and Amino Acid Carrier Proteins in Muscle Tissue

As shown in **Table 6**, the phosphorylation level of p70S6K, a downstream signaling molecule of the mTOR pathway, was enhanced in muscle tissues collected from mice in almost all treatment groups except the ones supplied with an insufficient amount of protein. However, the magnitude of increase was far smaller compared to that of the mammary gland tissues. In addition, the phosphorylation levels of mTOR and 4EBP1 tended to be

Table 4. Hormone and glucose levels in the blood.

	A	B	C	D	E	SEM	P
Insulin	21.31	13.57	41.06	53.96	38.58	13.44	0.23
IGF-1	102.84[a]	66.98[b]	46.48[b]	39.01[b]	47.10[b]	11.01	<0.01
GH	3.70	3.99	3.33	2.45	1.61	0.93	0.41
PRL	1.12[ab]	0.67[b]	1.91[ab]	1.90[ab]	3.50[a]	0.82	0.21
Glu	7.61	6.86	8.48	7.84	7.34	0.78	0.69

Note: The experimental data are expressed using the mean and SEM. Different letters in superscript following the values in the same row of the table ((a), (b), (c)) indicate statistically significant differences ($P < 0.05$).

Table 5. Protein expression of the mTOR pathway and amino acid transporter in mammary tissue.

	A	B	C	D	E	SEM	P
mTOR	1.00	0.77	0.75	0.77	0.93	0.09	0.26
4E	1.00	0.68	0.73	0.66	0.92	0.19	0.66
p70S6k	1.00	0.74	0.83	0.64	0.73	0.13	0.39
P-mTOR/mTOR	1.00	1.65	3.02	2.21	2.12	0.57	0.28
P-4E/4E	1.00	2.22	3.87	3.44	1.88	0.92	0.23
P-p70/p70	1.00[b]	1.75[a]	1.89[a]	1.58[ab]	1.39[ab]	0.20	0.04
ASCT2	1.00	0.67	0.72	0.68	0.79	0.15	0.57
CAT1	1.00[b]	1.17[ab]	1.22[ab]	1.51[a]	1.43[a]	0.10	0.03

Note: The experimental data are expressed using the mean and SEM. Different letters in superscript following the values in the same row of the table ((a), (b), (c)) indicate statistically significant differences ($P < 0.05$).

Table 6. Protein expression of the mTOR pathway and amino acid transporter in muscle tissue.

	A	B	C	D	E	SEM	P
mTOR	1.00	0.88	0.73	0.67	0.59	0.17	0.49
4E	1.00	0.83	0.79	0.88	0.86	0.18	0.72
p70	1.00	1.16	1.10	1.30	1.13	0.10	0.35
P-mTOR/mTOR	1.00	1.35	1.35	1.38	1.70	0.35	0.74
P-4E/4E	1.00[b]	1.09[ab]	1.11[ab]	1.26[a]	1.17[ab]	0.06	0.16
P-p70/p70	1.00[bc]	1.29[b]	1.80[a]	0.83[c]	1.09[bc]	0.14	<0.01
ASCT2	1.00[a]	0.74[b]	0.86[ab]	0.92[ab]	0.80[b]	0.05	0.04

Note: The experimental data are expressed using the mean and SEM. Different letters in superscript following the values in the same row of the table ((a), (b), (c)) indicate statistically significant differences ($P < 0.05$).

increased. The magnitude of increase was smaller compared with that of the mammary gland tissues. The expression level of the Met carrier protein ASCT2 was reduced in all of the treatment groups ($P < 0.05$), and the largest reduction was observed in the starved group.

The results show that when experiencing dietary amino acid deficiency, lactating mice enhance muscle tissue degradation to preferentially meet the needs of lactation. In mammary gland tissue, the amount of utilized amino acid transporters is elevated, the phosphorylation level of the mTOR pathway is enhanced and the total amount of proteins synthesized is increased. In muscle tissue, the protein phosphorylation level is also increased. However, the amount of utilized amino acid transporters is reduced, the total amount of proteins synthesized is decreased, and protein degradation is enhanced.

Dietary amino acids and energy affect the activity of the ubiquitin-proteasome pathway, which is responsible for muscle tissue degradation. Adequate dietary amino acids and energy may enhance the activity of the pathway.

Hormones significantly affect the protein metabolism in mammary gland and muscle tissues. Among the hormones, the effect of insulin-like growth factors is especially remarkable.

4. Discussion

4.1. Changes in Specialized Proteins and Expression of the Ubiquitin System in Mammary Gland and Muscle Tissues

The mammary gland displays the highest level of differentiation and the strongest metabolic activity throughout the lactating period [1]. The mammary gland is also one of the two types of tissues that utilize most of the nutrients in the maternal body. As the lactation period starts, the overall nutrient distribution and metabolism of the animals change significantly to meet the needs of the mammary gland. During the lactation period, the nutritional needs of the animals rise to a higher level to support the production of milk. The majority of animal species meet the increasing demand for nutrients by increasing food intake or utilizing nutrients stored in the body. In addition, the metabolism of major nutrients is often altered to provide sufficient nutrients to the mammary gland. In early lactation, many animal species use the body's reserves rather than adjust the food intake to meet the demands of lactation [2]. Protein degradation in muscle tissue is a common metabolic adaptation mechanism employed by animals to provide the required amino acids for the production of milk proteins [1]. Peragon *et al.* and Hayase *et al.* reported that the protein turnover in animal organs and tissues is affected by the protein content in the diet [3]. Studies have shown that when the usable energy is sufficient and not restricted by environmental factors, dietary proteins are utilized preferentially to synthesize the somatic proteins, which increase as amino acid intake increases. The continuous increase in amino acid intake results in a decreased protein deposition rate in the body. Low-protein diets reduce the relative rate of total protein synthesis and significantly enhance the rate of total protein reutilization, thereby promoting protein deposition [4].

In the present study, lactating mice were exposed to amino acid deficiency-induced nutritional stress. No significant decrease in casein secretion was detected in the short term even though the nutrition or energy supply is lacking. On the contrary, the expression of the casein gene was upregulated, which suggested that mammary gland tissue might achieve protein turnover and ensure the priority of lactation through the degradation of muscle tissues. The level of casein secretion was slightly higher in mice supplied with a sufficient amount of protein compared to the mice supplied with a low amount of protein. Judging from the changes in the expression level of specialized genes, there was no clear evidence that the amount of protein provided post starvation would affect the level of casein synthesis. The expression levels of the casein gene were significantly decreased in mice from both the low protein and the high protein groups compared to the mice from the starved group, while the expression level of the casein gene was lower in starved mice compared to the mice supplied with only energy. The expression level of the MHC2α gene, which encodes one of the myosin heavy chain isoforms, was decreased in the muscle tissues ($P < 0.05$), indicating that the protein content of the muscle tissues was reduced. However, the results were not sufficient to prove whether the decrease was due to elevated protein degradation or due to reduced protein synthesis. Research conducted by Varshavsky *et al.* showed that the ubiquitin-proteasome proteolytic pathway is the primary pathway of muscle protein degradation in various consumptive diseases (including starvation, infections, diabetes, burns and metabolic acidosis) [5]. The main components of the ubiquitin pathway are the ubiquitins and the 26S proteasome complex. The 20S proteasome is the catalytic core of the 26S proteasome complex. Therefore, this study examined the mRNA expression of the components related to the ubiquitin-proteasome pathway. The results showed that the expression levels of PolyUbC, ubiquitin-conjugating enzyme E2$_{14k}$ and the C2 subunit of the 20S proteasome were all upregulated ($P < 0.01$). Previous studies have demonstrated that the expression of genes in the ubiquitin system is positively correlated with the activity of the system. The inhibition of expression of the subunit genes significantly reduces the content and activity of the proteasomes in cells [6]. The findings described above provide a powerful explanation for our results that protein degradation was elevated in muscle tissues.

A study performed by Emery *et al.* showed that if the net energy provided by grain or roughage increases by 4.18 MJ, the total milk protein content will increase correspondingly by 0.015 units. Furthermore, each additional 1 MJ of metabolic energy provided by the diet will result in an increase of 0.03 units in total milk protein content [7]. The above findings indicate that milk protein content is positively correlated with energy intake (r = 0.42). Sporndly *et al.* have identified a positive correlation between milk protein content and metabolizable energy intake (r = 0.42, r = 0.31), suggesting that milk protein content is primarily affected by dietary energy levels [8]. The present study showed that the expression level of the casein gene was the highest in mammary gland tissue collected from mice supplied with energy only in comparison to mice from the control group and other treatment groups. Our result was consistent with the findings of the above studies. The mRNA expression of the specialized genes in muscle tissue was examined. and the results showed that when the lactating mice were provided only with sufficient energy, the protein content in the muscle tissue decreased significantly ($P < 0.05$). The magnitude of the decrease was larger than that of the group of mice provided with protein. The results indicated that compared with the protein factor, the energy factor may exert a more significant effect on protein turnover and metabolism in the mammary gland and muscle tissues.

In animals, the efficiency of protein turnover and metabolism is significantly affected by the level of dietary energy intake. Kita *et al.* conducted a study in which the protein level was kept constant and the metabolizable energy level was adjusted gradually from a state of deficiency to a state that met the needs of the animals. Kita *et al.* [9] found that the rates of whole-body protein synthesis and degradation were elevated in the animals. When dietary energy level was further increased to exceed the needs of the animals, the protein synthesis rate remained constant. In contrast, insufficient dietary energy intake resulted in limited protein synthesis in the animal's body. However, the mechanisms by which energy intake affects protein turnover are not yet clear. Wu *et al.* has proposed that as the protein deposition rate increases, the energy cost per gram of protein deposition will increase accordingly. Insufficient energy intake has little effect on the protein synthesis rate, protein synthesis capability and protein synthesis efficiency in animal tissues and the body. However, insufficient energy intake results in an enhanced rate of muscle protein degradation, which provides amino acids for oxidative reaction and energy production. In the present study, the mRNA expression levels of the factors related to the ubiquitin-proteasome pathway were significantly increased ($P < 0.01$). Except for PolyUbC, the mRNA expression levels of the other examined factors increased the most in mice provided with only energy, suggesting that sufficient energy would promote the activity of the ubiquitin-proteasome proteolytic pathway. In addition, significant differences were observed in the mRNA expression of factors related to the ubiquitin-proteasome pathway between different treatment groups. These results suggested that compared with the starvation treatment, the supply of protein may enhance the activity of the ubiquitin-proteasome proteolytic pathway and muscle tissue degradation and the magnitude of enhancement may be larger when adequate amounts of protein were provided in comparison to an insufficient protein supply.

4.2. Changes in Hormone Levels

In the present study, the blood hormone levels of lactating mice were examined, and the results showed that the level of GH was slightly elevated in the blood of the mice from the starved group. However, the difference was not statistically significant. Analysis of the expression of the casein gene showed that its expression level was increased in the starved group. A significant number of studies have confirmed that GH exerts a strong lactation-promoting effect and is capable of enhancing milk yield in dairy cows [10] [11]. Sakamoto *et al.* [12] found that in the absence of prolactin and insulin, GH acts directly on secretory epithelial cells in mammary glands and increases the expression of casein at both the gene and protein levels. Molento *et al.* found that the unique nutritional distribution function of GH in the body allows more nutrients to be allocated to the mammary gland [13]. GH promotes the secretion of IGF-1 [14]. In dairy cows, the blood level of IGF-1 is often positively correlated with milk yield [15]. Using mammary tissues or mammary epithelial cells of dairy cows as experimental models, Sakamoto *et al.* demonstrated at the cell and tissue levels that GH promotes the synthesis of αs casein and the expression of the β-casein gene [12]. Furthermore, studies conducted by Glimm *et al.* and Baumrucker *et al.* confirmed the presence of GH and IGF-1 receptors in the mammary tissue of dairy cows [16] [17]. Therefore, GH may exert its effect either by directly acting on mammary glands or by stimulating the secretion of IGF-1, thus indirectly affecting mammary glands.

A study by Prosser and Davis showed that the infusion of IGF-1 into the external pudendal artery significantly increased blood flow in mammary glands and elevated the secretion of mammary gland milk [18]. In addition, a study performed by Burgos *et al.* showed that IGF-1 promotes protein synthesis in the mammary epithelial cells of dairy cows [19]. Dohm *et al.* found that IGF-1 displays a strong promoting effect on the development and anabolism of skeletal muscles and other organs [4]. IGF-1 exerts its effects on skeletal muscle through IGF-1 receptors. By binding to its receptors, IGF-1 promotes the proliferation and differentiation of skeletal muscle cells, increases amino acid and glucose uptake in skeletal muscle cells, stimulates protein synthesis in skeletal muscle and inhibits protein degradation, thereby enhancing the net protein deposition in skeletal muscle. Studies have also shown that patients with protein malnutrition tend to have low levels of IGF-1. Liu *et al.* found that the IGF-1 concentration in bovine blood is related to dietary nutrient levels and dietary intake. The IGF-1 concentration is positively correlated with the concentration of casein in the diet. Some scholars have reported that the main factor affecting the blood concentration of IGF-1 is the crude protein level, and the response of IGF-1 to the crude protein level is affected by the metabolizable energy concentration in the diet. A study conducted by Conlon *et al.* showed that that plasma IGF-1 concentration is strongly correlated with the plasma concentrations of nutrients [20]. The plasma IGF-1 concentration is decreased in fasting table poultry, and this decrease is accompanied by a reduced rate of pectoralis muscle protein synthesis. The plasma IGF-1 concentration returns to normal after supplementary feeding. Broiler chickens at 7 days of age were given intramuscular injections of IGF-1 (35 mg/chicken). At 6 h after injection, the relative rate of pectoral muscle protein synthesis was significantly elevated, and the relative rate of the protein degradation was reduced, resulting in increased daily weight gain and nitrogen deposition. Comparing the two treatment groups in the present study that were supplied with proteins, the high protein group showed a IGF-1 level higher than that of the low protein group, which is consistent with the findings described above. Breier *et al.* conducted a study of beef cattle and found that the plasma concentration of IGF-1 decreases only when the cattle are in a state of negative energy balance [21]. A study conducted by Williams *et al.* showed that improvement of dietary energy levels leads to a linear increase in the blood concentrations of insulin and IGF-1 in primiparous heifers [22]. The present study showed that IGF-1 levels were markedly decreased in starved mice and in mice supplied with energy only ($P < 0.01$). In addition, the degradation of muscle tissue was increased. These results were consistent with the findings of the previous studies described above. However, the present study failed to detect any increase in the IGF-1 level in mice supplied with energy in comparison to the starved mice, which is inconsistent with the general theory.

Spomdly *et al.* utilized the hyperinsulinemic-euglycemic clamp technique to study the function of insulin [8]. The results have shown that the application of insulin leads to significantly increased milk protein content and yield. In nutritionally adequate cattle, the milk protein yield is increased by 25%. These results suggest that insulin is a major endocrine regulatory factor controlling milk protein synthesis. In the present study, all of the treatment groups except for the starved group exhibited increased insulin content. However, no statistically significant differences were detected between the groups. A study performed by Canfield and Butler showed that insulin is an important hormone regulating carbohydrate, fat and protein metabolism and maintaining stable blood sugar levels [11]. Insulin usually reflects the comprehensive balance between feed intake and milk yield. The insulin concentration is greatly affected by the energy levels. Insulin is a hormone that reflects the energy status of the body. In the present study, the changes in the insulin levels were not statistically significant. However, compared with the normal control group, the blood level of insulin was decreased after starvation and increased when sufficient energy was supplied, indicating that insulin reflected the energy status of the body.

4.3. Phosphorylation Levels of the Effectors of the mTOR Pathway and Expression Levels of Carrier Proteins in Mammary Gland and Muscle Tissues

Studies have shown that once phosphorylated and activated, mTOR controls the translation of mRNAs in a specific subgroup through two disparate downstream pathways, the 4E-BP1 and the p70S6K pathways, and subsequently increases protein synthesis. In the present study, the phosphorylation levels of mTOR and 4EBP1 were elevated in mammary gland tissue. However, the changes were not statistically significant. In contrast, the downstream signaling molecule of mTOR, p70S6K, demonstrated a markedly increased phosphorylation level ($P < 0.05$). These results were consistent with the findings described previously that the expression of the casein gene was upregulated. Similarly, the phosphorylation levels of mTOR and 4EBP1 were also elevated in muscle tissue, but the differences were statistically insignificant. In addition, the increase in the muscle tissue was significantly smaller than that in the mammary gland tissue. The phosphorylation level of p70S6K was markedly elevated, whereas it was significantly decreased when an insufficient amount of protein was supplied ($P < 0.01$).

Research conducted by Humphrey *et al.* indicated that the adaptive response of animal tissues to different dietary components and nutrient levels is primarily reflected by changes in the type and amount of the transporters of the nutrients in the body. The chemical composition of the diet directly or indirectly affects the expression of the transporters [23]. As an increasing number of cDNA sequences encoding mammalian amino acid transporters have been cloned, many studies have focused on the regulatory effect of dietary nutrient composition on the expression of amino acid transporters. Dietary nutrient levels, especially the protein (amino acid) levels, affect the regulation of amino acid transporter expression. To maintain cell survival under the conditions of amino acid deficiency, protein catabolism is increased in muscle cells, amino acid biosynthesis is elevated and an increasing amount of amino acids is transported across the membrane into the cells. In addition, the synthesis of the transporter protein CAT-1 is enhanced. The levels of insulin and other hormones significantly affect the expression of the amino acid transporters. Simmons *et al.* treated quiescent muscle cells with a 10-fold increase of interleukin-1 beta (IL-1β) and interferon gamma (IFN-γ) and found that the expression level of CAT-1 mRNA was elevated. Under the action of cytokines, the expression level of CAT-1 mRNA was also increased. Shi *et al.* employed an animal model to investigate for the first time the effect of daily diet on the level of CAT-1 expression in pig intestine. Studies have shown that compared with a high protein diet, a low protein diet has a bigger impact on the relative expression level of CAT-1 mRNA in the intestine of fattening pigs, especially in the jejunum. Using an in vitro culture method, Zhi *et al.* found that the abundance of CAT-1 mRNA expression increases as the lysine concentration increases. The difference was highly significant and dose-dependent. The present study showed that the expression of the Lys/Arg transporter CAT-1 was drastically elevated in mammary gland tissue ($P < 0.05$). Moreover, the increase in CAT-1 expression was more significant in mice supplied with protein after starvation compared to mice supplied with energy.

In a study that employed BeWo cells as the experimental model, it was shown that changes in the substrate concentration affect the mRNA expression of a number of amino acid transporters. However, the tendency to increase or decrease varies among the transporters. Jones *et al.* found that essential amino acid deficiency in the body leads to a significantly decreased expression of sodium-coupled neutral amino acid transporter 1 (SNAT1) mRNA within 1 h. However, no obvious changes in sodium-coupled neutral amino acid transporter 2 (SNAT2) mRNA expression are detected within 1 h. In contrast, the level of SNAT2 mRNA increases at or after 3 h. Furthermore, the level of SNAT2 mRNA expression is markedly elevated when the supply of amino acids increases [24]. Lys and Met are two major limiting amino acids for growth and milk protein synthesis. The present study showed that the expression level of the Met transporter protein ASCT2 was significantly reduced in muscle tissue ($P < 0.05$). These results indicated that the amount of transporter protein was decreased, which might lead to declined protein synthesis in the muscle tissue. Compared with the starved group, mice that were given dietary protein showed a slightly decreased level of ASCT2. The results were consistent with findings from previous studies showing that the substrate concentration affects the expression of amino acid transporters.

Energy metabolism is a very complex process. The mTOR signaling pathway is involved in the regulation of energy homeostasis. Energy-producing substances participate in energy regulation primarily through the liver kinase B1 (LKB1)-adenine monophosphate-activated protein kinase (AMPK)-tuberous sclerosis complex (TSC)-mTOR signaling pathway. AMPK is a sensor of cellular energy levels. Intracellular energy deficiency activates the AMPK protein. Activated AMPK inhibits mTOR activity and subsequently initiates ATP synthesis and prevents ATP consumption, ceasing cell growth. When sufficient energy is available, AMPK functions as a "switch" to shut down the energy supply and ensures that the energy is released and utilized to promote cell growth. In addition, changes in the activation state of AMPK affect the activity and phosphorylation level of p70S6K, a downstream signaling molecule of mTOR, which will further affect mRNA translation in somatic animal cells and control protein synthesis. The hypothalamus senses changes in energy balance through the mTOR pathway and controls food intake through feedback mechanisms, thus contributing to the achievement of energy homeostasis in the body. Abnormal mTOR signaling leads to disorders of energy metabolism. Excessive food intake-induced obesity has been observed in TSC1-knockout mice. Sobolewska *et al.* found that IGF-1 and epidermal growth factor (EGF) activate mTOR in bovine mammary epithelial cells, whereas the inhibition of mTOR by rapamycin abolishes the inhibitory effect of IGF-1 and EGF on autophagy [25]. AMPK achieves its role as a sensor of cellular energy status through the negative regulation of mTOR. Bolster *et al.* found that the injection of rats with energy-providing substances does not alter AMPKα1 activity in gastrocnemius muscle. However, AMPKα2 activity was significantly enhanced [26]. Compared with the control group, muscle protein synthesis was reduced by 45% in the treatment group because the downregulation of mTOR by AMPK directly inhibits translation initiation and protein synthesis. Kimura *et al.* [27] treated human corneal epithelial cells with AMPK activator and found that the activity and phosphorylation of p70S6K, a downstream signaling factor of mTOR, are suppressed. In addition, changes in glucose concentration also regulate the activity of AMPK and p70S6K. In the present study, p70S6K phosphorylation in both types of tissue was elevated in the starved group in comparison with the normal treatment group. However, the magnitude of increase was significantly lower in the muscle tissue compared to that in the mammary gland tissue. Compared with the starved group, mice supplied with sufficient energy showed an increased level of p70S6K phosphorylation in both types of tissues ($P <$ 0.05, $P < 0.01$), which is consistent with previously published results.

5. Conclusions

When experiencing dietary amino acid deficiency, lactating mice enhance muscle tissue degradation to preferentially meet the needs of lactation. In mammary gland tissue, the amount of utilized amino acid transporters is elevated, the phosphorylation level of the mTOR pathway is enhanced and the total amount of proteins synthesized is increased. In muscle tissue, the protein phosphorylation level is also increased. However, the amount of utilized amino acid transporters is reduced, the total amount of proteins synthesized is decreased, and protein degradation is enhanced.

Dietary amino acids and energy affect the activity of the ubiquitin-proteasome pathway, which is responsible for muscle tissue degradation. Adequate dietary amino acids and energy may enhance the activity of the pathway.

Hormones significantly affect the protein metabolism in mammary gland and muscle tissues. Among the hormones, the effect of insulin-like growth factors is especially remarkable.

Acknowledgements

Financial support was provided by the fund for Modern Agro-industry Technology Research System of China (CARS-37, Modern Agro-industry Technology Research System of Shandong (SDAIT-12-011-06)), Shandong province science technology development plan (2012NC11103), natural science fund of China (31072050) (31372340) and cattle breed project of Shandong province.

References

[1] Bauman, D.E. (2000) Ruminant Physiology: Digestion, Metabolism, Growth and Reproduction. CAB International, Souse Africa, 311-328.

[2] Vernon, R.G. (1998) Homeorhesis. In: *Research Reviews, Hannah Yearbook*, Hannah Research Institute, Ayr, UK, 64-73.

[3] Peragón, J., Barroso, J.B., García-Salguero, L., *et al.* (1994) Dietary Protein Effects on Growth and Fractional Protein Synthesis and Degradation Rates in Liver and White Muscle of Rainbow Trout. *Aquaculture*, **124**, 35-46. http://dx.doi.org/10.1016/0044-8486(94)90352-2

[4] Dohm, G.L., Elton, C.W., Raju, M.S., *et al.* (1990) IGF-I–Stimulated Glucose Transport in Human Skeletal Muscle and IGF-I Resistance in Obesity and NIDDM. *Diabetes*, **39**, 1028-1032. http://dx.doi.org/10.2337/diab.39.9.1028

[5] Varshavsky, A. (1997) The N-End Rule Pathway of Protein Degradation. *Genes to Cells*, **2**, 13-28. http://dx.doi.org/10.1046/j.1365-2443.1997.1020301.x

[6] Grune, T., Blasig, I.E. and Sitte, N. (1998) Peroxynitrite Increases the Degradation of Aconitase and Other Cellular Proteins by Proteasome. *Journal of Biological Chemistry*, **273**, 10857-10862. http://dx.doi.org/10.1074/jbc.273.18.10857

[7] Emery, R.S. (1978) Feeding for Increased Milk Protein. *Journal of Dairy Science*, **61**, 825-828. http://dx.doi.org/10.3168/jds.S0022-0302(78)83656-X

[8] Sporndly, E. (1989) Effects of Diet on Milk Composition and Yield of Dairy Cows with Special Emphasis on Milk Protein Content. *Swedish Journal of Agricultural Research*, **19**, 99-106.

[9] Wu, X.L. and Ying, F. (2002) Research Method and Model of Animal Protein Business Turnover. *Journal of Nuclear Agriculture Science*, **16**, 156-161.

[10] Lough, D.S., Muller, L.D., Kensinger, R.S., *et al.* (1989) Effect of Exogenous Bovine Somatotropin on Mammary Lipid Metabolism and Milk Yield in Lactating Dairy Cows. *Journal of Dairy Science*, **72**, 1469-1476. http://dx.doi.org/10.3168/jds.S0022-0302(89)79256-0

[11] Canfield, R.W. and Butler, W.R. (1990) Energy Balance and Pulsatile LH Secretion in Early Postpartum Dairy Cattle. *Domestic Animal Endocrinology*, **7**, 323-330. http://dx.doi.org/10.1016/0739-7240(90)90038-2

[12]   Sakamoto, K., Komatsu, T., Kobayashi, T., Rose, M.T., Aso, H., Hagino, A. and Obara, Y. (2005) Growth Hormone Acts on the Synthesis and Secretion of α-Casein in Bovine Mammary Epithelial Cells. *Journal of Dairy Research*, **72**, 264-270. http://dx.doi.org/10.1017/S0022029905000889

[13]   Molento, C.F.M., Block, E., Cue, R.I. and Petitclerc, D. (2002) Effects of Insulin, Recombinant Bovine Somatotropin, and Their Interaction on Insulin-Like Growth Factor-I Secretion and Milk Protein Production in Dairy Cows. *Journal of Dairy Science*, **85**, 738-747. http://dx.doi.org/10.3168/jds.S0022-0302(02)74131-3

[14]   Bauman, D.E. (1999) Bovine Somatotropin and Lactation: From Basic Science to Commercial Application. *Domestic Animal Endocrinology*, **17**, 101-116. http://dx.doi.org/10.1016/S0739-7240(99)00028-4

[15]   Rose, M.T., Weekes, T.E.C. and Rowlinson, P. (2005) Correlation of Blood and Milk Components with the Milk Yield Response to Bovine Somatotropin in Dairy Cows. *Domestic Animal Endocrinology*, **28**, 296-307. http://dx.doi.org/10.1016/j.domaniend.2004.12.001

[16]   Glimm, D.R., Baracos, V.E. and Kennelly, J.J. (1990) Molecular Evidence for the Presence of Growth Hormone Receptors in the Bovine Mammary Gland. *Journal of Endocrinology*, **126**, R5-R8. http://dx.doi.org/10.1677/joe.0.126R005

[17]   Baumrucker, C.R. and Erondu, N.E. (2000) Insulin-Like Growth Factor (IGF) System in the Bovine Mammary Gland and Milk. *Journal of Mammary Gland Biology and Neoplasia*, **5**, 53-64. http://dx.doi.org/10.1023/A:1009515232450

[18]   Prosser, C.G., Davis, S.R., Farr, V.C., Moore, L.G. and Gluckman, P.D. (1994) Effects of Close-Arterial (External Pudic) Infusion of Insulin-Like Growth Factor-II on Milk Yield and Mammary Blood Flow in Lactating Goats. *Journal of Endocrinology*, **142**, 93-99. http://dx.doi.org/10.1677/joe.0.1420093

[19]   Burgos, S.A. and Cant, J.P. (2010) IGF-1 Stimulates Protein Synthesis by Enhanced Signaling through mTORC1 in Bovine Mammary Epithelial Cells. *Domestic Animal Endocrinology*, **38**, 211-221. http://dx.doi.org/10.1016/j.domaniend.2009.10.005

[20]   Conlon, M.A. and Kita, K. (2002) Muscle Protein Synthesis Rate Is Altered in Response to a Single Injection of Insulin-Like Growth Factor-I in Seven-Day-Old Leghorn Chicks. *Poultry Science*, **81**, 1543-1547. http://dx.doi.org/10.1093/ps/81.10.1543

[21]   Breier, B.H., Bass, J.J., Butler, J.H. and Gluckman, P.D. (1986) The Somatotrophic Axis in Young Steers: Influence of Nutritional Status on Pulsatile Release of Growth Hormone and Circulating Concentrations of Insulin-Like Growth Factor 1. *Journal of Endocrinology*, **111**, 209-215. http://dx.doi.org/10.1677/joe.0.1110209

[22]   Williams, N.G., Interlichia, J.P., Jackson, M.F., Hwang, D., Cohen, P. and Rodgers, B.D. (2011) Endocrine Actions of Myostatin: Systemic Regulation of the IGF and IGF Binding Protein Axis. *Endocrinology*, **152**, 172-180. http://dx.doi.org/10.1210/en.2010-0488

[23]   Humphrey, B.D., Stephensen, C.B., Calvert, C.C. and Klasing, K.C. (2004) Glucose and Cationic Amino Acid Transporter Expression in Growing Chickens (*Gallus gallus domesticus*). *Comparative Biochemistry and Physiology Part A: Molecular & Integrative Physiology*, **138**, 515-525. http://dx.doi.org/10.1016/j.cbpb.2004.06.016

[24]   Jones, H.N., Ashworth, C.J., Page, K.R. and McArdle, H.J. (2006) Cortisol Stimulates System A Amino Acid Transport and SNAT2 Expression in a Human Placental Cell Line (BeWo). *American Journal of Physiology-Endocrinology and Metabolism*, **291**, E596-E603. http://dx.doi.org/10.1152/ajpendo.00359.2005

[25]   Sobolewska, A., Gajewska, M., Zarzyńska, J., Gajkowska, B. and Motyl, T. (2009) IGF-I, EGF, and Sex Steroids Regulate Autophagy in Bovine Mammary Epithelial Cells via the mTOR Pathway. *European Journal of Cell Biology*, **88**, 117-130. http://dx.doi.org/10.1016/j.ejcb.2008.09.004

[26]   Bolster, D.R., Crozier, S.J., Kimball, S.R. and Jefferson, L.S. (2002) AMP-Activated Protein Kinase Suppresses Protein Synthesis in Rat Skeletal Muscle through Down-Regulated Mammalian Target of Rapamycin (mTOR) Signaling. *Journal of Biological Chemistry*, **277**, 23977-23980. http://dx.doi.org/10.1074/jbc.C200171200

[27]   Kimura, N., Tokunaga, C., Dalal, S., Richardson, C., Yoshino, K., Hara, K., *et al.* (2003) A Possible Linkage between AMP-Activated Protein Kinase (AMPK) and Mammalian Target of Rapamycin (mTOR) Signalling Pathway. *Genes to Cells*, **8**, 65-79. http://dx.doi.org/10.1046/j.1365-2443.2003.00615.x

2

Glyphosate Effects on Sugarcane Metabolism and Growth

Caio Antonio Carbonari, Giovanna Larissa Gimenes Cotrick Gomes,
Edivaldo Domingues Velini, Renato Fernandes Machado, Plinio Saulo Simões,
Gabrielle de Castro Macedo

Department of Crop Science, College of Agricultural Sciences, São Paulo State University (UNESP), Botucatu, Brazil
Email: carbonari@fca.unesp.br

Abstract

Glyphosate is the most widely used herbicide in the world. In sugarcane, it is used as a herbicide when applied at its field rate, but it is also used as ripener when applied as low doses. However, the effects of glyphosate on plant metabolism and sugarcane growth are not fully understood. This study aimed to evaluate the metabolic changes and the effects on sugarcane plant growth caused by the application of different doses of glyphosate. Sugarcane plants were grown in a greenhouse and subjected to glyphosate applications at doses of 7.2; 18; 36; 72; 180; 360 and 720 g a.e. ha^{-1}. Plants grown without an herbicide application were used as a control. Plants from each treatment were collected at 2, 7, 14, and 21 days after treatment (DAT) application to quantify the levels of shikimic acid, quinic acid, shikimate-3-phosphate, glyphosate, α-amino-3-hydroxy-5-methyl-4-isoxazolepropionic acid (AMPA), phenylalanine, tyrosine, and tryptophan. Visual evaluations of plant intoxication were performed at the same time as the collection of plants, and the quantification of their shoot dry biomass was performed at 21 DAT. At doses of glyphosate greater than 72 g a.e. ha^{-1}, increases in the levels of shikimic acid, quinic acid, and shikimate-3-phosphate occurred and AMPA was detected in the plants. Initially, glyphosate caused increases in the plant levels of phenylalanine and tyrosine at doses of 72 and 180 g a.e. ha^{-1}, although a decrease in the levels of aromatic amino acids subsequently occurred at and above the doses of 72 or 180 g a.e. ha^{-1}. The doses ranging from 7.2 to 36 g a.e. ha^{-1} promoted an increase in plant shoot biomass, and doses greater than 72 g a.e. ha^{-1} caused significant reductions in dry mass.

Keywords

EPSPS, AMPA, Shikimic Acid, Herbicide, Sugarcane, Ripener

1. Introduction

Brazil is the world's largest sugarcane (*Saccharum* spp.) producer, with a planted area of approximately 9.09 million hectares and a mean yield of 72.444 kg·ha^{-1} [1]. Sugarcane is a semi-perennial plant requiring a tropical or sub-tropical climate. With a C4 metabolism, this crop has high photosynthetic efficiency and high water use efficiency [2]. The cultivation of sugarcane is one of the best alternatives for the sustainable production of large amounts of biomass that may be converted into various products, especially sugar and ethanol.

Glyphosate plays a key role in global agriculture and in sugarcane cultivation as well because this herbicide is used for managing weeds, for managing the sugarcane ratoon itself, and at low doses, for improving the quality of raw materials by acting as a ripener, stopping flowering and optimizing the maturation potential of sugarcane varieties [3]-[6].

The glyphosate mechanism of action is the enzymatic inhibition of EPSPS (5-enolpyruvylshikimate-3-phosphate (EPSP) synthase, E.C. 2.5.1. 19), which catalyzes the reaction of shikimate-3-phosphate (S3P) with phosphoenolpyruvate (PEP), forming 5-enolpyruvylshikimate-3-phosphate (EPSP) and inorganic phosphorus (Pi) [7]. The enzymatic inhibition of EPSPS by glyphosate affects the shikimic acid metabolic pathway, which generates the three aromatic amino acids phenylalanine, tyrosine, and tryptophan [8].

The shikimic acid pathway, the main pathway for the production of aromatic amino acids, is a metabolic pathway of plants and microorganisms only and is not present in animals [9]. In plants, this pathway is presumably confined to the plastids [10].

These three aromatic amino acids and other intermediate compounds of the shikimic acid pathway are precursors of a wide variety of plant secondary metabolites [11]. Thus, this pathway is eminently important for the synthesis of numerous compounds of commercial interest and also originate various compounds involved in growth regulation or plant defense, especially condensed tannins, anthocyanins, vitamin E, indole acetic acid, salicylic acid, flavones, isoflavones, phenylpropanoids, and coumarins, compounds that are fundamental to plant growth and development [6] [12] [13]. Furthermore, intermediate pathways may produce substrates for other metabolic pathways, including the biosynthesis of quinic acid and derivatives thereof, including chlorogenic acid [9].

The process of regulation of the shikimic acid pathway by glyphosate upon its application to plants is unclear, and it is not known whether the mechanisms of control in various plant species are similar, although the available data indicate they are not similar [13]. A key metabolic alteration triggered in plants upon glyphosate application or drift is the accumulation of shikimic acid. Various authors have been able to correlate glyphosate plant intoxication with shikimic acid accumulation [14]-[21]. Quinic acid, a compound with a similar structure to shikimic acid, can also accumulate in plants exposed to glyphosate [15] [21]-[23]. Thus, this study aimed to evaluate the effects of the application of various glyphosate doses on the metabolic changes and growth of sugarcane plants.

2. Materials and Methods

2.1. Plant Growth and Glyphosate Application

Stem cuttings of the sugarcane variety SP801842 collected in the field, from an area of cash crops, were planted in pots containing 3 L of substrate and maintained in a greenhouse. Sugarcane plants received an application of the herbicide glyphosate when they had six fully expanded leaves. In a controlled environment (laboratory), a boom sprayer equipped with four XR 11002 VS nozzles, spaced 0.5 m apart, and placed 0.5 m above the plants was used for applications. The working pressure of the device was 2.0 kgf·cm^{-2}, with a 3.6 km·h^{-1} speed and a 200 L·ha^{-1} consumption of spraying volume. The glyphosate doses of 7.2, 18, 36, 72, 180, 360, and 720 g a.e. ha^{-1} were applied, and control plants were maintained without receiving an herbicide application. Treatments were arranged in a completely randomized design with four replicates.

2.2. Plant Evaluation and Sample Collection

All leaves from a single plant per replicate of each treatment were collected at 2, 7, 14, and 21 days after treatment (DAT) application, always at the same time. The plant material was washed three times in 50 mL of distilled water following collection to remove any herbicide residues that were deposited on leaves and unabsorbed.

All plant material was stored in paper bags and dried in a forced-air oven at 40°C for 72 hours. The samples were then stored in an ultrafreezer (−80°C) for the subsequent extraction and quantification of compounds.

Visual evaluations of plant intoxication were performed at 21 DAT; a score of 0 corresponded to no injury, and that of 100 corresponded to plant death. The dry biomass of plant shoots was quantified at 21 DAT, by weighing after drying in a forced-air oven.

2.3. Extraction and Quantification of Compounds

The dried plant material was macerated in a mortar containing liquid nitrogen, and approximately 100 mg of sample was weighed into and stored in a 15 mL centrifuge tube. Next, 10 mL of water that had been acidified to pH 2.5 was added to the tube containing the sample [16]. The tubes were stirred to homogenize the dry sample with the water.

The tubes were placed in an ultrasound bath with a 42-KHz ultrasonic frequency for 30 minutes [24]. Subsequently, they were centrifuged at 4000 rpm for 10 minutes at 20°C. The supernatant was collected and filtered using a 0.45 μm Millex HV filter with a 13 mm Durapore membrane and stored in a 9 mm (2 mL) amber glass vial for subsequent quantification by liquid chromatography–tandem mass spectrometry (LC-MS/MS).

The mass spectrometer was a triple quadrupole instrument, and infusions were performed to optimize its conditions, that is, direct injections of 1 mg·L^{-1} analytical standard solution of each compound were individually introduced into the spectrometer. The ionization source mode (Electrospray ionization, ESI) was chosen based on the infusion procedure, which produces analyte ions in the liquid phase prior to entering the mass spectrometer. The negative ionization mode was used for the following compounds: shikimic acid, quinic acid, shikimate-3-phosphate, glyphosate, and α-amino-3-hydroxy-5-methyl-4-isoxazolepropionic acid (AMPA). The positive ionization mode was used for the three aromatic amino acids (phenylalanine, tyrosine, and tryptophan).

A chromatographic column (Gemini 5 μ C18 110 Å (150 mm × 4.6 mm)) was used to separate the compounds for quantification in the negative ionization mode, and 5 mM ammonium acetate in water (Phase A) and 5 mM ammonium acetate in methanol (Phase B) were used as the mobile phases at a flow rate of 0.5 mL·min^{-1}. The gradient employed consisted of 0 - 1 minutes 30% Phase B and 70% Phase A; 1 - 5 minutes 50% Phase B and 50% Phase A; 5 - 8.5 minutes 75% Phase B and 25% Phase A; 8.5 - 15 minutes 90% Phase B and 10% Phase A; 15 - 18 minutes 30% Phase B and 70% Phase A. A Synergi 2.5 μ Fusion RP 110 Å chromatographic column was used to separate the compounds for quantification in the positive ionization mode, with the same mobile phases and flow rates as described for the negative ionization mode. The gradient employed consisted of 0 - 2 minutes 10% Phase B and 90% Phase A; 2 - 4 minutes 40% Phase B and 60% Phase A; 4 - 12 minutes 95% Phase B and 5% Phase A; 12 - 15 minutes 10% Phase B and 90% Phase A. The retention times of each compound in the chromatographic column were 3.86 minutes for shikimic acid, 3.79 minutes for quinic acid, 3.58 minutes for shikimate-3-phosphate, 3.10 minutes for glyphosate, 3.69 minutes for AMPA, 9.71 minutes for phenylalanine, 6.84 minutes for tyrosine, and 10.31 minutes for tryptophan.

2.4. Data Analysis

The data for the various parameters evaluated were subjected to analysis of variance using the F test, and the means were compared using the t test (p ≤ 0.05). The standard errors of each mean (mean ± standard error) were assessed. Regression analysis was performed for the glyphosate and AMPA concentration data using a quadratic equation. A logistic equation was used for the shikimic acid, quinic acid and shikimate-3-phosphate concentration and plant intoxication data, and regression analysis was performed for the plant dry mass accumulation data, fitting the Lorentzian model. The regression procedure was performed using Sigma Plot version 13.0 (Systat Software, Inc., Richmond, CA, USA). The regression equations and corresponding parameters are presented in the figures.

3. Results and Discussion

The highest levels of glyphosate in leaf tissues were observed at 2 DAT in plants subjected to the dose of 720 g·ha^{-1}. Over the course of the other periods evaluated, for the 720 g a.e. ha^{-1} dose, the level of glyphosate gradually decreased and was very low at 21 DAT; consequently, the levels of AMPA, which is the main metabolite of glyphosate, increased during this time (**Figure 1**). For doses of 360 g a.e. ha^{-1} and below, the levels of glyphosate in the plants at 21 DAT were similar to those observed at 2 DAT, which may be related to slower

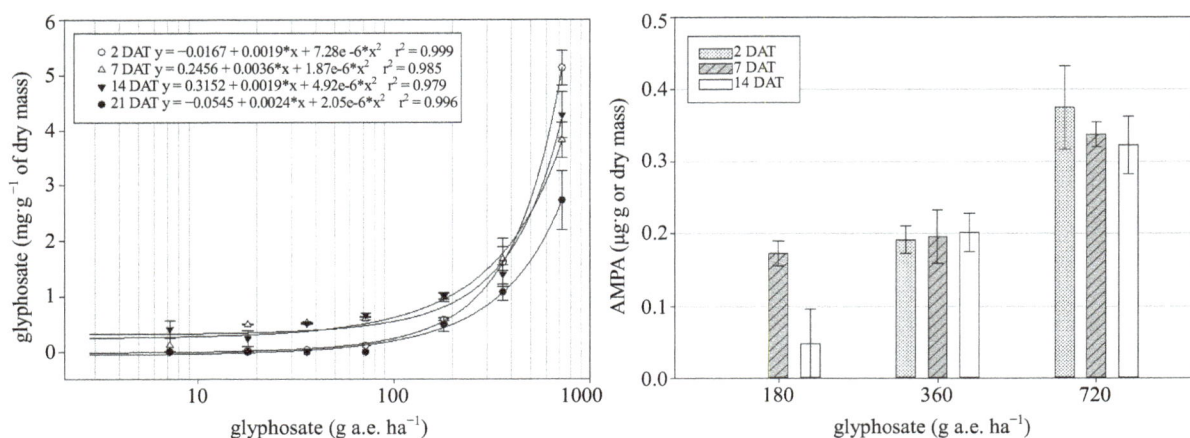

Figure 1. Glyphosate and AMPA concentrations in sugarcane plants (internal) at 2, 7, 14, and 21 days after treatment (DAT) applications of the herbicide glyphosate.

absorption at lower doses, given the lower herbicide concentration in the preparation and the slower rate of diffusion into the leaves, or to greater root exudation at the higher dose as a result of the translocation of greater amounts of herbicide through the plant, or even to the metabolism of glyphosate in the plants.

The presence of AMPA (**Figure 1**) was only detected at doses greater than 72 g a.e. ha^{-1}, and the plant concentrations of AMPA increased starting at this dose. There were no significant differences among the periods evaluated, except at the dose of 180 g·ha^{-1} at 7 DAT. The presence of AMPA may be related to the metabolism of the glyphosate herbicide in sugarcane plants or to the absorption of AMPA metabolite present on the surface of leaves as the result of epiphytic microbial degradation of glyphosate [17]. The detection of AMPA in leaves, stems, and seeds from various crops, including soybean resistant to glyphosate, following its application suggests that glyphosate oxidoreductase (GOX) or a similar type of enzyme catalyzes this reaction [17] [25] [26].

No increases in the plant levels of shikimic acid were observed in plants at or under the dose of 72 g a.e. ha^{-1} for any period evaluated when compared to non-treated plants (**Figure 2**). Accumulations of shikimic acid were observed above that dose and the greatest accumulations of shikimic acid, corresponding to the doses tested, were observed at 2 DAT, which was the best time to characterize sugarcane plant intoxication by glyphosate. A similar performance to that observed in this study was also reported for young and adult *Citrus limonia* leaves in which shikimic acid had accumulated to high concentrations at 2 DAT and then subsequently decreased in concentration, indicating a transient effect of the herbicide at sublethal doses [27]. Other authors have reported that the shikimic acid level following glyphosate application may change with time, as noted for young *Abutilon theophrasti* leaves [28], wheat grains [29], and horseweed leaves [30].

The sugarcane plants did not accumulate high levels of shikimic acid, even at the dose of 720 g a.e. ha^{-1}, which indicates that this dose was not sufficient to cause high levels of injury to these plants and characterizes them as highly tolerant to the herbicide glyphosate. In contrast, shikimic acid accumulated rapidly in adult *Beta vulgaris* L. leaves, reaching a concentration 80-fold greater than the control by 24 hours following the application [31]. High shikimic acid concentrations have been recorded in several studies, including 0.17 mg·g^{-1} of *A. theophrasti* dry mass following the application of glyphosate [32], an increase in the shikimic acid concentration from 0.4 to 40 µmol·g^{-1} fresh mass (100-fold increase) in young leaves of soybean non-resistant to glyphosate, and an increase from 0.4 to 12.8 µmol·g^{-1} (32-fold increase) in maize non-resistant to glyphosate [33].

The concentrations of quinic acid also changed in the shikimic acid pathway at doses of 72 g a.e. ha^{-1} and above (**Figure 2**). This compound followed a similar pattern as shikimic acid, although it was a less sensitive indicator of glyphosate intoxication than the former. High correlations between the levels of shikimic and quinic acids and glyphosate in maize plants have been reported, indicating that quinic acid can be a good indicator of glyphosate-intoxicated plants [34].

Apparently, quinic acid may act as a reserve compound in the shikimic acid pathway, although its physiological role is not completely understood [15]. A 1.4-fold quinic acid accumulation in pea leaves (*Pisum sativum* L.) at 15 days after treatment with glyphosate was observed [15] because of the accumulation of compounds in the shikimic acid pathway, and a similar result was observed for shikimic acid, protocatechuic acid, and gallic acid

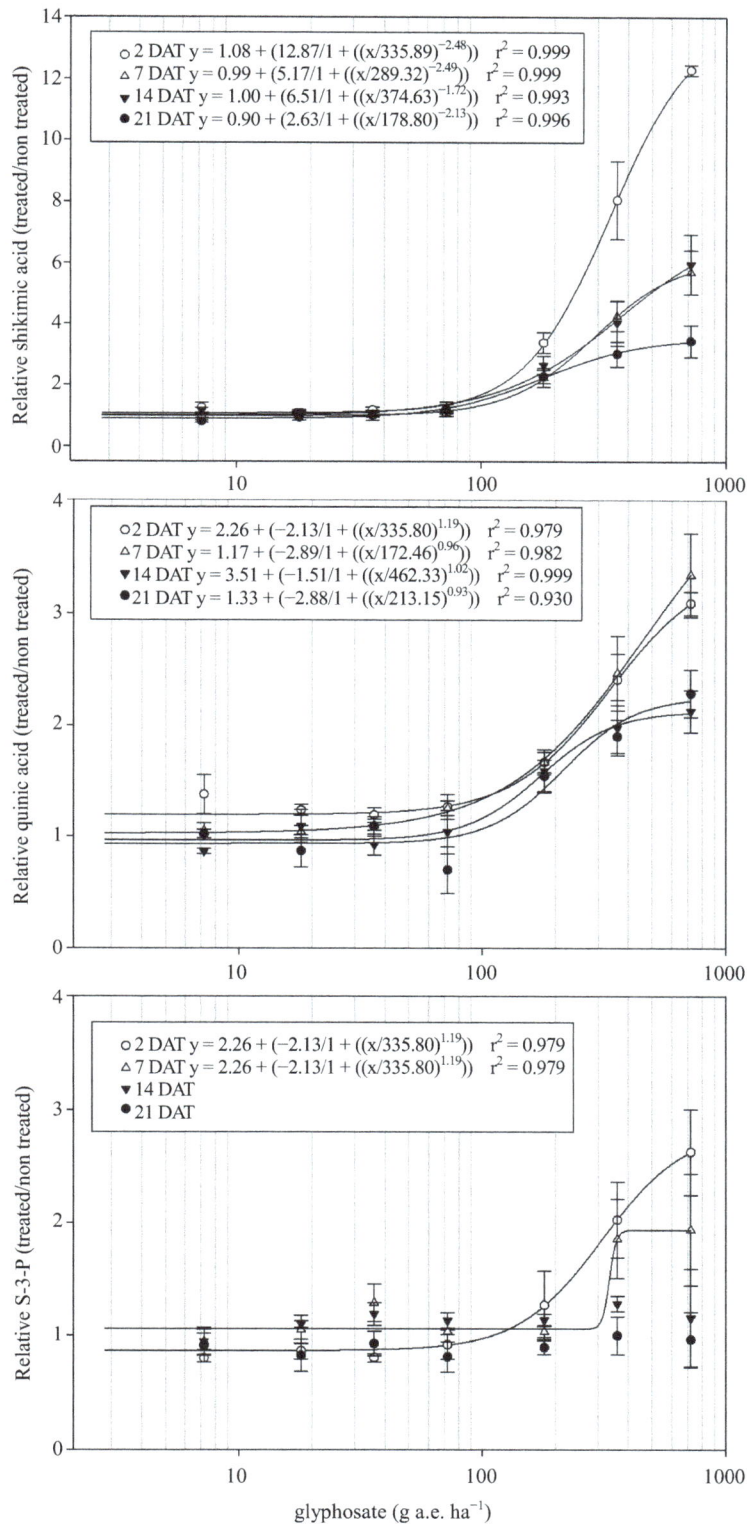

Figure 2. Relative (treated/non-treated) concentrations ± the standard error of shikimic acid, quinic acid, and shikimate-3-phosphate in sugarcane plants 2, 7, 14, and 21 days after applying various doses of glyphosate (days after treatment, DAT).

[15]. Similarly, shikimate-3-phosphate had accumulated at 2 and 4 days after the application of doses greater than 72 g a.e. ha^{-1} because this compound is the substrate directly used in the reaction catalyzed by EPSPS (**Figure 2**). The quinic acid and shikimate-3-phosphate acid exhibited dynamics very similar to those of shikimic acid in sugarcane plants, although the relative increases were smaller.

The levels of phenylalanine and tyrosine had increased compared to the control at 2 DAT for the glyphosate dose of 360 g a.e. ha^{-1}, and there was a nearly 2-fold increase in these amino acids relative to the control at the glyphosate dose of 72 g a.e. ha^{-1} (**Table 1**). The correlation between the phenylalanine and tyrosine levels in the leaf tissue may be related to the formation of these two amino acids from the same precursor, prephenate, following the branching of the shikimic acid pathway. There were small variations in tryptophan in plants subjected to various doses of glyphosate during this same period, and the levels of tryptophan were greater than or equal to the control at the majority of doses (**Table 1**). A possible explanation for this observation is that tryptophan is the aromatic amino acid that is least sensitive to glyphosate inhibition [34]. Compared to non-treated plants, an increase in tryptophan concentration was observed in *Cyperus rotundus* seedlings 3 DAT with glyphosate [35]. The levels of aromatic amino acids were analyzed in *Nicotiana plumbaginifolia* cells 4 days after supplementing the culture media with 100 µM glyphosate, and decreases of 59% and 77% in the tyrosine and phenylalanine concentrations, respectively, were observed, while the tryptophan level only decreased by 13% [36].

At 14 and 21 DAT, small increases in the concentrations of the 3 aromatic amino acids compared to the controls were observed at the glyphosate doses of 18 g·ha^{-1} for tryptophan and 36 g·ha^{-1} for the other 2 amino acids (**Table 1**). Decreasing trends in the levels of the 3 amino acids levels occurred at the dose of 72 g·ha^{-1} and

Table 1. Relative (treated/non-treated) concentrations of phenylalanine, tyrosine, and tryptophan in sugarcane plants at 2, 7, 14, and 21 days after treatment (DAT) application.

Glyphosate	Days after treatment (DAT)			
(g a.e. ha^{-1})	2	7	14	21
	Relative phenylalanine (treated/non-treated)			
7.2	1.30 ± 0.16	0.98 ± 0.12	1.07 ± 0.11	0.85 ± 0.06
18	1.28 ± 0.05	0.94 ± 0.12	1.13 ± 0.13	1.08 ± 0.17
36	1.13 ± 0.07	1.39 ± 0.36	1.14 ± 0.21	1.23 ± 0.10
72	1.77 ± 0.34	0.75 ± 0.07	0.5 ± 0.08	1.05 ± 0.29
180	1.42 ± 0.53	0.62 ± 0.04	0.43 ± 0.03	0.68 ± 0.02
360	1.31 ± 0.38	0.95 ± 0.05	0.57 ± 0.16	0.86 ± 0.09
720	0.93 ± 0.14	1.01 ± 0.13	0.55 ± 0.18	0.71 ± 0.06
	Relative tyrosine (treated/non-treated)			
7.2	1.33 ± 0.16	0.65 ± 0.09	1.05 ± 0.16	0.99 ± 0.07
18	1.28 ± 0.09	0.53 ± 0.04	0.77 ± 0.08	1.44 ± 0.42
36	0.97 ± 0.06	0.54 ± 0.02	0.95 ± 0.17	1.68 ± 0.17
72	1.96 ± 0.29	0.46 ± 0.03	0.61 ± 0.08	0.98 ± 0.20
180	1.66 ± 0.49	0.34 ± 0.03	0.45 ± 0.02	0.61 ± 0.05
360	1.34 ± 0.32	0.55 ± 0.02	0.50 ± 0.15	0.78 ± 0.14
720	0.80 ± 0.09	0.54 ± 0.05	0.56 ± 0.12	0.87 ± 0.15
	Relative tryptophan (treated/non-treated)			
7.2	1.18 ± 0.11	0.86 ± 0.07	1.10 ± 0.15	1.00 ± 0.12
18	1.10 ± 0.07	1.11 ± 0.08	1.27 ± 0.14	1.38 ± 0.09
36	0.97 ± 0.05	1.12 ± 0.10	1.09 ± 0.15	1.36 ± 0.04
72	1.17 ± 0.11	0.86 ± 0.06	0.77 ± 0.03	1.02 ± 0.14
180	1.04 ± 0.17	0.76 ± 0.03	0.84 ± 0.08	0.73 ± 0.02
360	1.23 ± 0.04	0.96 ± 0.08	0.63 ± 0.09	0.77 ± 0.11
720	1.14 ± 0.09	0.73 ± 0.07	0.76 ± 0.03	0.79 ± 0.11

above at 7, 14, and 21 DAT. The levels of phenylalanine and tyrosine slightly increased again at the dose of 180 g·ha^{-1} and above, albeit still below the control levels. This slight increase in the levels of amino acids in plant tissues subjected to the greatest doses of glyphosate at 7, 14, and 21 DAT may be related to protein degradation and the release of these amino acids in tissues. Aromatic amino acids are used not only for protein synthesis in plants but also as precursors of a large number of secondary metabolites [12].

A marked increase in the concentration of phenylalanine was reported for *Brassica napus* plants in response to concentrations of 1 μM and 10 μM glyphosate, although the concentration tended to decrease to levels lower than in non-treated plants at higher glyphosate concentrations [19]. Although glyphosate is responsible for blocking the biosynthesis of aromatic amino acids, it often fails to produce a clear decrease in the levels of phenylalanine, tyrosine, and tryptophan when the concentrations of plants exposed to glyphosate are compared to the concentrations of control plants.

A transient effect of glyphosate on the total levels of aromatic amino acids was also observed in *Citrus limonia* plants subjected to various doses of glyphosate, with decreases at 2 DAA and increases starting at 4 DAA, regardless of the glyphosate dose evaluated [27]. A decrease in the levels of aromatic amino acids (the sum of phenylalanine, tyrosine, and tryptophan in relation to total amino acids) occurred in pea plants treated with glyphosate from the first day after the treatment, although the levels of amino acids increased again after this initial transient drop [15].

Plant intoxication symptoms were observed at the doses of 72 g a.e. ha^{-1} and above at 21 DAT (**Figure 3**). The symptoms were very severe at the two highest doses, significantly compromising plant development. In addition, the increases in the levels of shikimic acid, quinic acid, and shikimate-3-phosphate compared to the non-treated plants at the same doses indicates the absence of negative effects in this regard at lower doses.

The dry mass of the plants was significantly reduces at doses of 72 g a.e. ha^{-1} and above, and there were signs of injury to leaves (**Figure 3**). However, plants produced greater biomass compared to the control treatment at doses ranging from 7.2 to 36 g a.e. ha^{-1} at 21 DAT. The stimulation of growth of a number of species subjected to low doses of glyphosate has been reported and discussed by various authors [37]-[39]. Glyphosate applications at the dose of 1.8 g a.e. ha^{-1} reportedly provided an increase in sugarcane shoot and root dry mass compared to plants that received no glyphosate application [40].

4. Conclusion

At doses of glyphosate greater than 72 g a.e. ha^{-1}, increases in the levels of shikimic acid, quinic acid, and shikimate-3-phosphate occurred, and AMPA was detected in the plants. Initially, glyphosate caused increases in the levels of phenylalanine and tyrosine in plants at doses of glyphosate of 72 and 180 g a.e. ha^{-1}, although a subsequent decrease over time in the levels of these aromatic amino acids occurred at these doses. The doses between 7.2 and 36 g a.e. ha^{-1} promoted an increase in plant shoot biomass, while doses of glyphosate greater than 72 g a.e. ha^{-1} caused significant reductions in dry mass.

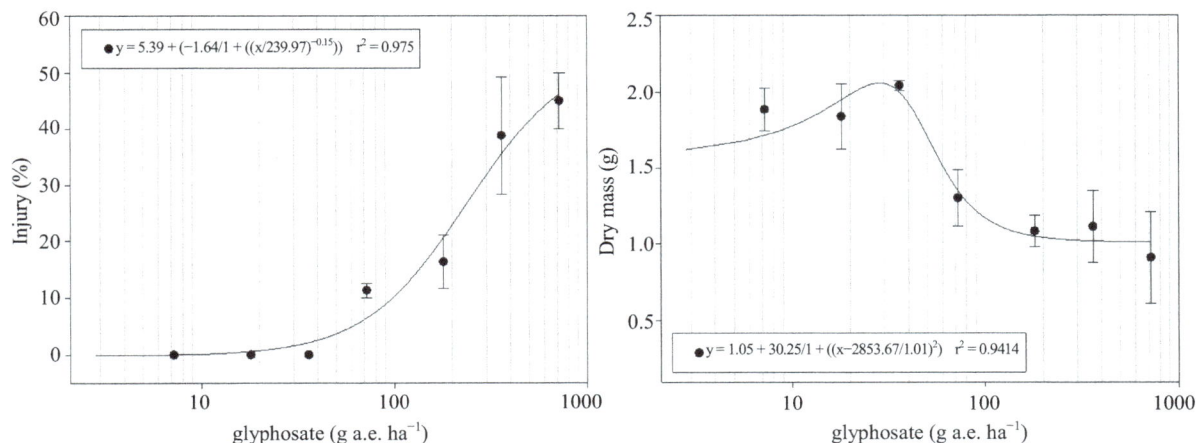

Figure 3. Injury percentages and dry masses of sugarcane plant shoots 21 days after applying various doses of glyphosate (DAT).

Acknowledgements

This research was funded by the São Paulo Research Foundation (FAPESP).

References

[1] CONAB (2014) Acompanhamento da safra brasileira de cana-de-açúcar [Monitoring of the Brazilian Sugarcane Harvest]. Conab, Brasília.

[2] Casagrande, A.A. and Vasconcelos, A.C.M. (2008) Fisiologia da parte aérea. In: Dinardo-Miranda, L.L., Vasconcelos, A.C.M. and Landell, M.G.A., Eds., *Cana-de-Açúcar*, Instituto Agronômico, Campinas, 57-78.

[3] Silva, M.A., Carlin, S.D. and Caputo M.M. (2006) Tipos de colheita e épocas de aplicação de glifosate na erradicação de ratoons de cana-de-açúcar [Harvest Types and Times of Glyphosate Application in the Eradication of Sugarcane Ratoons]. *Pesquisa Agropecuária Brasileira*, **41**, 43-49. http://dx.doi.org/10.1590/S0100-204X2006000100007

[4] Netto, J.M. (2006) Maturatores e reguladores vegetais na cultura da sugarcane [Maturators and plant growth regulators of the sugarcane crop]. In: Egato, S.V., Pinto, A.S. Jendiroba, E. and Nóbrega, J.C.M., Eds., *Atualização em produção de cana-de-açúcar [Update on the Sugarcane Production]*, CP, Piracicaba, 307-318.

[5] Meschede, D.K., Sanomya, R., Carbonari, C.A. and Velini, E.D. (2011) Respostas fisiológicas da cana-de-açúcar ao uso do glyphosate como maturador [Physiological Responses of Sugarcane to the Use of Glyphosate as a Ripener]. In: Velini, E.D., Meschede, D.K., Carbonari, C.A. and Trindade, M.L.B., Eds., *Glyphosate*, Fepaf, Botucatu, 445-459.

[6] Velini, E.D., Trindade, M.L.B., Barberis, L.R.M. and Duke, S.O. (2010) Growth Regulation and Other Effects of Herbicides. *Weed Science*, **58**, 351-354. http://dx.doi.org/10.1614/WS-D-09-00028.1

[7] Franz, J.E., Mao, M.K. and Sikorski, J.A. (1997) Glyphosate: A Unique Global Herbicide. ACS monograph, Washington DC.

[8] Duke, S.O. (1988) Glyphosate. In: Kearney, P.C. and Kaufman, D.D., Eds., *Herbicides: Chemistry, Degradation, and Mode of Action*, Dekker, New York, 1-70.

[9] Herrmann, K.M. and Weaver, L.M. (1999) The Shikimate Pathway. *Annual Review of Plant Physiology and Plant Molecular Biology*, **50**, 473-503. http://dx.doi.org/10.1146/annurev.arplant.50.1.473

[10] Weber, A.P.M., Schwacke, R. and Flugge, U.I. (2005) Solute Transporters of the Plastid Envelope Membrane. *Annual Review of Plant Biology*, **56**, 133-164. http://dx.doi.org/10.1146/annurev.arplant.56.032604.144228

[11] Dewick, P.M. (1998) The Biosynthesis of Shikimate Metabolites. *Natural Products Reports*, **15**, 17-58. http://dx.doi.org/10.1039/a815017y

[12] Herrmann, K.M. (1995) The Shikimate Pathway: Early Steps in the Biosynthesis of Aromatic Compounds. *The Plant Cell*, **7**, 907-919. http://dx.doi.org/10.1105/tpc.7.7.907

[13] Velini, E.D., Carbonari, C.A., Trindade, M.L.B., Gomes, G.L.G.C., Meschede, D.K. and Duke, S.O. (2011) Modo de ação do Glyphosate [Glyphosate Mechanism of Action]. In: Velini, E.D., Carbonari, C.A., Meschede, D.K. and Trindade, M.L.B., Eds., *Glyphosate*, Fepaf, Botucatu, 39-66.

[14] Reddy, K.N., Bellaloui, N. and Zablotowicz, R.M. (2010) Glyphosate Effect on Shikimate, Nitrate Reductase Activity, Yield, and Seed Composition in Corn. *Journal of Agricultural and Food Chemistry*, **58**, 3646-3650. http://dx.doi.org/10.1021/jf904121y

[15] Orcaray, L., Igal, M., Marino, D., Zabalza, A. and Royuela, M. (2010) The Possible Role of Quinate in the Mode of Action of Glyphosate and Acetolactate Synthase Inhibitors. *Pest Management Science*, **66**, 262-269. http://dx.doi.org/10.1002/ps.1868

[16] Matallo, M.B., Almeida, S.D.B., Cerdeira, A.L., Franco, D.A., Blanco, F.M.G., Menezes, P.T.C., Luchini, L.C., Moura, M.A.M. and Duke, S.O. (2009) Microwave-Assisted Solvent Extraction and Analysis of Shikimic Acid from Plant Tissues. *Planta Daninha*, **27**, 987-994. http://dx.doi.org/10.1590/S0100-83582009000500012

[17] Reddy, K.N., Rimando, A.M., Duke, S.O. and Nandula, V.K. (2008) Aminomethylphosphonic Acid Accumulation in Plant Species Treated with Glyphosate. *Journal of Agricultural and Food Chemistry*, **56**, 2125-2130. http://dx.doi.org/10.1021/jf072954f

[18] Buehring, N.W., Massey, J.H. and Reynolds, D.B. (2007) Shikimic Acid in Field-Grown Corn (*Zea mays*) Following Simulated Glyphosate Drift. *Journal of Agricultural and Food Chemistry*, **55**, 819-824. http://dx.doi.org/10.1021/jf062624f

[19] Petersen, I.L., Hansena, H.C.B., Ravn, H.W., Sorensen, J.C. and Sorensen, H. (2007) Metabolic Effects in Rapeseed (*Brassica napus* L.) Seedlings after Root Exposure to Glyphosate. *Pesticide Biochemistry and Physiology*, **89**, 220-229. http://dx.doi.org/10.1016/j.pestbp.2007.06.009

[20] Feng, C.C., Tran, M., Chiu, T., Sammons, R.D., Heck, G.R. and CaJacob, C.A. (2004) Investigations into Glypho-

sate-Resistant Horseweed (*Conyza canadensis*): Retention, Uptake, Translocation, and Metabolism. *Weed Science*, **52**, 498-505. http://dx.doi.org/10.1614/WS-03-137R

[21] Harring, T., Streibig, J.C. and Husted, S. (1998) Accumulation of Shikimic Acid: A Technique for Screening Glyphosate Efficiency. *Journal of Agricultural and Food Chemistry*, **46**, 4406-4412. http://dx.doi.org/10.1021/jf9802124

[22] Ossipov, V.I. and Aleksandrova, L.P. (1982) Spatial Organization of Quinic and Shikimic Acid Biosynthesis in the Autotrophic Cell of *Pinus sylvestris* Needles. *Soviet Plant Physiology*, **29**, 289-292.

[23] Orcaray, L., Zulet, A., Zabalza, A. and Royuela, M. (2012) Impairment of Carbon Metabolism Induced by the Herbicide Glyphosate. *Journal of Plant Physiology*, **169**, 27-33. http://dx.doi.org/10.1016/j.jplph.2011.08.009

[24] Gomes, G.L.G.C. (2011) Alterações metabóLicas de Plantas de Milho Submetidas à Aplicação de Glyphosate e Fosfito [Metabolic Changes of Maize Plants Subjected to an Application of Glyphosate and Phosphite]. MSC. Thesis, Faculdade de Ciências Agronômicas, Universidade Estadual Paulista, Botucatu [School of Agricultural Sciences, São Paulo State University, Botucatu].

[25] Duke, S.O., Rimando, A.M., Pace, P.F., Reddy, K.N. and Smeda, R.J. (2003) Isoflavone, Glyphosate, and Aminomethylphosphonic Acid Levels in Seeds of Glyphosate-Treated, Glyphosate-Resistant Soybean. *Journal of Agricultural and Food Chemistry*, **51**, 340-344. http://dx.doi.org/10.1021/jf025908i

[26] Arregui, M.C., Lenardón, A., Sanchez, D., Maitre, M.I., Scotta, R. and Enrique, S. (2004) Monitoring Glyphosate Residues in Transgenic Glyphosate-Resistant Soybean. *Pest Management Science*, **60**, 163-166. http://dx.doi.org/10.1002/ps.775

[27] Gravena, R., Victoria Filho, R., Alves, P.L., Mazzafera, P. and Gravena, A.R. (2009) Low Glyphosate Rates Do Not Affect *Citrus limonia* (L.) Osbeck Seedlings. *Pest Management Science*, **65**, 420-425. http://dx.doi.org/10.1002/ps.1694

[28] Becerril, J.M., Duke, S.O. and Lydon, J. (1989) Glyphosate Effect on Shikimate Pathway Products in Leaves and Flowers of Velvetleaf. *Phytochemistry*, **28**, 695-699. http://dx.doi.org/10.1016/0031-9422(89)80095-0

[29] Bresnahan, G.A., Manthey, F.A., Howatt, K.A. and Chakraborty, M. (2003) Glyphosate Applied Preharvest Induces Shikimic Acid Accumulation in Hard Red Spring Wheat (*Triticum aestivum*). *Journal of Agricultural and Food Chemistry*, **51**, 4004-4007. http://dx.doi.org/10.1021/jf0301753

[30] Mueller, T.C., Massey, J.H., Hayes, R.M., Main, C.L. and Stewart Jr., C.N. (2003) Shikimate Accumulates in both Glyphosate-Sensitive and Glyphosate-Resistant Horseweed (*Conyza canadensis* L. Cronq.). *Journal of Agricultural and Food Chemistry*, **51**, 680-684. http://dx.doi.org/10.1021/jf026006k

[31] Geiger, D.R., Tucci, M.A. and Serviates, J.C. (1987) Glyphosate Effects on Carbon Assimilation and Gas Exchange in Sugar Beet Leaves. *Plant Physiology*, **85**, 365-369. http://dx.doi.org/10.1104/pp.85.2.365

[32] Fuchs, M.A., Geigera, D.R., Reynoldsb, T.L. and Bourqueb, J.E. (2002) Mechanisms of Glyphosate Toxicity in Velvetleaf (*Abutilon theophrasti* Medikus). *Pesticide Biochemistry and Physiology*, **74**, 27-39. http://dx.doi.org/10.1016/S0048-3575(02)00118-9

[33] Singh, B.K. and Shaner, D.L. (1998) Rapid Determination of Glyphosate Injury to Plants and Identification of Glyphosate-Resistant Plants. *Weed Technology*, **12**, 527-530.

[34] Amrhein, N., Deus, B., Gehrke, P. and Steinrücken, H.C. (1980) The Site of the Inhibition of the Shikimate Pathway by Glyphosate.II. Interference of Glyphosate with Chorismate Formation *in Vivo* and *in Vitro*. *Plant Physiology*, **66**, 830-834. http://dx.doi.org/10.1104/pp.66.5.830

[35] Wang, C.Y. (2001) Effect of Glyphosate on Aromatic Amino Acid Metabolism in Purple Nutsedge (*Cyperus rotundus*). *Weed Technology*, **15**, 628-635. http://dx.doi.org/10.1614/0890-037X(2001)015[0628:EOGOAA]2.0.CO;2

[36] Forlani, G., Lejczak, P. and Kafarski, P. (2000) The Herbicidally Active Compound *N*-2-(5-Chloropyridyl) Aminomethylene Bisphosphonic Acid Acts by Inhibiting both Glutamine and Aromatic Amino Acid Biosynthesis. *Australian Journal of Plant Physiology*, **27**, 677-683.

[37] Schanbenberger, O., Tharp, B.E., Kells, J.J. and Penner, D. (1999) Statistical Tests for Hormesis and Effective Dosage in Herbicide Dose Response. *Agronomy Journal*, **91**, 713-721. http://dx.doi.org/10.2134/agronj1999.914713x

[38] Cedergreen, N., Streibig, J.C., Kudsk, P., Mathiassen, S.K. and Duke, S.O. (2007) The Occurrence of Hormesis in Plants and Algae. *Dose-Response*, **5**, 150-162. http://dx.doi.org/10.2203/dose-response.06-008.Cedergreen

[39] Velini, E.D., Alves, E., Godoy, M.C., Meschede, D.K., Souza, R.T. and Duke, S.O. (2008) Glyphosate Applied at Low Doses Can Stimulate Plant Growth. *Pest Management Science*, **64**, 489-496. http://dx.doi.org/10.1002/ps.1562

[40] Silva, M.A., Aragão, N.C., Barbosa, M.A., Jeronimo, E.M. and Carlin, S.D. (2009) Efeito Hormótico de Gliphosate no Desenvolvimento Inicial de Cana-de-Açúcar [Hormetic Effect of Glyphosate on the Initial Development of Sugarcane]. *Bragantia*, **68**, 973-978. http://dx.doi.org/10.1590/S0006-87052009000400017

3

Molecular Regulation of the Metabolic Pathways of the Medicinal Plants: *Phyla dulcis*

Godson O. Osuji*, Aruna Weerasooriya, Peter A. Y. Ampim, Laura Carson, Paul Johnson, Yoonsung Jung, Eustace Duffus, Sela Woldesenbet, Sanique South, Edna Idan, Dewisha Johnson, Diadrian Clarke, Billy Lawton, Alfred Parks, Ali Fares, Alton Johnson

Plant Systems Research Unit, College of Agriculture and Human Sciences, Prairie View A & M University, Prairie View, USA
Email: *goosuji@pvamu.edu, cropyielddoublingbiotechnology@yahoo.com

Abstract

Phyla (*Lippia*) *dulcis* contains hernundulcin sesquiterpene zero-caloric sweetener that is about a thousand times sweeter than sucrose, and also bitter constituents including camphor and limonene. There is yet no simple method to remove the undesirable constituents. The yield of sweetener hernundulcin is very low, and there is no simple method to maximize its composition. The aim of the project was to characterize the mRNA targets that regulate the primary and terpenoid metabolic enzymes of *P. dulcis*. Restriction fragment differential display polymerase chain reaction of *P. dulcis* glutamate dehydrogenase-synthesized RNA showed that many mRNAs encoding β-caryophyllene, (+)-epi-α-bisabolol, bicyclogermacrene, bifunctional sesquiterpene, and geraniol synthases shared sequence homologies with ribulose-1,5-bisphophatase carboxylase, granule-bound starch synthase, pyruvate kinase, glucose-6-phosphate dehydrogenase, and phosphoenol pyruvate carboxylase. Sequence similarities between mRNAs encoding primary metabolic enzymes and terpene synthases suggested that photosynthesis could regulate terpenoid metabolism in order to increase the yield of sweetener hernundulcin.

Keywords

Hernundulcin Sweetener, Primary Metabolism, Terpene Synthase mRNA, Glutamate Dehydrogenase

---

*Corresponding author.

1. Introduction

Phyla (*Lippia*) *dulcis* (Verbenaceae) is a Central American plant used traditionally by Aztac peoples as herbal sweetener [1]. Herbal ingredients in dietary supplements for control of diabetes and obesity are gaining popularity and have a huge market [2]. However, more scientific studies on these medicinal plants are needed in order to bring them to commercial products. One of the predispositions to obesity is the intake of high caloric foods. Therefore more research was focused on the chemistry of zero-calorie sugar substitutes. There are over ~100 medicinal plant-derived sweet compounds of 20 major structural types that have been reported, and are isolated from more than 25 different families of green plants [1]. The Central American plant *Phyla dulcis* has two sesquiterpene sweetener constituents: hernandulcin and 4β-hydroxyhernandulcin which are 1000 times sweeter than sucrose [3]. As such, they have potential for use as natural low calorie sweeteners in the dietary management of diabetes/obesity. However, other compounds identified in *Phyla* extracts are undesirable and include camphor, limonene, terpineol, α-pinene, α-copaene, trans-caryophyllene, δ-cadinene, and α-bisabolol [4]. Efforts are in progress to remove the camphor from leaf extract through hydro-distillation [4], supercritical fluid extraction technology [5]; microbial degradation of the camphor [6]; hernandulcin production in yeast [7] [8]; and/or production of hernandulcin by hairy root/shoot culture of *P. dulcis* [9]. *Phyla* species are characterized by variability in the chemical compositions of their monoterpenes, and sesquiterpenes depending on the origin of plant materials, and the stage of maturity of the plant part selected for analysis. Various metabolic variants (chemotypes) of *Lippia alba* have been identified [4]. But the molecular regulation that conferred the biochemical characteristics on the chemotypes was not studied. *Phyla* species abound in terpene and sesquiterpene synthases [7] [10] [11]. Therefore it is anticipated that some of the regulatory targets would be associated with the mRNAs encoding the monoterpene and sesquiterpene synthases. Earlier results demonstrated the successes in the utilization of some environmental conditions (mineral salts, and nucleotide solutions) to alter the yields of fatty acids, resveratrol, amino acids, cellulose, proteins, and biomass feedstock metabolic pathways of crops including sweetpotato, soybean, peanut, and cowpea [12]-[14]. The mechanism is that the stoichiometric mineral ion, and nucleotide mixes induced the glutamate dehydrogenase (GDH) to isomerize and to synthesize some RNAs which silence mRNAs homologous to them [12]-[17]. The research approach [13] has explained many hitherto inexplicable biological phenomena including the production of arachin-free peanut [14], metabolic detoxification of xenobiotics in plants [15], doubling of peanut yield [16], and of ultra-high resveratrol peanut [17]. GDH is the target site of the action of nucleophiles including nucleotides, mineral ions etc. [18] [19]. Such plant-based systems research approaches have not been applied to *Phyla* species. With the perfection of the genetic basis of yeast fermentation production of sesquiterpenes [8] accompanied by the detailed analytical chemistry of terpenes [6] [7] [10], it is logical to focus research attention on potential agricultural technologies for production of high-hernandulcin *P. dulcis* metabolic variants. *Phyla* sweetener industry generates about $1.5 billion [2] [20]. Wherefore, the proof of the biochemical protocols for the GDH-based plants system research concept is the demonstration of the RNA synthetic activity [21] of *P. dulcis* GDH and characterization of the metabolic functions of the RNA as presented hereunder.

2. Materials and Methods

2.1. Cultivation of Medicinal Plants *Phyla dulcis*

Stem cuttings from *P. dulcis* (Trev.) Mold. (Verbenaceae) growing in a peat moss potting medium in plastic containers in a greenhouse were planted on raised beds in March-April, 2013 in the medicinal plants garden of Prairie View A & M University Research Farm, and watered by drip irrigation as necessary without fertilizer treatment. The soil at the site is characterized as a fine-loamy, siliceous, thermic Typic Paleudalf. The weather conditions throughout the *Phyla* establishment were monitored at the USDA-NRCS Scan Station on the Prairie View A & M University farm a few meters from the *Phyla* plot. The *Phyla* established rootings quickly and commenced good vegetative growth. In late April, green and young leaves were harvested from many healthy plant stands, frozen in dry ice and transported to storage in −80°C freezer. The *P. dulcis* continued to grow in the plots, and in June-July the intense summer light and heat of Texas induced the purple coloration of the older leaves.

2.2. Purification and Assay of GDH

GDH was extracted with Tris-HCl buffer solution containing RNAse A and DNase 1, and purified by electrophoresis as described before [21] [22] from *P. dulcis* green leaves harvested from the medicinal plants garden. RNA synthetic activity of GDH isoenzymes [12] was assayed in combined deamination and amination substrate solutions of 0.1 M Tris-HCl buffer solution (pH 8.0) containing the four NTPs (0.6 mM each), $CaCl_2$ (3.5 mM), L-glu (3.23 µM), NAD^+ (0.375 µM), NH_4Cl (0.875 mM), α-ketoglutarate (10.0 mM), NADH (0.225 mM), 5 Units RNase inhibitor, 1 Unit DNase 1, and 5 µg of actinomycin D. Reaction was started by adding 0.2 mL of whole gel-eluted GDH charge isomers containing 3 - 6 µg protein per mL. Final volume of the reaction was brought to 0.4 mL with 0.1 M Tris-HCl buffer pH 8.0. Reactions were incubated at 16°C overnight and stopped by phenol-chloroform (pH 5.5) extraction of the enzyme. RNA was precipitated with ethanol, and dissolved in minimum volume of molecular biology quality water. RNA yield and quality were determined by photometry and by agarose gel electrophoresis. Assays were carried out in duplicate to verify the reproducibility of the results.

2.3. Complementary DNA Synthesis, Cloning and Characterization

cDNAs were synthesized with 2 µg of each product RNA synthesized by the whole gel-eluted GDH charge isomers using random hexamer primer. Restriction fragment PCR amplification; adapter ligation; sequencing gel fractionation; and purification of cDNA fragments [12] [13] were conducted according to the methods of Display Systems Biotech, Vista, CA, USA. Selected cDNA fragments were subcloned into pCR4-TOPO vector and transformed into TOP10 One Shot Chemically Competent *Escherichia coli* (Invitrogen, Carlsbad, CA), followed by overnight growth on selective plates. Up to ten positive transformant colonies were picked per plate and cultured overnight in LB medium containing 50 µg/mL of kanamycin. Plasmid DNA was purified with a plasmid kit (QiaGen mini kit, Madison, WI). The insert cDNA was sequenced with T3 and T7 primers by Functional Biosciences, Inc. (Madison, WI, USA).

To characterize the GDH-synthesized RNAs, the cDNA sequences were used as queries to search the NCBI nucleotide-nucleotide (excluding ESTs) BLAST (blastn), and non-redundant protein translation (blastx) databases for *Phyla dulcis* and related taxids. Complementary DNAs that displayed the highest alignment scores with mRNAs encoding the enzymes of primary and natural products (secondary) metabolism were selected.

3. Results and Discussion

3.1. Cultivation of *P. dulcis* in Texas, USA

Phyla dulcis, prostate perennial medicinal herb with many branches, originally a South American sweet herb has been established in the medicinal plants garden of the University, Waller County, Texas, USA. The weather conditions for March and April 2013 (**Table 1**) showed that rainfall decreased but temperatures increased during the period of the experiment. The weather conditions are important for reporting experimental conditions and for future field plot establishment of the species. Under the intensive light, heat and humidity conditions of Texas summer, the older leaves turned purple (**Figure 1**) suggesting that the photosynthetic pathways could be subject to environmental regulation. There is no literature record on the sustainable cultivation of the species in the USA, therefore environmental research is in progress for identifying best management strategies (fertilization, plant protection, irrigation etc.).

3.2. *Phyla dulcis* GDH Activity

Rotofor isoelectric focusing (IEF) of *P. dulcis* GDH extracts gave a single horizontal row of isoenzymes covering from Rotofor chambers (fractions) 4 to 12 on native PAGE (figures not shown) unlike that of peanut [22]. RNA synthetic assays of the whole-gel eluted isoenzymes gave a series of predominantly low molecular weight

Table 1. Field weather conditions from transplanting to harvesting of the *Phyla dulcis* leaves[†].

Month	Rainfall (mm)	Maximum daily temperature (°C)	Minimum daily temperature (°C)	Relative humidity (%)	Solar radiation (lang)	Wind speed (mph)
March	0.61 ± 2.38[‡]	21.3 ± 4.6	7.4 ± 5.7	79.2 ± 14.9	371.6 ± 102.0	7.7 ± 2.7
April	3.5 ± 6.9	24.0 ± 4.2	12.2 ± 5.3	89.5 ± 9.1	353.8 ± 146.6	7.8 ± 2.9

[†]The weather data were obtained from the USDA-NRCS Scan Station on the Prairie View A & M University farm a few meters from the *Phyla* plot; [‡]Monthly mean and standard deviation.

(<500 nucleotides long) RNAs on agarose gels (figures not shown) irrespective of the pI values of the isoenzymes. Therefore, the acidic isoenzymes (Rotofor fractions 4 to 6) were combined, neutral isoenzymes (Rotofor fractions 7 and 8) were combined, and basic isoenzymes (Rotofor fractions 9 to 12) were combined and the three composite samples were applied for the double differential display analyses.

3.3. Differential Display of GDH-Synthesized RNAs of *P. dulcis*

The purpose of the differential display RF-PCR of the GDH-synthesized RNAs was to permit easy molecular biology amplification, isolation, and bioinformatics characterization of the cDNA fragments homologous to *P. dulcis* mRNAs as were done previously [21]. The double differential display patterns of the cDNAs (**Figures 2-4**) showed that the RNAs synthesized by the acidic, neutral, and basic isoenzymes of *Phyla* GDH were structurally different isomers in agreement with the binomial subunit compositions in the hexameric isoenzymes [21]-[25]. All the 64 display PROBES of Display Systems Biotech, Vista, CA, USA were studied. Based on the subsets of cDNA fragments obtained, the PCR priming by display PROBES 1, 4, and 18 (**Figures 2-4**) showed that the neutral isoenzymes of GDH were more active in RNA synthesis than the acidic and basic isoenzymes. The display patterns obtained in replicate RF-PCR experiments showed complete identity per display PROBE. Similarly, the differential band patterns for GDH-synthesized RNAs were different from those for mRNAs [26]. Therefore the synthesis of RNA by *P. dulcis* GDH was specific and reproducible reactions. cDNAs of GDH-synthesized RNAs are important Northern hybridization tools for monitoring and quantitation of the abundances of mRNAs that are homologous to them [12]-[17].

3.4. Messenger RNA Targets of *P. dulcis* GDH-Synthesized RNAs

To assign functions to the cDNA fragments, their sequences were used to search the GenBank databases with the BLASTN etc. algorithms. An overview of the mRNA targets homologous to the differential cDNA fragments (**Figures 2-4**) showed that overwhelmingly the mRNAs encoding the enzymes of primary metabolism were the targets of the RNAs synthesized by the acidic GDH isoenzymes; whereas predominantly the mRNAs encoding the enzymes of natural products metabolism were the targets of the RNAs synthesized by the neutral and basic GDH isoenzymes. These are important molecular differences and similarities that would allow environmental conditions to be focused either on the primary or terpenoid metabolism of the plant species.

Differential cDNA band 1.02 (**Figure 2**) yielded several isomeric cDNAs (**Table 2**). They showed sequence homologies with mRNAs encoding *Phyla* primary metabolic enzymes including dehydroquinate dehydratase, small subunit of ribulose-1,5-bisphophatase carboxylase, cytochrome P-450 reductase, granule-bound starch synthase, pyruvate kinase, glucose-6-phosphate dehydrogenase, protoporphyrinogen oxidase, phosphoenol pyruvate carboxylase, quinolinate phosphirobosyltransferase, photosystem II protein, and coumarate: coenzyme A ligase. The mechanism of GDH-synthesized RNA is that they silence mRNAs homologous to them [16] [24]. All the mRNAs homologous to cDNA fragments 1.02 (**Figure 2**) have different molecular weights therefore making them very easy to identify on Northern blot analyses. This is a considerable advantage in target mRNA profiling and modeling of biochemical pathways [14] [17]. Differential cDNA fragment 1.03 (**Figure 2**) was homologous to mRNA encoding peroxidase. The metabolic probes embodied by the cDNA fragments 1.02 and

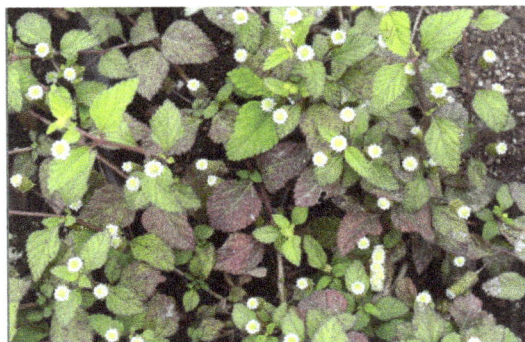

Figure 1. *Phyla dulcis* growing in field plot in Texas summer conditions. There are green leaves, and older leaves that are purple.

Lippia Primary Metabolic Targets

For cDNA fragments in band 1.02

* **Dehydroquinate dehydratase**
* **Ribulose - 1,5-biphosphatase carboxylase**
* **Grannule-bound starch synthase**
* **Pyruvate kinase**
* **Glucose-6-phosphate dehydrogenase**
* **Protoporphyrinogen oxidase**
* **Cytochrome P-450 reductase**
* **PEP carboxylase**
* **Quinolinate phosphirobosyltranferase**
* **Coumarate:coenzyme A ligase**
* **Photosystem II protein**

For cDNA fragments in band 1.03a

Peroxidase

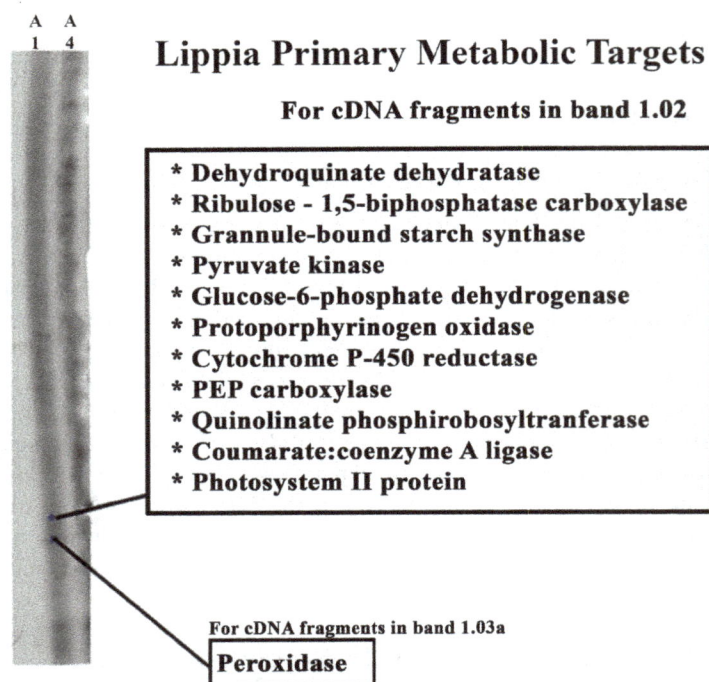

Figure 2. Differential display of RNA synthesized by the GDH of *P. dulcis*. The RNA synthesized by the acidic isoenzymes (whole gel purified Rotofor fractions 4-6 were combined = A) was used. After cDNA preparation, the restriction fractions were amplified by Display System's Double Differential-PCR method and fractionated on sequencing PAGE. Lanes A1, A4 were for display PROBEs 1 and 4 respectively as PCR primers. The indicated fragments were sequenced.

Lippia Natural Products Metabolic Targets

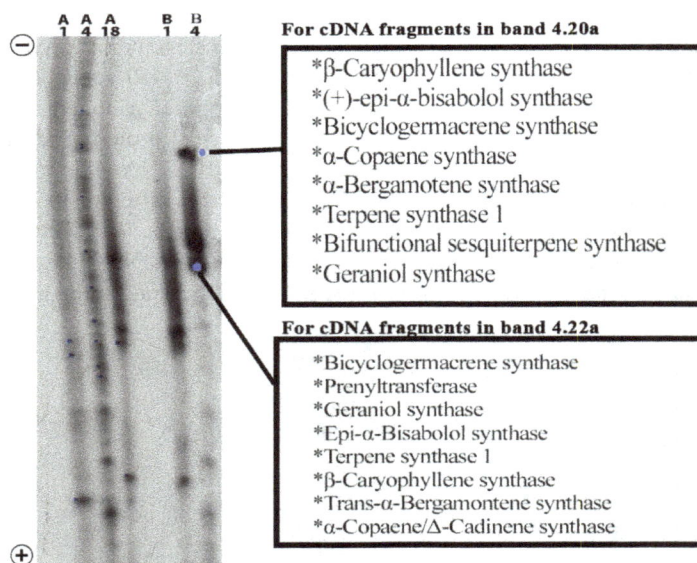

For cDNA fragments in band 4.20a

* *β-Caryophyllene synthase
* *(+)-epi-α-bisabolol synthase
* *Bicyclogermacrene synthase
* *α-Copaene synthase
* *α-Bergamotene synthase
* *Terpene synthase 1
* *Bifunctional sesquiterpene synthase
* *Geraniol synthase

For cDNA fragments in band 4.22a

* *Bicyclogermacrene synthase
* *Prenyltransferase
* *Geraniol synthase
* *Epi-α-Bisabolol synthase
* *Terpene synthase 1
* *β-Caryophyllene synthase
* *Trans-α-Bergamontene synthase
* *α-Copaene/Δ-Cadinene synthase

Figure 3. Differential display of RNA synthesized by the GDH of *P. dulcis*. The RNA synthesized by the acidic isoenzymes (whole gel purified Rotofor fractions 4-6 were combined = A), and neutral isoenzymes (whole gel purified Rotofor fractions 7 & 8 were combined = B) were used. After cDNA preparation, the restriction fractions were amplified by display System's Double Differential-PCR method and fractionated on sequencing PAGE. Lanes A1, A4, A18 were for display PROBEs 1, 4 and 18 respectively as PCR primers for the acid isoenzyme synthesized RNA; lanes B1, and B4 were for display PROBES 1 and 4 respectively for the neutral isoenzyme synthesized RNA. The indicated fragments were sequenced.

Lippia Natural Products Metabolic Targets

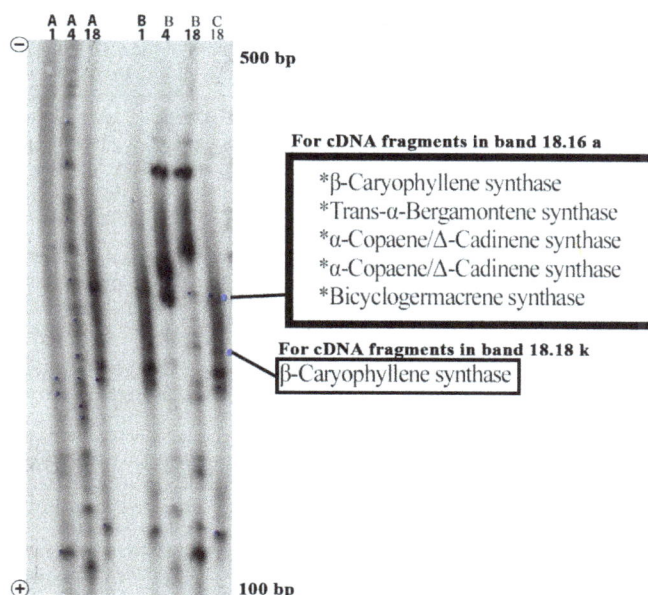

Figure 4. Differential display of RNA synthesized by the GDH of *P. dulcis*. The RNA synthesized by the acidic isoenzymes (whole gel purified Rotofor fractions 4-6 were combined = A), neutral isoenzymes (whole gel purified Rotofor fractions 7&8 were combined = B), basic isoenzymes (whole gel purified Rotofor fractions 9-12 were combined = C) were used. After cDNA preparation, the restriction fractions were amplified by display System's Double Differential-PCR method and fractionated on sequencing PAGE. Lanes A1, A4, A18 were for display PROBEs 1, 4 and 18 respectively as PCR primers for the acid isoenzyme synthesized RNA; lanes B1, B4, and B18 were for display PROBES 1, 4, and 18 respectively for the neutral isoenzyme synthesized RNA; lane C18 was for display PROBE 18 for the basic isoenzyme synthesized RNA. The indicated fragments were sequenced.

1.03 constitute important molecular tools for monitoring and regulating *P. dulcis* mRNA targets in photosynthesis (**Figure 1**). The dual importance of GDH-synthesized RNAs is that *in vivo* they silence mRNAs homologous to them; and *in vitro* they serve as reliable probes in Northern hybridization analyses [12]-[16].

Complementary DNA fragments 4.20 (**Figure 3**) showed sequence homologies with mRNAs encoding *Phyla* terpenoid metabolic enzymes including β-caryophyllene synthase, (+)-epi-α-bisabolol synthase, bicyclogermacrene synthase, α-copaene/δ-cadinene synthases, trans-α-bergamotene synthase, terpene synthase 1, bifunctional sesquiterpene synthase, and geraniol synthase (**Table 2**). These are some of the terpene synthases that have been characterized before [7] [11]; and the encoding mRNAs are related to the enzymes that synthesize some of the undesirable secondary metabolites of *Phyla* [4] [10]. Complementary DNA fragments 4.22 (**Figure 3**) similar to fragments 4.20 showed sequence homologies with mRNAs encoding *Phyla* terpenoid metabolic enzymes including in addition prenyltransferase (**Table 2**). All the mRNA homologous to cDNA fragments 4.20 and 4.22 possess different molecular weights therefore making them very easy to profile on Northern blot analyses. The metabolic probes embodied by cDNA fragments 4.20 and 4.22 constitute important molecular tools for monitoring and regulating *Phyla* biochemical targets in the study of the effects of agronomic management factors (fertilization, irrigation, pesticide tolerance) on secondary metabolism.

RNAs synthesized by the basic isoenzymes of *Phyla* GDH (**lane C-18** of **Figure 4**) gave differential cDNA fragmentation patterns similar to those of the RNAs synthesized by the neutral isoenzymes (**lanes B-1**, **B-4**, **B-18** of **Figure 4**). Complementary DNA fragments 18.16 (**Figure 4**) shared sequence homologies with mRNAs encoding β-caryophyllene synthase, α-copaene/δ-cadinene synthases, and trans-α-bergamotene synthase, bicyclogermacrene synthase (**Table 2**) all of which are molecular targets in natural products metabolism. Complementary DNA fragments 18.18 (**Figure 4**) shared sequence homology with mRNAs encoding β-caryophyllene synthase (**Table 2**) therefore it will complement fragments 18.16 in Northern profiling of *Phyla* total RNAs. RNA differential display (**Figures 2-4**) is a sensitive, reproducible, and versatile technology for profiling different RNAs simultaneously [26].

Table 2. Some cDNA sequences of the RNAs synthesized by the GDH of medicinal plant *Phyla dulcis*, their homologous mRNAs, and the encoded enzymes.

Enzymes and mRNA accessions	cDNA sequences of the GDH-synthesized RNAs homologous to the mRNAs
a 3-dehydroquinate dehydratase/shikimate dehydrogenase isoform ID: gb|AY578144.1|	gggtgcatagcggcgcgaattcgcccttactggtctcgtagactgcgtacccgataatcctcagcaaat gacaacgtggctggccgggcaagcctcggaccccgtaaagcgcgcgtccttgttgacgcacttttccc tcaaggatcaagctgacagaacgttttcagacggcgtacgtcagaccctgcaggggatgggaaactg gtccgatgcgcaggcatcaggcaatgctttccttgcgagcctcaacggttgggtgccggatcgtttcatc gctgttgagcagttgcacggtgatcctttcggtcaggactcata
b chloroplast ribulose 1,5-bisphosphate carbox-ylase/oxygenase small subunit ID: gb|KM025319.1| c cytochrome P-450 reductase ID: emb|X96784.1|	tgagcgtattgcggncgcgnnatcgcccttgatgagtcctgaccgatataacgcgaagaaccttacca ggccggtacgcagtctacgagaccagtagcgatgagtcctgaccgggtacgcagtctacgagaccag tagtacgcagtctacgagaccagtagtacgcagtctacgagaccagttgtatgctgtttactggatgctttt gggcctggtagactgttccgtttagtgtaggtttgttgtgaacttggtgtggtgag
d grannule-bound starch synthase ID: gb|EF584735.1|	ccttactggtctcgtagactgcgtacccggtcaggactcatcagtcaggactactggtctcgtagactgc gtacccggtcaggactcatcgctatatcggtcaggactcatcaa
e pyruvate kinase (plastid isozyme) ID: emb|Z28374.1|	tattttcttattcggcgccatactctctctctgtgctcacagaccgcgcaatactggtcgcgactcactact aatgggcccggaaagggtcttcgcgatatatcagtcacgactacatcaccttatagaccacgactcatc acatcagtcatgactcatcatatcagtaatgatcataatattggtcacgactcatcaagggagaattctatt aaacctgcaggactaccctctttaatgatggttaattatgatcttgtagta
f cytosolic glucose-6-phosphate dehydrogenase ID: emb|AJ001769.1|	caggtgatagcggncgcgnattcgcccttgatgagtcctgaccgatatagcgatgagtcctgaccgat atagtgatgagtcctgaccgatatgctttctccaggcgtaaaaaagcccgctcaattggcgggctgcta ttcttcggtcgggtacgcagtctacgagaccagta
g protoporphyrinogen oxidase ID: gb|AF044128.1|AF044128	gggaatagcggatgcgcatgcgcactctctggtgtcgtagactgcctacccggttaggactcatcctta ctggtcgtgaagactgcgaactctgtgaggactcatcatcactggtctcgtagactgcgtacccggtca ggactcatcggtactggtctcgtagacagcttaccggcctgggaaggttcttcgtgttatatcggtcatga ttcatcaagcgcgaattctcc
h phosphoenolpyruvate carboxylase ID: sp|P27154.1	ggcgtattagcggcgcgaattcgcccttactggtctcgtagactgcgtaatcggtcaggactcatcacta ctggtctcgtagactgcgtaccactggtctcgtagactgcgtactactggtctcgtagactgcatatcggt caggactcatca
i photosystem II protein N: ID: NP_054528.1	ccttactggtctcgtagactgcgtacccggtcaggactcatcagtcaggactactggtctcgtagactgc gtacccggtcaggactcatcgctatatcggtcaggactcatca
j 4-coumarate:coenzyme A ligase. ID: dbj|D43773.1|	gtgcaatacggncgcgaattcgcccttactggtctcgtagactgcgtacccgatcaggactcatcgctat atcggtcaggctcatcactatatcggtcaggactcatca
k peroxidase ID: dbj|AB044154.1|	ggggaaaaaacgggcgcgaattcgcccttactggtctcgtagactgcgatatcggtcaggactcatc actactggtctcgtagactgcgtacccggtcaggactcatcgctactggtctcgtagactgcgtacccgg tcaggactcatcgctatatcggtcaggactcatcatatcggtcaggactcatcaagggcgaattcgtttaa acctgcaggactagtccctttagtgagggttaattctgagcttggcgtaatcatggtcatagctgtttcctgt gtgaaattg
l beta-caryophyllene synthase <u>ID:</u> gb|JQ731634.1 m (+)-epi-alpha-bisabolol synthase <u>ID:</u> sp|J7LH11.1| n Bicyclogermacrene synthase ID: gb|JQ731633.1 o alpha-copaene/delta-cadinene synthase <u>ID:</u> gb|JQ731632.1| p trans-alpha-bergamotene synthase <u>ID:</u> gb|JQ731635.1| q Bifunctional sesquiterpene synthase 1 <u>ID:</u> sp|J7LP58.1| r geraniol synthase <u>ID:</u> gb|ADK62524.1	gaggtaatagcggcgcgaattcgcccttactggtctcgtagactgcgtacccgatgcagaaggcggga aaacatgaaatgagcgtcaagcaggccgtgaaggttgccgagcttttgaagtgcaacccgatggaggt tatctgcggggtgatgtttcaccaggacgtaatggagcgggatttctggacggacattttccagcagaca gtcaccgaaaacgaccgccgccactacttcaagaaggtttaggcaggctttcggtcaggactcata
s prenyltransferase alpha-subunit ID: emb|CDI30233.1|	ctggtctcgtagactgcgtacccgatgcagaaggcgggaaaacatgaaatgagcgtcaagcaggccg tgaaggttgccgagcttttgaagtgcaacccgatggaggttatctgcggggtgatgtttcaccaggacgt aatggagcgggatttctggacggacattttccagcagacagtcaccgaaaacgaccgccgccactact tcaagaaggtttaggcaggctttcggtcaggactcataaagggcgaattcgtttaaacctgcaggact

3.5. Structure of RNAs Synthesized by *Phyla* GDH

The GDH-synthesized RNAs that were homologous to mRNAs encoding *Phyla* primary metabolic enzymes displayed extensive sequence similarities. The cDNA fragment (**Table 2**) homologous to the mRNA encoding granule-bound starch synthase shared 8-fold plus/minus sequence matches with the cDNA fragment (**Table 2**) homologous to the mRNA encoding glucose-6-phosphate dehydrogenase; 5-fold plus/minus sequence matches with the cDNA fragment (**Table 2**) homologous to the mRNA encoding protoporphyrinogen oxidase; but 4-fold plus/plus sequence matches with the cDNA fragment (**Table 2**) homologous to the mRNA encoding 4-coumarate: coenzyme A ligase. The RNAs synthesized by GDH are isomeric in structure similar to the binomial subunit structure of the enzyme's hexamers [25]. Structural similarities between a GDH-synthesized RNA and several mRNAs in different biochemical pathways constitute the channels of cross-talks that differentially regulate or synchronize metabolism [12]-[16] through coordinate silencing as distinct from coordinate expression of transcripts. GDH is present in the cytoplasm, chloroplast, and mitochondria [27] thereby enabling the RNA it synthesizes to regulate different metabolic pathways.

There were also structural similarities between the RNAs synthesized by the acidic, neutral, and basic isoenzymes of *P. dulcis* GDH. The cDNA fragment (**Figure 2**) homologous to the mRNA encoding dihydroquinate dehydratase (**Table 2**) shared 3-fold matches two of which were plus/minus and the remaining one was plus/plus sequence matches with the cDNA fragment (**Table 2**) homologous to the mRNA encoding β-cryophyllene synthase, a natural products metabolic enzyme. The cDNA fragment (**Table 2**) homologous to the mRNA encoding granule-bound starch synthase (primary metabolism) shared 5-fold plus/plus sequence matches with the cDNA fragment (**Table 2**) homologous to the mRNA encoding bifunctional sesquiterpene synthase, a natural products metabolic enzyme. The geographic positioning of the cDNA fragments on the sequencing gel (**Figures 2-4**) whereby those resulting from the cathodal GDH isoenzymes (north side of the gel) regulated those from the anodal isoenzymes (south side) and *vice versa*; and those from the acidic GDH isoenzymes (west side) regulated those from the neutral and basic isoenzymes (east side) and *vice versa* describe the fidelity of the GDH-synthesized RNAs in the silencing of mRNAs *in vivo*, and the fool-proof characteristics of the cDNA fragments as Northern probes. The plus and minus strands of a cDNA fragment as two-probes-in-one potentially assure that the target mRNA will not be missed during Northern hybridization reaction. Furthermore, the multiple internal sequence repeats in the GDH-synthesized RNA assure tenacious crisscross binding of the cDNA fragment to the homologous mRNA thereby maximizing specificity and stringency through liquefaction reaction during Northern hybridization. Single-stranded nucleic acid probes lack the crisscross tenacious binding specificity and stringency embodied by GDH-synthesized RNAs. Geographic positioning on the sequencing gel landscape of the RNAs synthesized by GDH (**Figures 2-4**) would permit the biochemical selection of specific metabolic chemotypes of *P. dulcis* as was in the case of peanut [12]-[17]. Therefore, photosynthetic processes regulate secondary metabolism, suggesting that environmental conditions would be able to differentiate the metabolism of terpenoids to produce several *Phyla* chemotypes. Aside from the general fact that the initial substrates for secondary metabolism are sourced from primary metabolism, the cross-connections at the mRNA level (coordinated silencing) between primary and secondary metabolic pathways could potentially provide a practical approach for molecular regulation of terpenoid accumulation. The superimposition of a rainbow of environmental conditions on *Phyla* growth and development may manipulate the inter-mRNA cross-talks to the extent that special metabolic chemotypes arise some of which could be high hernundulcin thus illuminating possible alternative chemical treatment approaches [5] [6] for the cultivation of the medicinal plants.

By knocking down biomass and fatty acid metabolic pathways, GDH-synthesized RNAs enhanced the production of arachin-free low linoleic acid [14], and ultra-high resveratrol [17] peanut kernels. Similar technologies could be readily patterned for knocking down aspects of *Phyla* photosynthetic or monoterpene metabolism in order to enhance sesquiterpene accumulation. Several poor or disaster-afflicted rural communities exist worldwide [28]. Governments and humanitarian agencies are reaching out to alleviate the sociological and agricultural stresses of those communities. *Phyla dulcis* now grows luxuriantly in USA (**Figure 1**). *Phyla* species are money-makers [2] for small-scale farmers promoting rural economy in South Africa, India, China, and South America. High hernundulcin metabolic variants of the medicinal plants could enable limited resource farmers to increase their farm income thereby promoting rural economy world-wide besides complementing the industrial production of hernundulcin [1] [8] [9]. One of the major predispositions to obesity is the consumption of high calorie food. Sugar is one of the high calorie ingredients added in to food. The zero-calorie hernundulcins could possess the potential to minimize sugar intake while offering sweet taste to sweet-consumers. High-hernundulcin *Phyla*-based natural sweetener, similar to stevia could be popular in the health-conscious market place.

4. Conclusion

Phyla dulcis contains hernundulcin sesquiterpene zero-caloric sweetener and also bitter constituents including camphor, limonene, terpineol, α-pinene, α-copaene, trans-caryophyllene, δ-cadinene, and α-bisabolol. There is yet no simple method to remove the undesirable components. Therefore, R & D are being focused to plant-based zero-caloric sweeteners. The aim was to characterize the mRNA targets that regulate the primary and terpenoid metabolic enzymes. Restriction fragment differential display polymerase chain reaction methodology showed that the RNAs synthesized by the glutamate dehydrogenase (GDH) of *Phyla dulcis* shared extensive sequence homologies with many mRNAs encoding dehydroquinate dehydratase, ribulose-1,5-bisphophatase carboxylase, granule-bound starch synthase, pyruvate kinase, glucose-6-phosphare dehydrogenase, protoporphyrinogen oxidase, cytochrome P-450 reductase, phosphoenol pyruvate carboxylase, quinolinate phosphirobosyltransferase, photosystem II protein, and coumarate:coenzyme A ligase in primary metabolism; and also β-caryophyllene synthase, (+)-epi-α-bisabolol synthase, bicyclogermacrene synthase, α-copaene/δ-cadinene synthases, trans-α-bergamotene synthase, terpene synthase 1, bifunctional sesquiterpene synthase, and geraniol synthase in terpenoid metabolism. GDH-synthesized RNAs are important because *in vivo* they coordinately silence appropriate mRNAs homologous to them, and their cDNAs are applied *in vitro* as high specificity maximum stringency probes to profile mRNA responses to environmental changes affecting primary metabolism and the accumulation of secondary metabolites. The extensive sequence similarities between GDH-synthesized RNA and several mRNAs encoding photosynthetic enzymes and terpene synthases suggested that secondary metabolism of *Phyla dulcis* could be regulated by photosynthesis at the mRNA level, an emerging subject that has not been widely exploited in plant biotechnology.

5. Ethical Compliance

The authors declare no conflict of financial interests. The research project was approved by the Institutional Review Board of the University; Prairie View A & M University, Texas A & M University, and USDA-NIFA Plan of Work; and supported by NIFA-USDA Allen Fund.

Acknowledgements

USDA/NIFA Evans Allen funds made to PVAMU supported this project including salaries and stipends in full for the authors, materials and supplies, costs for manuscript preparation and journal publication.

References

[1]   Kim, N. and Kinghorn, A.D. (2002) Highly Sweet Compounds of Plant Origin. *Archives Pharmacy Research*, **25**, 725-746. http://dx.doi.org/10.1007/BF02976987

[2]   Husain, A. (1991) Economic Aspects of Exploitations of Medicinal Plants. In: Akerele, O.V. and Heywood, S.H., Eds., *Conservation of Medicinal Plants*, Cambridge University Press, Cambridge. http://dx.doi.org/10.1017/CBO9780511753312.009

[3]   Kinghorn, A.D., Pan, L., Fletcher, N. and Chai, H. (2011) The Relevance of Higher Plants in Lead Compound Discovery Programs. *Journal Natural Products*, **74**, 1536-1555. http://dx.doi.org/10.1021/np200391c

[4]   Lopez, M.A., Stashenko, E.E. and Fuentes, J.L. (2011) Chemical Composition and Antigenotoxic Properties of *Lippia alba* Essential Oils. *Genetics Molecular Biology*, **34**, 479-488. http://dx.doi.org/10.1590/S1415-47572011005000030

[5]   De Oliveira, P.F., Machado, R.A.F., Bolzan, A. and Barth, D. (2012) Supercritical Fluid Extraction of Hernandulcin from *Lippia dulcis* Trev. *The Journal of Supercritical Fluids*, **63**, 161-168. http://dx.doi.org/10.1016/j.supflu.2011.12.003

[6]   Eaton, R.W. and Sandusky, P. (2009) Biotransformations of 2-Methylisoborneol by Camphor-Degrading Bacteria. *Applied Environmental Microbiology*, **75**, 583-588. http://dx.doi.org/10.1128/AEM.02126-08

[7]   Attia, M., Kim, S. and Ro, D. (2012) Molecular Cloning and Characterization of (+)-epi-α-Bisabolol Synthase, Catalyzing the First Step in the Biosynthesis of the Natural Sweetener, Hernandulcin, in *Lippia dulcis*. *Archives Biochemistry Biophysics*, **527**, 37-44. http://dx.doi.org/10.1016/j.abb.2012.07.010

[8]   Takahashi, S., Yeo, Y., Greenhagen, B.T., McMullin, T., Song, L., Maurina-Brunker, J., Rosson, R., Noel, J.P. and Chappell, J. (2007) Metabolic Engineering of Sesquiterpene Metabolism in Yeast. *Biotechnology Bioengineering*, **97**, 170-181. http://dx.doi.org/10.1002/bit.21216

[9]   Kinghorn, A.D., Chin, Y., Pan, L. and Jia, Z. (2010) Comprehensive Natural Products Chemistry II: Chemistry and Biology. In: Mander, L., Liu, H. and Verpoorte, R., Eds., *Development and Modification of Bioactivity*, Elsevier, Oxford, Vol. 3, 269-315.

[10] Degenhardt, J., Kollner, T.G. and Gershenzon, J. (2009) Monoterpene and Sesquiterpene Synthases and Origin of Terpene Skeletal Diversity in Plants. *Phytochemistry*, **70**, 1621-1637. http://dx.doi.org/10.1016/j.phytochem.2009.07.030

[11] Yeo, Y., Nybo, S.E., Chittiboyina, A.G., Weerasooriya, A.D., Wang, Y., Gongora-Castillo, E., *et al.* (2013) Functional Identification of Valerena-1,10-Diene Synthase, a Terpene Synthase Catalyzing a Unique Chemical Cascade in the Biosynthesis of Biologically Active Sesquiterpenes in *Valeriana officinalis*. *The Journal of Biological Chemistry*, **288**, 3163-3173. http://dx.doi.org/10.1074/jbc.M112.415836

[12] Osuji, G.O., Brown, T.K. and South, S.M. (2010) Optimized Fat and Cellulosic Biomass Accumulation in Peanut through Biotechnology. *International Journal of Biochemistry and Biotechnology*, **6**, 451-472.

[13] Osuji, G.O., Brown, T.K., South, S.M., Duncan, J.C., Johnson, D. and Hyllam, S. (2012) Molecular Adaptation of Peanut Metabolism to Wide Variations of Mineral Ion Concentration and Combination. *American Journal Plant Sciences*, **3**, 33-50. http://dx.doi.org/10.4236/ajps.2012.31003

[14] Osuji, G.O., Brown, T.K., South, S.M., Johnson, D. and Hylam, S. (2012) Molecular Modeling of Metabolism for Allergen-Free Low Linoleic Acid Peanuts. *Applied Biochemistry and Biotechnology*, **168**, 805-823. http://dx.doi.org/10.1007/s12010-012-9821-6

[15] Osuji, G.O., Brown, T.K. and South, S.M. (2008) Discovery of the RNA Synthetic Activity of GDH and Its Application in Drug Metabolism Research. *The Open Drug Metabolism Journal*, **2**, 1-13. http://dx.doi.org/10.2174/1874073100802010001

[16] Osuji, G.O., Brown, T.K., South, S.M., Duncan, J.C. and Johnson, D. (2011) Doubling of Crop Yield through Permutation of Metabolic Pathways. *Advances in Bioscience and Biotechnology*, **2**, 364-379. http://dx.doi.org/10.4236/abb.2011.25054

[17] Osuji, G.O., Johnson, P., Duffus, E., Woldesenbet, S., Idan, E., Johnson, D., South, S.M., Clarke, D.A., Brown, T.K. and Kirven, J.M. (2015) Metabolic and RNA Profiling of Peanut for Modeling the Resveratrol Biosynthetic Pathway. *Applied Biochemistry and Biotechnology*, Accepted for Publication.

[18] Osuji, G.O., Reyes, J.C. and Mangaroo, A.S. (1998) Glutamate Dehydrogenase Isomerization: A Simple Method for Diagnosing Nitrogen, Phosphorus, and Potassium Sufficiency in Maize (*Zea mays* L.). *Journal of Agricultural and Food Chemistry*, **46**, 2395-2401. http://dx.doi.org/10.1021/jf971065x

[19] Osuji, G.O., Haby, V.A. and Chessman, D.J. (2006) Metabolic Responses Induced by Serial Harvesting of Alfalfa Pasture Established on Amended Acid Soils. *Communications in Soil Science and Plant Analysis*, **37**, 1281-1301. http://dx.doi.org/10.1080/00103620600623608

[20] Kinghorn, A.D. and Soejarto, D.D. (2002) Discovery of Terpenoid and Phenolic Sweeteners from Plants. *Pure and Applied Chemistry*, **74**, 1169-1179. http://dx.doi.org/10.1351/pac200274071169

[21] Osuji, G.O., Konan, J. and M'Mbijjewe, G. (2004) RNA Synthetic Activity of Glutamate Dehydrogenase. *Applied Biochemistry Biotechnology*, **119**, 209-228. http://dx.doi.org/10.1007/s12010-004-0003-z

[22] Osuji, G.O., Braithwaite, C., Fordjour, K., Madu, W.C., Beyene, A. and Roberts, P.S. (2003) Purification of Glutamate Dehydrogenase Isoenzymes and Characterization of Their Substrate Specificities. *Preparative Biochemistry and Biotechnology*, **33**, 13-28. http://dx.doi.org/10.1081/PB-120018366

[23] Osuji, G.O. and Madu, W.C. (1995) Ammonium Ion-Dependent Isomerization of Glutamate Dehydrogenase in Relation to Glutamate Synthesis in Maize. *Phytochemistry*, **39**, 495-503. http://dx.doi.org/10.1016/0031-9422(94)00976-Z

[24] Osuji, G.O., Brown, T.K. and South, S.M. (2009) Nucleotide-Dependent Reprogramming of mRNAs Encoding Acetyl Coenzyme A Carboxylase and Lipoxygenase in Relation to Fat Contents of Peanut. *Journal of Botany*, **2009**, Article ID: 278324. http://www.hindawi.com/journals/jb/2009/278324.html

[25] Osuji, G.O. and Brown, T. (2007) Environment-Wide Reprogramming of mRNAs Encoding Phosphate Translocator and Glucosyltransferase in Relation to Cellulosic Biomass Accumulation in Peanut. *The ICFAI Journal of Biotechnology*, **1**, 35-47.

[26] Liang, P. (2002) A Decade of Differential Display. *Biotechniques*, **33**, 338-346.

[27] Osuji, G.O. and Madu, W.C. (2015) Glutamate Dehydrogenase. In: D'Mello, J.P.F., Eds., *Amino Acids in Higher Plants*, CABI Publishers, Oxford, 1-29. http://dx.doi.org/10.1079/9781780642635.0001

[28] Douglas, J.B. (2013) USDA Texas Farm Service Agency Emergency Loans Available to 207 Counties in Texas. http://sweetwaterreporter.com/content/fsa-emergency-loans-available

4

Chemical Composition of the Essential Oil and Nitrogen Metabolism of Menthol Mint under Different Phosphorus Levels

Marco A. A. Souza[1], Osmário J. L. Araújo[1], Diego M. C. Brito[1]*, Manlio S. Fernandes[2], Rosane N. Castro[1], Sonia R. Souza[1]

[1]Department of Chemistry, Universidade Federal Rural do Rio de Janeiro, Seropédica, Brazil
[2]Soil Department, Universidade Federal Rural do Rio de Janeiro, Seropédica, Brazil
Email: *diegobioquimica@hotmail.com

Abstract

The purpose of this work was to evaluate the effects of different phosphorus levels (0.05, 0.5, 1 and 2 mM) under nitrogen metabolism and the essential oil profile of menthol mint (*Mentha arvensis* L.). The relationship between the leaf maturity and the essential oil profile was also explored. The experiment was conducted in a hydroponic system located in a grow chamber during 41 days and after the harvest, nitrate reductase activity, and the NO_3^--N, amino-N, and soluble sugars levels of each plant part were evaluated. Also the essential oil from young leaves (6th to 8th node) and adult leaves (3rd to the 5th node) was analyzed. An uptake mechanism related to the increase in fresh weight of the roots was promoted with the use of low P levels (0.05 and 0.50 mmol·L^{-1}). With 1 mmol·L^{-1} P plants showed in all parts an increased nitrate reductase activity and high levels of nitrate and amino-N in leaves. Plants submitted to the lowest P level (0.05 mmol·L^{-1}) presented high levels of menthol. In leaves from 6th to 8th node (mature leaves) menthol level was approximately 87% of the essential oil however leaves from the 3rd to the 5th node (young leaves) showed high levels of pulegone, that can be toxic for humans. The results indicate that the essential oil quality in menthol mint is influenced by the leaf maturity and the P levels. Also it was showed that the oil extracted from mature leaves of plants under low P levels has the best commercial profile.

Keywords

Mentha arvensis L., Lamiaceae, Gas Chromatography, Hydropony, Menthol

---

*Corresponding author.

1. Introduction

The production of essential oil from menthol mint (*Mentha arvensis* L.) is the second largest of the world, reaching 18,000 tonnes by year [1]. Chemically, the essential oils of plants are composed mainly of terpenoids and also phenylpropanoids such as the monoterpenes that are generally the most abundant [2]. In menthol mint monoterpenes constitutes approximately 90% of the essential oil and menthol represents 70% - 95% of the monoterpenes (**Figure 1**) [3].

In vegetal nutrition studies hydropony is a high utility tool since it allows that the nutrient supply be provided in an almost constant tax and an easier manipulation of nutrients compared with the conventional method [4]. Furthermore the use of nutrient solutions excludes some influence factors in metabolism, as soil-associated diseases and weeds [5]. Accordingly, the use of hydroponic system allows a more precise evaluation about interactions between nutrients and metabolic processes in plants.

Phosphorus is a nutrient largely used in energy transfer processes in cells, mainly as a component of ATP [6]. In plant nutrition, phosphorus (P) has been shown to be related with dry and fresh weight production and also in variations in the quality of essential oils of various aromatic species [7]. Thus, the aim of this study was to evaluate the effects of different levels of P in the nutrient solution in nitrogen metabolism and in the composition of essential oils of menthol mint plants.

2. Materials and Methods

2.1. General Informations and Seedling Production

Seedlings of menthol mint (*Mentha arvensis* L.) were propagated in a greenhouse at the Chemistry Department of Universidade Federal Rural do Rio de Janeiro (UFRRJ). Also, samples of the plants used in this experiment were subjected to herborization and registered in the herbarium (RBR) of the Botany Department of UFRRJ under number (RBR)-32886. The plants were produced from cuttings with approximately 15 cm in length of the middle third of the shoots treated with 2% sodium hypochlorite (10 min), washed with distilled water and fixed on polystyrene support. Two-thirds of the bottom of the cuttings were immersed in a nutrient solution modified with 15 mmol·L^{-1} NO_3^--N at 1/2 strength under constant aeration [8]. After two weeks, the seedlings were standardized by root size and number of leaves.

2.2. Description of the Hydroponic System and Treatments

The seedlings were placed in 2-cm Styrofoam plates thick with the help of synthetic foam and then placed on pots (1.8 L) connected by caliber flexible tubes to an electromagnetic air compressor (Resun, model OC-003) with a flow rate of 65 L·min^{-1}, programmed to 15 min of activity per hour. This hydroponic system was placed on benches of a growth chamber with photosynthetic photon density of 200 μmol·m^{-2}·s^{-1} and a 12 h photoperiod at 25°C. The plants were cultivated for 41 days in a nutrient solution modified with 15 mmol·L^{-1} NO_3^--N at 1/2 strength with different P doses, as described in **Table 1** [8]. Every day, the pH of the nutrient solution was measured and adjusted to 5.8 and the volume was adjusted to 1.6 L per pot. The nutrient solution was replaced weekly.

2.3. Fresh Weight, Soluble Fractions and Nitrate Reductase Analyses

Roots, stems and leaves were separated and used for fresh weight analysis. Moreover 1 g samples from median-portion of each plant part (3rd and 4th nodes of leaves) were powdered in 10 mL of 80% ethanol, filtered, parti-

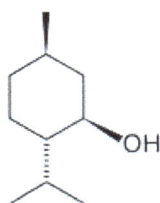

Figure 1. Structure of menthol.

Table 1. Composition of the nutrient solutions used for the cultivation of menthol mint (*Mentha arvensis* L.) during 41 days in growth chamber. A 1/2 strength nutrient solution [8] modified with 15 mmol L^{-1} NO$_3^-$-N was used as a source of other nutrients.

Macronutrients	Levels (mmol·L^{-1})			
N-NO$_3^-$	15.00	15.00	15.00	15.00
N-NH$_4^+$	-	-	-	-
P	**0.05**	**0.50**	**1.00**	**2.00**
K	6.00	6.00	6.00	6.00
Ca	5.00	5.00	5.00	5.00
Mg	2.00	2.00	2.00	2.00
S-SO$_4$^{a}	2.48	2.25	2.00	2.00
Micronutrients	Levels (mmol·L^{-1})			
Fe	89.61	89.61	89.61	89.61
Mn	9.11	9.11	9.11	9.11
B	16.30	16.30	16.30	16.30
Zn	0.76	0.76	0.76	0.76
Cu	0.31	0.31	0.31	0.31
Mo	0.10	0.10	0.10	0.10

^{a}Changes in the concentration of sulfur were produced as a result of variation in the P levels.

tioned with chloroform, and the hydro-alcoholic phase was completed to 50 mL with 80% ethanol. This phase was used for amino-N [9], NO$_3^-$-N [10], ammonium [11] and soluble sugar [12] analyses. Also 0.2 g samples from median portion of each plant part (4th node of leaves) were used for the analysis of nitrate reductase activity [13].

2.4. Essential Oil Extraction and Analysis

Samples (3 g) from the upper leaves (3rd to 5th node) and lower leaves (6th to 8th node) were removed and immersed in 10 mL of dichloromethane for 48 h at 4°C. After this period the samples were filtered, the organic phase dried with anhydrous Na$_2$SO$_4$ and the extracts stored in a freezer (−20°C) for further analysis. A gas chromatograph (Hewlett-Packard 5890 Series II CA, USA) equipped with a flame ionization detection and a split/splitless injector, in a split ratio of 1:20 was used to separate and detect the constituents in the essential oil. The substances were separated into the fused silica capillary column CP-Sil-8CB [30 m × 0.25 mm (i.d.) × 0.25 µm (film thickness)]. Helium was used as the carrier gas at a flow rate of 1 mL·min^{-1}. The column temperature was programmed as follows: 60°C for 2 min followed by heating at 5°C·min^{-1} to 110°C, followed by heating at 3°C·min^{-1} to 150°C and finally followed by heating at 15°C·min^{-1} until 290°C and holding constant for 15 min. The injector temperature was 220°C and the detector temperature was 280°C.

The gas chromatography coupled with mass spectrometry (GC-MS) was used for the essential oil analysis using a Varian Saturn 2000 (Paolo Alto, CA). The flow of the helium gas carrier, the capillary column and the temperature conditions for the GC-MS analysis were the same as described for the GC. The temperature of the injector was 220°C and the temperature of the interface was 250°. Mass spectra were obtained with an ion trap detector operating at 70 eV, with 40 - 400 *m/z* mass range and scanning rate equal to 0.5 scan·s^{-1}. The identification of the oil constituents was based on comparisons of their GC retention indexes and their mass spectra with authentic standards [(−)-pulegone, (−)-menthone, (+)-neomenthol and (−)-menthol] from Sigma-Aldrich (USA), NIST database (2008) and retention index (RI) [14]. The RI was obtained from the co-injection of an alkane standard solution C8-C40 (Fluka, USA).

2.5. Experimental Design and Statistical

In the experiment each treatment was composed of four replicates arranged in a completely randomized experimental design and in each pot two plants were placed. The analysis of variance, standard deviation and the significance test (Fisher LSD, 5%) of the data were performed in SigmaStat 2.03 (Inc, Chicago, IL, USA). The Unscrambler® X version 0.0.0.42 was used for the principal component analysis (PCA) (©CAMO Software AS 2010, USA). The graphics were created in SigmaPlot 8.0 (Systat Software Inc., California, USA).

3. Results and Discussion

3.1. pH of the Nutrient Solutions

The variations in the pH of the nutrient solutions during the experiment showed two distinct phases (**Figure 2(A)**). In the first phase (from the 1st to 15th day) when the absorption of nutrients was not intense, an alkalinization of the nutrient solution was observed, always higher than the daily adjustment to pH 5.8. In the second phase (from the 16th to 41st) a strong variation in pH was observed, shifting from acid to alkaline depending on the elapsed time between the replacement of the nutrient solution. This unstable behavior may be associated with an increased influx of nutrients related to the growth of the root system.

The pH range which is suitable for a better development of crops generally lies between 5.5 and 5.8 and is mainly related to the availability of nutrients in the solution [15]. The pH of the nutrient solution undergoes con-

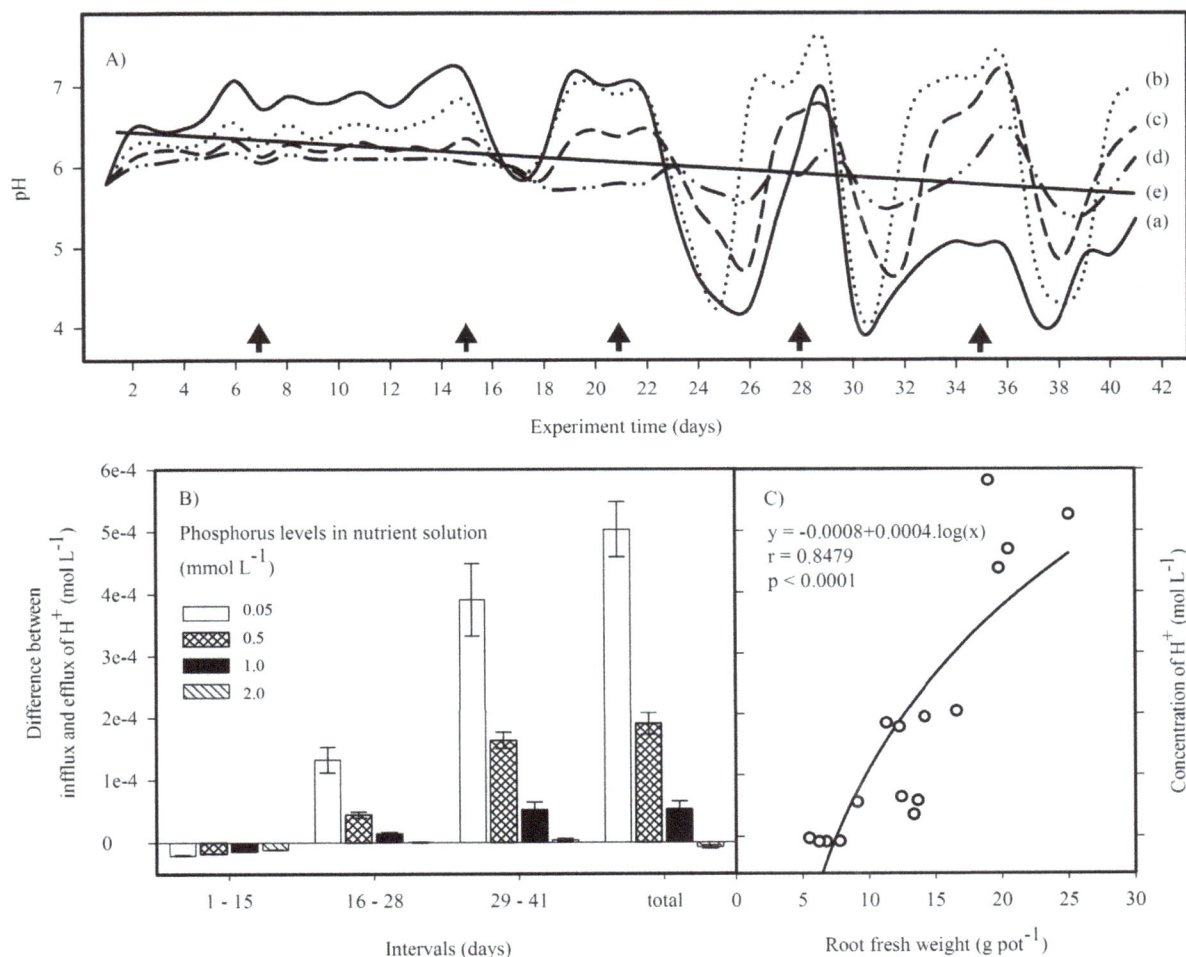

Figure 2. (A) pH values of the nutrient solutions with different levels of P during the cultivation of menthol mint (*Mentha arvensis* L.) for 41 days; lines (a) solid; (b) dotted; (c) dashed; (d) dotted-dashed respectively for 0.05, 0.50, 1.00 and 2.00 mmol·L⁻¹ of P in nutrient solutions and (e) linear regression of all points with r = 0.46 and P < 0.0001. Days when the nutrient solution was replaced are represented by ↑; (B) Difference between the infflux and efflux of H⁺; (C) Logarithmic correlation between the molar concentration of H⁺ in the nutrient solution and root production of menthol mint.

stant changes in response to the availability and influx of nutrients (symport or antiport) and the extrusion of H^+ [16]. Thus, the early absorption of phosphate and nitrate anions, caused the alkalinization of the nutrient solution, while later the lower levels of nutrients induces a second phase of extrusion of H^+ to the nutrient solution, leading to acidification of the nutrient solution. The intensity in which this pH oscillation occurs is the response of the plant to the availability of nutrients in the nutrient solution, as well as the demand that the plant exerts on them, as shown in **Figure 2(A)**.

Nutrient solutions with lower P doses (0.05 and 0.50 mmol·L^{-1}), especially the 0.05 mmol·L^{-1}, showed a high variation in pH with a great tendency to acidification in the course the experiment (**Figure 2(B)**). Since P is a macronutrient highly demanded the plant uses mechanisms to increase its uptake as increasing the production of roots and the extrusion of H^+, causing the acidification of the nutrient solution (**Figure 2(C)**) [16].

3.2. Biomass Production

A negative correlation between the P levels in the nutrient solution and the mass production of the roots was also observed (**Figure 3**). This result can be related to the fact that plants under low P doses are stimulated to produce more roots increasing the absorption area [17].

However, in studies with *Mentha piperita* L. an increase in roots production with the lower P dose in the nu-

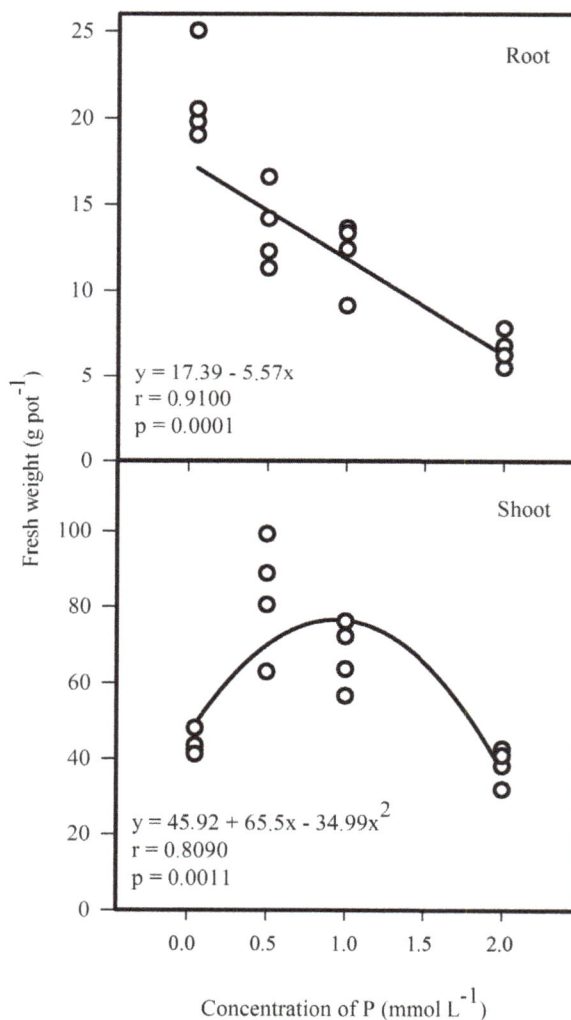

Figure 3. Correlation between fresh weight of roots and shoots of menthol mint (*Mentha arvensis* L.) under different levels of P (0.05, 0.5, 1 and 2 mmol·L^{-1}) in nutrient solution used in cultivation for 41 days.

trient solution was not observed [18]. It should be noted that the P dose at which the plants produced more shoot mass corresponds to only half of the higher P dose (2 mmol·L^{-1}) used in this research nutrient solution and in other solutions used in hydroponics for most crops [7] [19]-[21].

The plants grown in nutrient solution with 2 mmol·L^{-1} P had lower production of shoot weight and also showed early flowering and symptoms of toxicity (data not shown). Symptoms of toxicity caused by the excess in P are not well known [22]. However, it is known that above certain levels, this element causes nutritional antagonism [23]. Thus, the symptoms observed in plants under 2 mmol·L^{-1} P may be associated with the deficiency of other nutrients or also by influence of pH in the uptake of other nutrients.

3.3. Nitrogen Metabolism

The lowest percentage of soluble sugars was found in roots, stems and leaves of plants under 0.5 mmol·L^{-1} P (**Figure 4(A)**). However, the roots and leaves of these plants showed high contents of nitrate (**Figure 4(B)**). The leaves of plants under 0.5 and 1 mmol·L^{-1} P showed high levels of nitrate and amino-N (**Figure 4(B)** and **Figure 4(C)**).

The stem was the main site of nitrate accumulation in menthol mint (**Figure 4(B)**). In a previous study with plants of *Mentha piperita* was also observed that stem is the preferential organ for storage of this nutrient [7]. The nitrate accumulation in stem may be a plant evolutionary strategy to prevent the excess of nitrate in the leaves and to maintain the N supply for biochemical activities in low availability periods [15] [24] [25].

A higher nitrate reductase activity was detected in leaves of menthol mint plants. Plants under 0.5 and 1 mmol·L^{-1} P showed high nitrate reductase activity in roots and leaves (**Figure 4(D)**). Moreover, plants submitted to 1 and 2 mmol·L^{-1} P showed the highest activities of nitrate reductase in stem.

3.4. Essential Oil Composition and Principal Components Analysis (PCA)

Results showed in **Table 2** indicate that high levels of menthol were obtained from menthol mint plants submitted to the lowest P level (0.05 mmol·L^{-1}). To a better evaluation of the effect of the different P levels and position of the leaves over the chemical profile of the essential oil, a principal components analysis (PCA) was performed based on the percentages of the substances identified by GC-MS. This analysis provided a double-graphic of scores and loadings where the formation of clusters can be observed (**Figure 5**).

The analysis of the principal components revealed that the difference in maturity of the leaves is mainly represent for PC-1, with 48% of the total variability found in the chemical composition of the essential oils, while PC-2 with 22% of the variability, discriminate mainly the effect of different levels of P on essential oil composition (**Figure 5**).

Considering the distribution of the samples as a function of PC-1, it was found that the samples of essential oils extracted from young leaves in the left of the quadrant and extracted from mature leaves were grouped together in the right of the quadrant in **Figure 5**, between menthol and p-cymene, which contributed to the formation of this larger grouping. The PC-2 discriminated between the formation of cluster 1 with the higher levels of menthol and cluster 2 with the higher content of p-cymene.

In the left quadrant of **Figure 5** the samples were grouped only as a function of PC-2. In the upper left a greater presence of pulegone and menthone contributed to the formation of cluster 4, while in the lower left quadrant the presence of isomenthone contributed to the formation of clusters 3 and 5. However, cluster 5 showed lower contents of menthone and menthol and cluster 6 presented intermediate levels of substances that constitute the oil from menthol mint.

Also can be observed that the leaves from the 6th to the 8th node (mature leaves) showed an essential oil profile with more menthol than the essential oil from leaves from the 3rd to the 5th node (young leaves) (**Figure 5** and **Table 3**). This result indicates that the essential oil for mature leaves have the best commercial quality [3]. On the other hand, higher levels of ketone monoterpenes (pulegone, menthone and isomenthone) in the leaves from the 3rd to the 5th node (young leaves) is an indication that the essential oil has not matured, since those substances are intermediates in the biosynthesis of menthol [26]. In addition, a higher level of pulegone in the essential oil of leaves from the 3rd to the 5th node (young leaves) decreases the oil quality [27].

The leaves of plants in the genus *Mentha* have an age difference between the nodes of about 2.4 days [28]. Since the mature leaves are shaded, there may be a synergism caused by age and light intensity on the quality of essential oils. However, the age of the leaves seems to be a more plausible answer to explain the increase in the

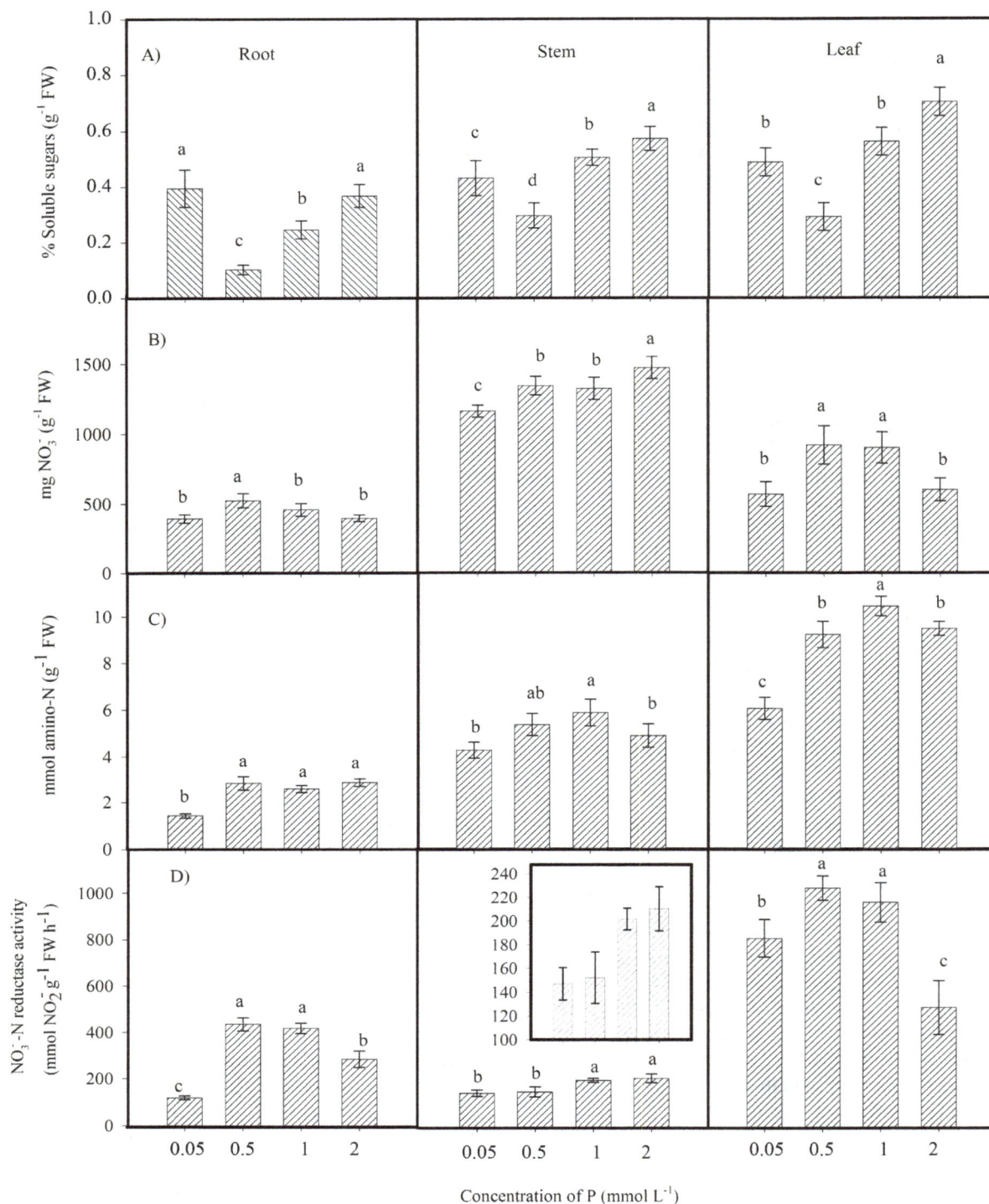

Figure 4. Soluble sugars (A); nitrate (B); amino-N (C); and nitrate reductase activity (D) in roots, stems and leaves of menthol mint (*Mentha arvensis* L.) cultivated for 41 days in nutrient solution with different P levels (0.05, 0.5, 1 and 2 mmol·L^{-1}). Different letters in the same plant part indicate significant difference (Fisher LSD, 5%). The bars represent the standard deviation.

concentration of menthol in the mature leaves observed in **Figure 5**, since that a significant production of menthol occurs late, at around 40 days after initiation of leaves and with a maximum increase of 2% menthol per day

Table 2. Percentages of the substances in the essential oil extracted from leaves of menthol mint (*Mentha arvensis* L.) plants cultivated under different P levels (0.05, 0.5, 1 and 2 mmol·L^{-1}) during 41 days in hydroponic system.

Essential oil composition (%)[a]				P levels (mmol·L^{-1})			
RT[b]	Substance	KI[c]	RI[d]	0.05	0.5	1.0	2.0
8.30	p-cymene	1026	1025	2.90 ± 0.63	2.29 ± 1.07	5.51 ± 1.07	4.36 ± 0.33
12.03	Menthone	1154	1166	2.32 ± 0.07	2.57 ± 0.03	2.68 ± 0.74	2.11 ± 0.20
12.32	Isomenthone	1164	1175	1.72 ± 0.07	1.60 ± 0.03	1.82 ± 0.04	1.76 ± 0.04
12.43	Neomenthol	1165	1179	1.56 ± 0.42	1.68 ± 0.02	1.76 ± 0.11	1.73 ± 0.08
12.69	Menthol	1173	1190	87.15 ± 1.09	83.70 ± 0.69	83.30 ± 0.59	81.74 ± 2.83
14.55	Pulegone	1237	1250	3.18 ± 0.62	7.24 ± 0.80	3.40 ± 1.09	7.31 ± 2.58
15.10	Piperitone	1252	1266	0.90 ± 0.20	0.91 ± 0.10	0.74 ± 0.19	0.54 ± 0.24
	Monoterpene ketone			8.12 ± 0.82	12.66 ± 0.57	8.64 ± 1.44	11.72 ± 1.81
	Monoterpene alcohol			88.71 ± 0.46	86.03 ± 0.44	85.06 ± 0.33	83.47 ± 1.67

[a]$\alpha = 0.95$. [b]RT = retention time. [c]KI = Kovats retention index (Adams, 1995). [d]RI = retention index.

Table 3. Percentages of the substances in the essential oil extracted from leaves at different positions of menthol mint (*Mentha arvensis* L.) plants cultivated under different P levels (0.05, 0.5, 1 and 2 mmol·L^{-1}) during 41 days in hydroponic system.

Essential oil composition (%)[a]				Leaf position at plant	
RT[b]	Substance	KI[c]	RI[d]	RT[b]	Substance
8.30	p-cymene	1026	1025	3.27 ± 1.00	4.38 ± 1.03
12.03	Menthone	1154	1166	3.58 ± 0.44	1.49 ± 0.84
12.32	Isomenthone	1164	1175	1.83 ± 0.05	1.51 ± 0.17
12.43	Neomenthol	1165	1179	1.71 ± 0.07	1.65 ± 0.21
12.69	Menthol	1173	1190	81.46 ± 2.25	86.87 ± 1.99
14.55	Pulegone	1237	1250	7.25 ± 2.19	3.47 ± 1.27
15.10	Piperitone	1252	1266	0.90 ± 0.40	0.62 ± 0.06
	Monoterpene ketone			13.56 ± 2.50	7.09 ± 2.12
	Monoterpene alcohol			83.17 ± 2.29	88.52 ± 2.01

[a]$\alpha = 0.95$. [b]RT = retention time. [c]KI = Kovats retention index (Adams, 1995). [d]RI = retention index.

after 30 days of leaf emergence [29].

4. Conclusion

Results showed that low P levels (0.05 and 0.50 mmol·L^{-1}) stimulated an uptake mechanism related to the increase in fresh weight of the roots and H$^+$ extrusion in menthol mint plants. With 1 mmol·L^{-1} P plants showed high levels of nitrate and amino-N in leaves and an increased nitrate reductase activity in all plant parts. This activity presented a negative correlation with the soluble sugars levels. High levels of menthol were obtained from plants submitted to the lowest P level (0.05 mmol·L^{-1}). In fact, menthol was the main component of the menthol mint oil, with approximately 87% in leaves from 6th to 8th node (mature leaves). However, leaves from the 3rd to the 5th node (young leaves) presented high levels of pulegone which presents a potential for toxicity to humans. Therefore, these results indicate that the harvesting period of menthol mint has a significant influence on its quality and that the essential oil from mature leaves has the best commercial profile.

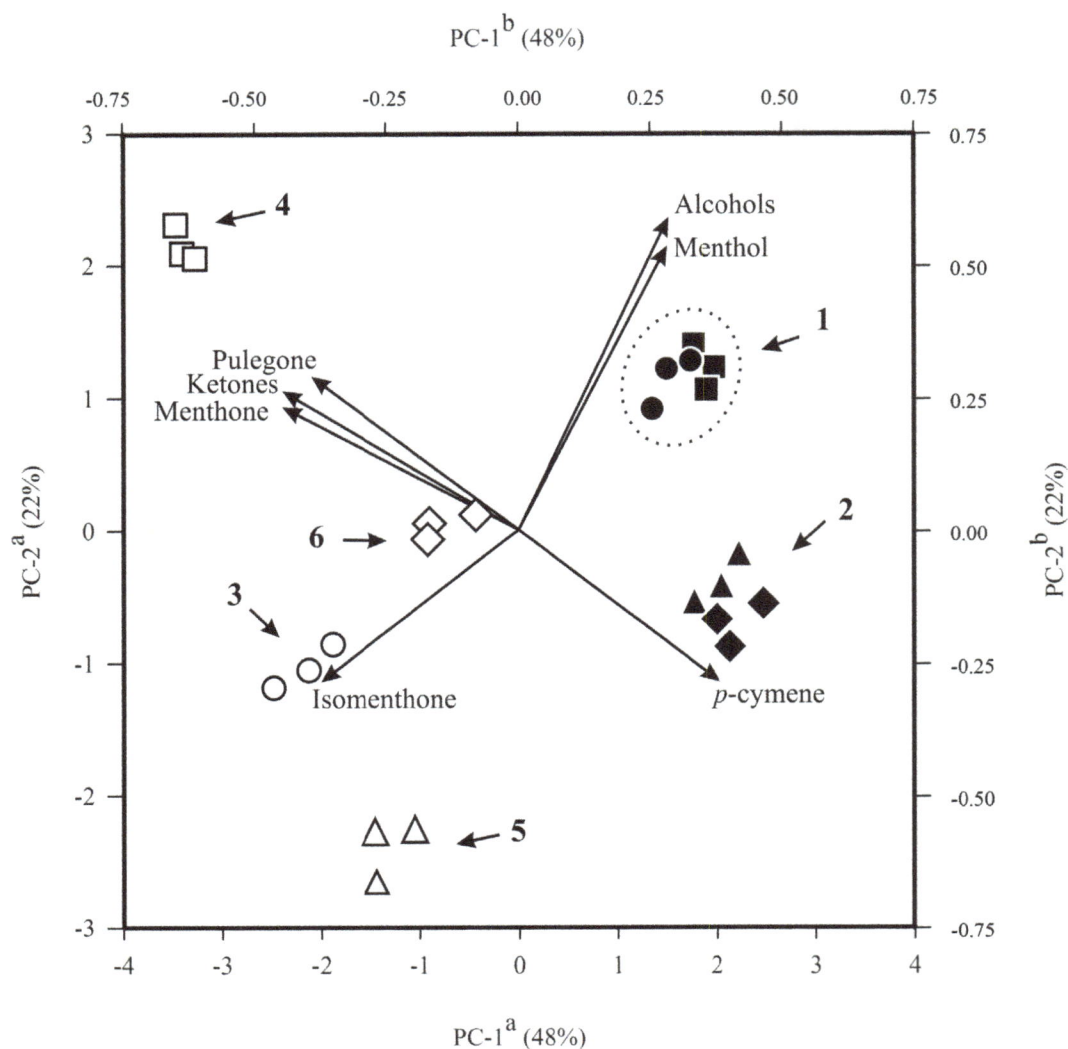

Figure 5. Principal component scatterplot of menthol mint (*Mentha arvensis* L.) cultivated for 41 days in hydroponic system with different P levels in nutrient solution. [a]Axes referring to 24 essential oil samples divided into four treatments with two cutting heights (scores) and represented by symbols as follows: nutrient solution with 0.05, 0.5, 1 and 2 mmol·L^{-1} P, respectively for (O, ●); (□, ■); (△, ▲) and (◇, ◆) of which the white and black symbols represent, respectively, leaves of 3rd to the 5th node and leaves of 6rd to the 8th node; [b]Axes referring to nine discriminant variables related to chromatographic profile (loadings) and represented as vectors from the origin. Arrows show the different clusters and the dotted line highlights the cluster with higher content of menthol in the essential oil. PC-1 and PC-2 represent respectively 48% and 22% of the total explained variance.

Acknowledgements

The authors acknowledge the financial support provided by Conselho Nacional de Desenvolvimento Científico e Tecnológico (CNPq), FAPERJ and CAPES. Technical support was provided by the Programa de Pós-Graduação em Química-UFRRJ.

References

[1]   Sanganeria, S. (2005) Vibrant India—Opportunities for the Flavor and Fragrance Industry. *Perfumer and Flavorist*, **30**, 24-34.

[2]   Sangwan, N.S., Farooqi, A.H.A., Shabih, F. and Sangwan, R.S. (2001) Regulation of Essential Oil Production in Plants.

Plant Growth Regulation, **34**, 3-21. http://dx.doi.org/10.1023/A:1013386921596

[3] Srivastava, R.K., Singh, A.K., Kalra, A.V., Tomar, K.S.R., Bansal, P., Patra, D.D., Chand, S., Naqvi, A.A., Sharma, S. and Kumar, S. (2002) Characteristics of *Mentha arvensis* Cultivated on Industrial Scale in the Indo-Gangetic Plains. *Industrial Crops and Products*, **15**, 189-198. http://dx.doi.org/10.1016/S0926-6690(01)00113-3

[4] Baligar, V.C. (1986) Interrelationships between Growth and Nutrient Uptake in Alfafa and Corn. *Journal of Plant Nutrition*, **9**, 1391-1404. http://dx.doi.org/10.1080/01904168609363536

[5] Sheikh, B.A. (2006) Hydroponics: Key to Sustain Agriculture in Water Stressed and Urban Environment. *Pakistan Journal of Agriculture, Agricultural Engineering and Veterinary Sciences*, **22**, 53-57.

[6] Araújo, A.P. and Machado, C.T.T. (2006) Fósforo. In: Fernandes, M.S., Ed., *Nutrição Mineral de Plantas*, Sociedade Brasileira de Ciência do Solo, Viçosa, 215-252.

[7] Souza, M.A.A., Araújo, O.J.L., Ferreira, M.A., Stark, E.M.L.M., Fernandes, M.S. and Souza, S.R. (2007) Produção de Biomassa e Óleo Essencial de Hortelã em Hidroponia em Função de Nitrogênio e Fósforo. *Horticultura Brasileira*, **25**, 41-48. http://dx.doi.org/10.1590/S0102-05362007000100009

[8] Hoagland, D.R. and Arnon, D.I. (1950) The Water-Culture Method for Growing Plants without Soil. *California Agricultural of Experimental*, **347**, 1-32.

[9] Yemm, E.W.E. and Cocking, E.C. (1955) The Determination of Amino-Acid with Ninhydrin. *Analytical Biochemistry*, **80**, 209-213.

[10] Cataldo, D., Harron, M., Scharader, L.E.E. and Youngs, V.L. (1975) Rapid Colorimetric Determination of Nitrate in Plant Tissue by Nitration of Salicylic Acid. *Communication in Soil Science and Plant Analysis*, **6**, 853-855. http://dx.doi.org/10.1080/00103627509366547

[11] Felker, P. (1977) Micro Determination of Nitrogen in Seed Protein Extracts. *Analytical Chemistry*, **49**, 1080-1080. http://dx.doi.org/10.1021/ac50015a053

[12] Yemm, E.W.E. and Willis, A.J. (1954) The Estimation of Carbohydrate in Plants Extracts by Anthrone. *Biochemistry*, **57**, 508-514.

[13] Jaworski, E.G. (1971) Nitrate Reductase Assay in Intact Plant Tissues. *Biochemical Biophysical Research Communication*, **43**, 1274-1279. http://dx.doi.org/10.1016/S0006-291X(71)80010-4

[14] Adams, R.P. (1995) Identification of Essential Oil Components by Gas Chromatography—Mass Spectroscopy. Allured Publishing, New York.

[15] Cometti, N.N., Furlani, P.R., Ruiz, P.R. and Fernandes, E.I.F. (2006) Soluções Nutritivas: Formulação e Aplicações. In: Fernandes, M.S., Ed., *Nutrição Mineral de Plantas*, Sociedade Brasileira de Ciência do Solo, Viçosa, 89-114.

[16] Fernandes, M.S. and Souza, S.R. (2006) Absorção de Nutrientes. In: Fernandes, M.S., Ed., *Nutrição Mineral de Plantas*, Sociedade Brasileira de Ciência do Solo, Viçosa, BR, 115-152.

[17] Epstein, E. and Bloom, A.J. (2005) Mineral Nutrition of Plants: Principles and Perspectives. Sinauer Associates Inc., Massachusetts.

[18] Rodrigues, C.R., Faquin, V., Trevisan, D., Pinto, J.E.B.P., Bertolucci, S.K.V., Rodrigues, T.M. (2004) Nutrição Mineral, Crescimento e Teor de Óleo Essencial da Menta em Solução Nutritiva sob Diferentes Concentrações de Fósforo e Épocas de Coleta. *Horticultura Brasileira*, **22**, 573-578. http://dx.doi.org/10.1590/S0102-05362004000300014

[19] Resh, H.M. (2004) Hydroponic Food Production: A Definitive Guidebook for the Advanced Home Gardener and the Commercial Hydroponic Grower. CRC Press, New Jersey.

[20] Haber, L.L., Luz, J.M.Q., Arvati, L.F.D. and Santos, J.E. (2005) Diferentes Concentrações de Solução Nutritiva para o Cultivo de *Mentha piperita* e *Melissa officinalis*. *Horticultura Brasileira*, **23**, 1006-1009. http://dx.doi.org/10.1590/S0102-05362005000400029

[21] Garlet, T.M.B., Santos, O.S., Medeiros, S.L.P., Garcia, D.C., Manfron, P.A. and Apel, M.A. (2007) Produção de Folhas, Teor e Qualidade do Óleo Essencial de Hortelã-Japonesa (*Mentha arvensis* L. forma piperascens Holmes) Cultivada em Hidroponia. *Revista Brasileira de Plantas Medicinais*, **9**, 72-79.

[22] Ceconi, D.E., Poletto, I., Lovato, T. and Muniz, M.F.B. (2007) Exigência Nutricional de Mudas de Erva-Mate (Ilex Paraguariensis A. St.-Hil.) à Adubação Fosfatada. *Ciência Florestal*, **17**, 25-32.

[23] Mota, J.H., Yuri, J.E., Resende, G.M., Oliveira, C.M., Souza, R.J., Freitas, S.A.C. and Rodrigues, J.C.J. (2003) Produção de Alface Americana em Função da Aplicação de Doses e Fontes de Fósforo. *Horticultura Brasileira*, **21**, 620-622. http://dx.doi.org/10.1590/S0102-05362003000400008

[24] Hirel, B., Le Gouis, J., Ney, B. and Gallais, A. (2007) The Challenge of Improving Nitrogen Use Efficiency in Crop Plants: Towards a More Central Role for Genetic Variability and Quantitative Genetics within Integrated Approaches. *Journal of Experimental Botany*, **58**, 1-19. http://dx.doi.org/10.1093/jxb/erm097

[25] Fageria, N.K., Baligar, V.C. and Li, Y.C. (2008) The Role of Nutrient Efficient Plants in Improving Crop Yields in the

Twenty First Century. *Journal of Plant Nutrition*, **31**, 1121-1157. http://dx.doi.org/10.1080/01904160802116068

[26] Croteau, R.B., Davis, E.M., Ringer, K.L. and Wildung, E.M. (2005) (−)-Menthol Biosynthesis and Molecular Genetics. *Naturwissenschaften*, **92**, 62-577. http://dx.doi.org/10.1007/s00114-005-0055-0

[27] Mahmoud, S.S. and Croteau, R.B. (2003) Menthofuran Regulates Essential Oil Biosynthesis in Peppermint by Controlling a Downstream Monoterpene Reductase. *Proceedings of the National Academy of Sciences of the United States of America*, **100**, 14481-14486. http://dx.doi.org/10.1073/pnas.2436325100

[28] Turner, G.W., Gershenzon, J.E. and Croteau, R.B. (2000) Development of Peltate Glandular Trichomes of Peppermint. *Plant Physiology*, **124**, 665-680. http://dx.doi.org/10.1104/pp.124.2.665

[29] Davis, E.D., Ringer, K.L., McConkey, M.E. and Croteau, R. (2005) Monoterpene Metabolism. Cloning, Expression and Characterization of Menthone Reductases from Peppermint. *Plant Physiology*, **137**, 873-881. http://dx.doi.org/10.1104/pp.104.053306

5

Monitoring Brain and Spinal Cord Metabolism and Function*

Pierre Pandin#, Marie Renard, Alessia Bianchini, Philippe Desjardin, Luc Van Obbergh

Department of Anesthesia & Critical Care, Erasmus Academic Hospital, Université Libre de Bruxelles, Brussels, Belgium
Email: #ppandin@ulb.ac.be, #Pierre.Pandin@erasme.ulb.ac.be

Abstract

Monitoring the metabolism and function of the central nervous system not only is an old idea but also is a topic that is of increasing interest to the technological evolution. Beside the optimization of cerebral and spinal cord perfusion and the preservation of vasoreactivity to ensure the viability of cerebral tissues and structures, we want to know more and more about the real intimate situation of these organs in real time at the patient's bedside. To this end, several tracks have been explored during the two last decades, leading to the development of numerous concepts and the conception of various monitoring systems. One of the main problems is to characterize the respective strong points and weaknesses of those ones and to conclude regarding their individual relevance and value in current clinical practice. It is more and more clear that the combination of different categories of monitoring is a way to try to find the most valuable technological compromise, to increase the chance of prediction or of early detection of intercurrent deleterious events corresponding to the concept of multimodality. The intraoperative period and the intensive care goals and targets are appreciably different. This is the reason for the attempt to define different and distinct sets of goals and targets for the intraoperative anesthetic setting and for the intensive care unit.

Keywords

Brain, Central Nervous System Monitoring, Metabolism, Function

1. Introduction

The most accurate possible monitoring of the metabolism and function of the central nervous system (CNS) re-

---

*Meeting at which this review has been presented: Annual meeting of the European Society of Anesthesia, EUROANAESTHESIA 2013, Barcelona, Spain, June 1st-4th 2013, Refresher Course 7RC2.
#Corresponding author.

mains a cornerstone that is a testament to the constant technological evolution. It makes possible the more and more adapted management of the brain and the spinal cord during either more and more complex and specific-neurosurgical interventions or more and more invasive investigations in neuro-intensive care unit (Neuro-ICU). For a long time now, the concept of active neuroprotection has been developed following the successive progress in the understanding of the complex interaction between the CNS, surgery, anesthesia, and/or a possible aggression (trauma, hemorrhage, ischemia, anoxia, edema, etc.). In the past, the pioneers used several rudimentary tools (for instance, the single trace analogue electroencephalogram), but unfortunately they were not integrated into the monitoring, and were without systematization or generalization (only used on a case-by-case basis). At the beginning of the nineties, a real neuro-monitoring culture emerged, as illustrated by the book edited by Peter Sebel and William Fitch, *Monitoring the central nervous system* [1]. Then, continuous efforts led to the conception of multimodal intraoperative monitoring (IOM), supported by pioneers as the American anesthesiologist Betty Grundy [2]-[4] and the English neurophysiologist Catherine Thornton [5] [6].

2. CNS: What Is Metabolism and What Is Function?

The specific functionality of well-defined neural loops or neural networks is now appreciated and their functioning seems to be governed by a biphasic on-off model [7] too often underestimated. Anesthesiologists and intensive care unit (ICU) specialists must change their mind about a more multimodal CNS monitoring for a more realistic vision of the function. Moreover, in the ICU, all the high-tech imaging innovations can give only a time to time idea of the neurological trend of the patients with sometime a lack a possible conclusion. On the other hand, in the operating room, the use of medical imaging remains limited for only very specific situations [8]. Alternatively, CNS follow-up regarding metabolism or function at the patient's bedside would be based on the combination of specific parameters not only regarding the experience of pioneers [9] [10] but also existing recommendations [11] [12] to depict with accuracy the topographical and temporal variability of the CNS [7].

3. Early Detection for Outcome Improvement But Not Any Old How…

Beside the early claimed dimension of global or segmental CNS investigation [13] [14], the early detection of the occurrence of possible troubles or abnormal events was advocated as well [2] [15], before permanent cerebral damage. The not only theoretical but desirable description of the fundamentals of this kind of monitoring is listed in **Table 1**. Their lack of materiality, fragility (micro or nanosignals respectively in μV and nV), and sensitivity to electromagnetic disturbances make recording difficult, while the frequent intricacy between what is metabolism and what is function is not so simple to interpret [16] [17]. From a practical point of view, the neuromonitoring of metabolism and function is more and more subdivided into two distinct entities: intraoperative neuro-monitoring and neuro-monitoring in the ICU (**Table 2**) considering the goals of the monitoring, and the possible accessibility of the CNS.

4. Temporal, Topographical, and Spatial Variations: The Brain Mapping Concept

The complexity of the CNS lies probably not only in its structural complexity but also in its spatial and temporal metabolic and functional variability in either awake or comatose/unconscious patients, under anesthesia or in ICU [18]-[25]. To take that into account, neuro-monitoring has not to be too excessively simplified [26]-[28] and limited only to the forehead, as accurately described by John in his "anaesthetic cascade" [19]. Moreover, resorting to standard tools and technologies makes it easier to discuss the case with the neuro-specialists regarding the patient's management and the different options.

5. Spontaneous Activities and Evoked Answers

Regarding CNS function, one other specificity lies in the difference between spontaneous activities (as a description of the neurological ambiance) and evoked responses (as the reaction capability of the CNS to stimulation) as listed in the **Table 3**. Briefly, the clinician has to use the optimal multimodal combination of monitoring following, first, the pathophysiological target and second, the local culture and know-how, and third, the availability of the potential tools [9] [14]. The ambient signals (**Table 2**) inform directly or not about the metabolic level, more or less directly linked to the regional functional level, but are nevertheless limited by the risk to be too cumulative and not discriminant enough [29]-[32]. To bypass this problem, one solution is to map the skull

Table 1. Theoretical description of the fundamentals of the ideal multimodal brain and spinal cord metabolism and function monitoring.

Theoretical description of the fundamentals of the ideal multimodal brain and spinal cord metabolism and function monitoring

Point 1: *Global or segmental investigation of the central nervous system (CNS) with the possibility of individual adaptation following each case request*

Point 2: *Similar physiological dimension of the neurological indicators in comparison to the physiological hemodynamic or respiratory parameters—no calculation, no index*

Point 3: *Early detection of possible deterioration of neural function before definitive damage, because the sooner neural dysfunction is detected, the more reversible it is (usefulness of trends)*

Point 4: *Multimodality*

Point 5: *Subclinical detection of physiological or pathophysiological changes before the occurrence of major and definitive consequences to guide the earliest possible intervention to reduce and/or inverse the neural suffering, to improve the vital and functional prognosis of the patients by limiting the impact on the brain, spinal cord, or both*

Point 6: *Monitoring the versatility of either cerebral pathophysiology (stroke, ischaemia, haemorrhage, seizures, etc.) or pharmacological interaction (anaesthesia, barbiturates, anti-epileptic drugs, etc.)*

Point 7: *Make as much as possible the distinction between the anesthesiology and the effects of surgery on the pathophysiological process*

Point 8: *Make concrete not only CNS metabolism but also CNS function to make easier the management of anesthetised patients during the intraoperative period or comatose patients during their intensive care unit stay*

Point 9: *Apply the precepts of telemedicine and telemonitoring*

Table 2. State of the art regarding the practice of neuro-monitoring during the intraoperative period vs. in the intensive care unit, based on differences in the practical conditions of realisation, goals and requests, and central nervous system accessibility (based on the literature, reflecting the actual worldwide practice "+++" corresponds to often used and/or even recommended monitoring, "++" is sometimes used and "+" matches for an occasional use. Alternatively, "-" corresponds to the lack of substantial clinical experience corresponding often to the impossibility of use, for several technical or practical reasons).

	Intraoperative neuro-monitoring (IONM)	Intensive care unit
Electrophysiology		
-Electroencephalogram	+++(continuous)	+++(discontinuous)
-Evoked potentials	+++(continuous)	++(discontinuous)
Cerebral biochemistry		
-Microdialysis	-	+++
Cerebral brain oxygen		
-SjvO2	+	+++
-PbtO2	+	+++
-SctO2 by NIRS	+++	++
Cerebral blood perfusion (CBF)		
-Regional CBF (TDF)	-	++
-Local CBF (LDF)	-	+
-TCD	++	+++

Table 3. Classification of central nervous system signals into spontaneous activities vs. evoked responses.

Signals	Spontaneous	Evoked
Basic principles	-Direct & immediate reading -Topographical correlation -Neural ambiance -More basic	-Indirect & immediate reading (specific treatment) -Anatomo-functional correlation -Neural state -More advanced
General vs. global	-Mapped EEG (cEEG, dEEG, CEEG, sEEG, qEEG, QEEG) -SvjO2 -SctO2 (NIRS)	-Mapped EP (brain or spinal cord) -Mapped SctO2 (NIRS) EROS
Regional vs. segmental	-Microdialysis -PbtO2 -lCBF -rCBF -TCD& microDoppler	-EP (SSEP, AEP, VEP, etc.)

Abbreviations: *EEG*: electroencephalogram; *cEEG*: computerised EEG; *dEEG*: digitised EEG; *CEEG*: continuous EEG; *sEEG*: simplified EEG; *qEEG* and *QEEG*: quantitative EEG; *EP*: evoked potentials; *SSEP*: somatosensory EP; *AEP*: auditory EP, *VEP*: visual EP; *SvJO2*: jugular venous oxygen saturation; *SctO2*:cerebral tissue oximetry; *NIRS*: near-infrared spectrometry; *EROS*: event-related evoked optical stimulation; *PbtO2*:brain tissue oxygen tension; *lCBF*: local cerebral blood flow; *rCBF*: regional cerebral blood flow; *TCD*: Transcranial Doppler.

surface with recording electrodes following a high enough resolution [24] [25], giving numerical or graphical trends [9] [14], useful for the early detection of potential neural degradation and to adapt the patient's management. Additionally, evoked responses can indicate the functional integrity or not of the neural networks [7] (audition, vision, somesthesia, motor function, nociception, etc.). Those ones, composed of neural loops through the different anatomical CNS levels, may help to locate the occurring problem and to assess the patient's prognosis [11]. In very disturbed and extreme conditions (brain death, deep hypothermia, etc.), the whole evoked responses are nearly completely depressed with a tremendous global decrease of CNS function, reversible or not.

6. Multimodal Neuro-Monitoring in Addition to the Usual Measurements

The combination of different neuro-parameters seems now to be logical regarding the capability to monitor the metabolism and/or the function of the brain and spinal cord, but the list of indicators to be combined is not yet fixed and depends on the specific clinical problem and situation of the patient. Moreover, the real impact on the final and the long-term outcome of neurological patients remains unclear, even if the preliminary but incomplete results seem to be interesting and convincing regarding a potential recommendation of the systematic use of neuro-monitoring [30] [31]. Monitoring of the central temperature, arterial and cerebral perfusion pressure, end tidal CO2, sequential arterial blood gas sampling, glycaemia follow-up, and, of course, monitoring of intracranial pressure (ICP) are currently recommended and always form part of CNS management, to maintain homeostasis, which indirectly preserves either the metabolism or function [33]. Therefore, multimodal neuro-monitoring must be a complement and not a replacement of what exists to achieve innovative solutions [33]. Until relatively recently, ICP remains a cornerstone in our practice when the brain is damaged [33]-[36]. Following the Monro-Kellie principle, the increase of intracranial volumes may result in brain herniation, reduction of cerebral blood flow (CBF), and of course, the rise of ICP is related to increased disability and mortality [37]. According to Treggiari's review [38], the raised but reducible ICP is associated with a three- to four-fold increase in the probability of death and/or poor neurological outcome, while a refractory ICP pattern is associated with a tremendous increase in the relative risk of death (odds ratio >100). One key point would be the aggressivity of the indications of ICP catheter insertion base on clinical (coma) and Computerized Tomography (CT) abnormality [38]. However, strong evidence seems to lack when ICP is considered to guide therapy in patients with acute brain injury [39] as illustrated by the recent Chesnut's [40] randomized controlled trial which demonstrated the lack of difference in 3- or 6-month outcomes in severe traumatic brain injury patients whose treatment was based on the ICP monitoring (strictly maintained below 20 mmHg) compared with those whose the follow-up was based on imaging (CTscan) and clinical examination without ICP monitoring. In this relatively controversial context, the spontaneous technological evolution gives to the clinicians a new opportunity to progressively monitoring the ICP by non-invasive methods as a sort of alternatives [41] [42]. The Transcranial Doppler (TCD) derived pulsatility index [41] [43], the intra-orbital optic nerve sonography [41] [44] [45] and the distorsion-product otoacoustic emissions (DPOAEs) monitoring [46] have valuable preliminary results although insufficient for now. Despite the actual controversy, the ICP monitoring remains a key element of therapeutic strategies when it rises, even if it is not excluded to have to reevaluate its real interest during the next years leading to the publication of updated recommendations of use. Less and less on its own side; the ICP monitoring is integrated more and more into multimodal neuro-monitoring [16].

7. Electrophysiology

7.1. Electroencephalogram (EEG) and Quantitative EEG (QEEG)

More functional than metabolic, EEG measures the electrical activity related to the function of the outermost brain layer: the cerebral cortex is composed of different lobes dedicated to distinct superior functions, with metabolic and functional variations [47] [48]. The mapped QEEG is able to detect the occurrence of abnormal increases or decreases (sudden or progressive) in brain electrical activity [9] [10], clinically significant or not, in comatose, sedated, anesthetised, or awake patients. QEEG has a dual value [9] [49], to detect an increase or depression of brain electrical activity. In 50% of cases, the seizures are nonconvulsive, completely silent or have an atypical clinical presentation [50] [51] potentially resulting in an increased secondary cerebral damage [52] and tissue loss [53] if they are not detected. The prevalence of nonconvulsive seizures varies between 4% to 30% [54] and is inextricably linked to sedation and anesthesia [55]. QEEG could have a real impact on not only the management of the prophylactic antiepileptic strategy, but also the final neurological outcome [56]. Within the QEEG-derived parameters, the variability in the alpha (awake) or the delta (coma or sleep) power may be helpful and relevant for the prediction of delayed ischemia in poor-grade subarachnoid haemorrhage [57] [58], to following the evolution in severe stroke patients [59], or to improve outcome in postanoxic comatose patients or after hypothermia [60]-[63]. Nevertheless, the implementation of QEEG in practice in anesthesia or critical care is challenging, requiring an interactive collaboration between anesthesiologists, ICU specialists and neurologists making supported by education and training of the participants on the ground (medical doctors, nurses), which is made easier in recent years by the development of telemedicine [64]-[68].

7.2. Evoked Potentials

The particularity of evoked potentials rests in their capability to monitor spinal cord function and indirectly monitor its metabolism [13]. By the judicious use of electrode montage, evoked potentials may inform about nervous conduction through the whole CNS until the different cerebral cortical lobes [69]-[71]. Similarly, their analysis may be global or segmental, and they can be divided into conduction index (subcortical) and in function index (cortical), as detailed in **Table 4** and **Table 5** [72]. Used worldwide, their usual indications are listed in **Table 6** [73]-[77]. Evoked potentials are usually affected by inhalational agents [73]-[75] in their amplitudes rather than their latencies, and changes in body temperature (hypothermia), nervous tissue perfusion, oxygenation and ventilation (either oxygen or carbon dioxide), and ICP (rise) may depress them [30] [78] [79]. Nevertheless and despite these influences, the evoked potentials monitoring is very valuable, remains advanced, but is more and more associated with EEG or QEEG in clinical practice and is accepted as the gold standard [75]. On the other hand, motor evoked responses or potentials (MEPs) give information about centrifugal nervous "conduction" [76] after typically, a transcranial stimulation (TcMEP). MEPsare globally less sensitive to intercurrent factors and particularly to the impact of anesthetic drugs making them a strong functional monitoring used during spine and spinal cord surgery. MEP monitoring provides excellent specificity and sensitivity whenever the motor tracts are involved in the pathological process, particularly in trauma medicine. The actual recommendation is to combine TcMEP monitoring electrophysiological modalities [75].

8. Microdialysis

Only cerebral microdialysis (MCD)provides brain metabolism monitoring, because it reflects the biochemistry (glucose, lactate, pyruvate, lactate/pyruvate ratio, glutamate, urea, and anecdotal aspartate) of the cerebral tissue where the specialised catheter tip is implanted, giving an idea of the composition of the extracellular fluid [80], the adequacy of the brain energy supply, and cellular function. During cerebral ischaemia, an elevated lactate/pyruvate ratio with an elevated glutamate and a low glucose indicate cellular hypoxia [81]. These metabolic

Table 4. Evoked potential-derived subcortical index of conduction [58].

Level of brain-stem lesion	SEPs	MLAEPs	BAEPs
1. MIDBRAIN	*Normal* P14 N20 *delayed or absent*	*Abnormal*	*Normal*
2. PONS	*Normal* P14 N20 *delayed or absent*	*Abnormal*	*Abnormal*
3. MEDULLA	*Absent* P14 N20 *delayed or absent*	*Normal*	*Normal*

SEPs: somatosensory evoked potentials; *MLAEPs*: midlatency auditory evoked potentials; *BAEPs*: brainstem auditory evoked potentials.

Table 5. Evoked potential-derived cortical index of function [58].

Index of Global Cortical Function (IGCF)	VEPs	SEPs
Grade 0	*Normal*	*Normal*
Grade 1	*Delayed peak III Peak VII present*	*Normal N20, P24, P27 N30 present*
Grade 2	*Delayed peak III Peak VII present*	*Normal N20, P24 N30 basent*
Grade 3	*Delayed peak III*	*Normal N20*
Grade 4	*No reproducible VEPs ERG present*	*P14 present*

VEPs: visual evoked potentials; *SEPs*: somatosensory evoked potentials; *ERG*: electroretinogram.

Table 6. Classical applications of sensory evoked potentials.

Classical applications of sensory evoked potentials (EPs) during the intraoperative period and/or intensive care unit stay
Somatosensory EPs

1) Invasive spine (arthrodesis) and spinal cord surgery for detection of either medullary or radicular syndrome (combined with motor EPs and/or evoked EMG)

2) Normothermic thoracic and thoracoabdominal aortic surgery for detection of cord ischaemia (compromised vascular supply—radicular anterior Adamkiewicz artery—combined with motor EPs)

3) Deep or intermediate hypothermia for neurosurgery (cerebral vascular bypass), cardiac, or major vascular surgery (combined with motor EPs)

4) Carotid endarterectomy (alternative to mapped EEG and QEEG, because less pharmacologically depressible)

5) Surgical peripheral nerve release (surgery guidance—possibly combined with motor EPs)

6) Post-anoxic comatose patients (prognosis dimension—outcome prediction)

7) Hypothermic comatose patients (prognosis dimension—outcome prediction)

8) Spinal cord post-trauma status (combined with motor EPs and/or evoked EMG)

Auditory EPs (short or midbrain latencies)

1) Intra and extracranial surgery of the auditory and/or the facial nerves (combined with facial evoked EMG—specific facial nerve monitoring)

2) Midbrain and/or spinal cord post-trauma status (combined with motor EPs and/or evoked EMG)

Auditory EPs (middle or early cortical latencies)

1) Post-anoxic comatose patients (prognosis dimension—outcome prediction)

2) Hypothermic comatose patients (prognosis dimension—outcome prediction)

Auditory EPs (long or late cortical latencies)

1) Postoperative, post-lesion, or post-trauma cognitive dysfunction

Visual EPs (cortical latencies)

1) Optic nerve, hypothalamic, pituitary gland, and diaphragma sellae surgery

2) Post-anoxic comatose patients (prognosis dimension—outcome prediction)

3) Hypothermic comatose patients (prognosis dimension—outcome prediction)

EMG: electromyogram; *EEG*: electroencephalogram; *QEEG*: quantitative electroencephalogram.

changes may occur before the usual cerebral physiological or pathophysiological changes [82] allowing earlier therapeutic adjustments. Some illustrative examples of successful MCD-motivated insulin therapy modifications have been published with the opportunity to determine individual optimal glycaemia threshold [80]-[85]. More and more often combined with the brain tissue oxygen tension (PbtO2), cerebral MCD is also able to optimise the Mean Arterial Pressure (MAP)/Cerebral Perfusion Pressure (CPP) [86] [87] and the transfusion thresholds [88] in patients at high risk of secondary brain ischaemia [89]. This has led to the establishment of guidelines in comatose patients for various problems [90] [91]. Moreover, a correlation has been demonstrated between variations in early biological markers and long-term outcome [92] supporting the concept of a possible influence of brain energy modulation on patient outcome. Despite these exciting results, MCD technology has an intrinsic limitation: the analysis is limited to the area surrounding the catheter tip, making this monitoring only local or even regional (**Table 2**). To bypass this problem, some successful experiences of multicatheter insertion have been reported, confirming the quality of the information provided by MCD, unfortunately too limited for now [93].

9. Brain Oxygen Monitoring

9.1. Jugular Venous Oxygen Saturation (SjvO2)

In this category of CNS monitoring, SjvO2 is the oldest since it was proposed in clinical practice from the 1940s. After a resurgence at the beginning of the 1990s, sustained by the availability of fibreoptic oximetric catheters, there has been a progressive lack of interest, which is related to the intrinsic weaknesses of this parameter and the concomitant emergence of new competitive technologies (see below). The difficulty of keeping the tip of the catheter in a good place (despite some attempts of ultrasound-guided optimisation, which was unfortunately not generalised), with the correlated high risk of displacement, particularly in awake but non-cooperative patients [94] [95]; the possibility of extracranial blood contamination; the lack of sensibility and specificity to detect limited brain ischaemia have often made the rational interpretation of SjvO2 too difficult and non-pertinen [96]. This is why, nowadays, SjvO2 is progressively competed by newer technologies.

9.2. Brain Tissue Oxygen Tension

The brain oxygen supply depends on cerebral blood flow (CBF), and the partial pressure of oxygen in brain tissue or brain oxygen (PbtO2 = product of CBF and cerebral arteriovenous oxygen tension difference) represents an effective indicator that is, nevertheless, more indicative of oxygen diffusion than cerebral metabolism [97]. PbtO2 is measured on-line via specific probes inserted in subcortical white matter, through multiple-lumen bolts adjacent to ICP monitors, but can also be measured in penumbral tissue, such as around haemorrhagic contusions or in areas at risk for secondary delayed vasospasm/ischaemia. Furthermore, PbtO2 is additional to ICP monitoring in guiding the management of CPP [98]. The response of PbtO2 to CPP/MAP increase allows the tailoring of the individual CPP threshold [98] [99]. Combined with TCD and neuroimaging, PbtO2 reactivity is adapted to manage delayed cerebral ischaemia in comatose patients with subarachnoid hemorrhage (SAH) when the classical influence factors are SaO2, ScO2, PvO2, and haemoglobinaemia, and while moderate hyperventilation [100], protective ventilation [101], and blood transfusion [102] may even be adjusted using PbtO2. Regarding neuro-trauma, a low PbtO2 without reactivity is a strong marker of poor outcome [103] and a discordant low PbtO2 may occur while ICP and CPP remain within the recommended thresholds [104]. This high intrinsic value has led to the recent incorporation of this topographical parameter into the recommendations for the brain injured patient [105] [106]. The progressive multiple parameter adjustment to increase PbtO2 has even been proposed as a useful way to identify "PbtO2 responders" with a better outcome [107]. However, despite this positive trend, the real impact on patient outcome of PbtO2-directed therapy remains controversial [105] [106] [108] and needs further investigations to clarify the vision. Nevertheless, the clinical relevance, safety, and effective documentation in the literature make the PbtO2 a quite systematically recommended parameter in routine CNS multimodal monitoring.

9.3. Cerebral Oximetry (SctO2) Using Near-Infrared Spectrometry (NIRS)

The measurement of SctO2 using NIRS technology [109]-[111] represents a newer alternative to PtbO2 for the direct measurement of cerebral tissue oxygenation. Different methodologies exist and are commercially available [112]: modified Beer-Lambert law, multidistance or spatially resolved spectroscopy, frequency-resolved (domain) spectroscopy, and time-resolved spectroscopy. Before being used for cerebral oximetry monitoring in anesthesia and in intensive care, NIRS was developed by neuroscientists and neurocognitivists for brain function investigation [113] [114]. Briefly, a rapid change in NIRS, recorded spontaneously or after stimulation, is directly correlated to the variation of function of the neural tissue just below the electrode, based on the "near-infrared window" concept [115] and the event-related evoked optical stimulation (EROS), a suitable and attractive method for the cognitive neurosciences [116].

In this context, NIRS has been topographically used in fundamental research, using relatively complex multiple electrode montages over the skull [117], corresponding to a new category of functional brain mapping, alone or combined with EEG [118], showing the complementarity of these technologies. Alternatively, for the intraoperative period or in the ICU, different dual-channel oximeters simplified for clinical practice (FORE-SIGHT device, CAS-Medical Systems, Brandford, CT, USA; INVOS series, Somanetics, Troy, MI, USA; and NIRO series, Hamamatsu Photonics K.K., Hamamatsu City, Japan) may be used.

Two electrodes disposed on the forehead of the patient would give information about oxygenation in the right and left cerebral hemispheres. Basically, NIR cerebral oximetry does not rely on pulsatile flow but measures a weighted average of arterial, capillary, and venous compartments (unfortunately, by cumulative assessment) in proportion to their relative intracranial volumes within the field of view [119]. It is measured following different physical methods (regional cerebral saturation by the INVOS series, tissue oxygenation index by the NIRO series, and $SctO_2$ by the FORE-SIGHT device), making sometimes difficult the comparison. For instance, despite normative values of $SctO_2$ of between 60% and 75% and a coefficient of variation for absolute baseline values of approximately 10% [120] being validated for the healthy brain, a wide intra- and inter-individual baseline variability remains a potential problem. The use of NIRS to guide the manipulation of systemic physiology to minimise the risk of cerebral hypoxia/ischaemia during carotid endarteriectomy (CEA) is an area where NIRS needs to be proved to have at least equivalent sensitivity and specificity to the other recommended modalities of monitoring [121]-[123]. NIRS has not been clearly proven to be superior for identifying critical cerebral ischaemia. The body of evidence suggests only a broad equivalence to other modalities, albeit with uncertainty as to the exact NIRS-derived threshold for the identification of critical ischaemia [124]-[126] (low positive predictive value). Regarding cardiac surgery, the absence of compelling data to support the use of NIRS-guided management strategies to reduce the incidence of postoperative cognitive dysfunction and stroke has not prevented NIRS from gaining popularity as a monitoring modality for the management of cerebral oxygenation during cardiac surgery [127] [128], particularly taking in account the significant associated over-cost (electrodes).

However, a recent review suggests that the neurocognitive decline after cardiac bypass surgery may not only be related to the intervention but may also reflect the natural decline of patients with multiple comorbidities raises an important question about the impact and value of neuro-monitoring, including NIRS, to guide treatment during cardiopulmonary bypass [129]. Otherwise, NIRS has been suggested for monitoring the healthy but at-risk brain during routine surgical procedures under general anesthesia, but always without real confirmation [130]. In this context, patients undergoing surgery in the beach chair position could take advantage of $SctO_2$ monitoring. Severe hypotension occurs in up to 20% of patients [131] and ischaemia-related cerebrovascular events have been reported [132]. It was first reported in an isolated case [133] [134] and then demonstrated by an observational study [135] of shoulder arthroscopy in a beach chair versus lateral decubitus position and using a FORE-SIGHT™ oximeter, which demonstrated cerebral desaturation in 80% of patients in the beach chair position compared with none in the lateral decubitus position. Nevertheless, there was no postoperative neurological impact, only a higher incidence of nausea and vomiting, supporting the hypothesis that brain oxygenation might be a surrogate of the adequacy of non-neurological organ perfusion.

Regarding brain injury in the ICU, the complex relationships between NIRS and other physiological variables (ICP, blood flow velocity, etc.) routinely used to assess cerebrovascular reactivity make it necessary to apply more complex analytical techniques to perform qualitative and quantitative analysis of cerebrovascular reactivity that is not available with other methods [136]. This way, NIRS might potentially provide the monitoring of cerebral autoregulation, although this is uncertain at present. However, compared with $PbtO_2$, NIRS lacks power for brain ischaemia detection in neuro-ICU [137]. For now, $PbtO_2$ remains the method of choice, but $SctO_2$ by NIRS is not necessarily inferior. The problem is trying to define the real interest and indications of this user-friendly, noninvasive monitoring modality. With several practical advantages in comparison to other neuro-monitoring techniques (invasive or minimally invasive), such as the capability to make measurements over multiple regions of interest simultaneously with high temporal resolution, NIRS might potentially monitor regional cerebral oxygenation, haemodynamics, and metabolism, and could guide therapeutic brain protection strategies. For now, mainly validated when ischemia occurs in normal and healthy brain monitoring without major neurological problem, it seems to suffer from a lack of concrete recommendations for use, bearing in mind that NIRS technology has the potential benefit of multiple recording sites either at the skull level (brain mapping similar to EEG and QEEG) or at extracranial sites for muscular oxygenation and metabolism follow-up [138] [139] or peripheral perfusion [140] [141].

To summarise (**Table 7**) regarding the three methodological options for brain oxygen monitoring, the maximal interest in SjVO2 was shown 10 to 15 years ago. It has been progressively replaced by the minimally invasive PbtO2 monitoring that is now more and more well established in clinical practice, while SctO2 by NIRS has not found its proper place in clinical practice in relation to its intrinsic practical advantages, and truly needs a clearer and objective definition of its recommended uses.

Table 7. The three methodological options regarding cerebral brain oxygen monitoring.

	Jugular venous oxygen saturation (SjvO2)	Brain tissue oxygen tension (PbtO2)	Cerebral oximetry using near-infrared spectrometry (SctO2 – NIRS)
Basic principle -indicator	Oxygen consumption —oxygen need—cerebral metabolism	Oxygen diffusion > cerebral metabolism	Oxygen consumption—oxygen need—cerebral metabolism in normal healthy brain
Applicability	Continuous at bedside	Continuous at bedside	Continuous at bedside
Application fields	Intraoperative ICU	Intraoperative ICU	Intraoperative ICU
Device	Invasive	Minimally invasive	Non-invasive (main advantage)
Limitations of use	-Catheter tip displacement -Compiled hemispheric measurement -Lack of detection of limited ischaemia -Extracranial blood pollution	-Local or regional measurement -Site-dependent measurement	-Mainly healthy brain monitoring -Inter- & intra-individual variability -Complex multi-factor brain pathophysiological process -Compiled hemispheric measurement -Desaturation ≠ real ischaemia and infarction -Specific SctO2 determination methodology of each device
Cost-investment	-Monitoring -Probe (reusable or single use)	-Monitoring -Probe (single use)	-Monitoring -Probe (single use)
Technical expertise, management & nursing	Advanced Time-consuming	Advanced Time-consuming	Basic (intuitive)
Specific infrastructure for insertion	Special need (invasive, ICU, or OR)	Special need (minimally invasive, OR)	No need
Ischaemia detection	Hemispheric (focal ischaemia undetected)	Local (insertion site-dependent)	Hemispheric
CPP correlation		CPP < 60 mmHg: PbtO2↓ CPP > 60 mmHg: PbtO2 ≈ or ↑	Variable (+/− more specific than SjvO2)
Numeric values	-Normal: 60% - 90% -Critical: 50% - 55% during 15 min = cerebral ischaemia	-Normal: 25 - 35 mmHg -Critical: <15 mmHg = ischaemia -<6 mmHg = infarction, even cerebral death	-Normal: 60% - 75% -Baseline variation: 10% -↓13%: ischaemic threshold -35% during 2 - 3 h: infarction
Thresholds correspondance	50%	8.5 mmHg	To be determined-variable (correct for internal carotid clamping, circulatory arrest)

ICU: intensive care unit; *OR*: operating room; *CPP*: cerebral perfusion pressure.

10. Cerebral Blood Perfusion

10.1. Regional Cerebral Blood Flow

PbtO2 (for the physiological definition, see the "Brain tissue oxygen tension" section) represents only an indirect assessment of the CBF influenced by external factors [98]. A recent technological alternative allows the direct measurement of regional blood flow (rCBF) via a thermal diffusion probe (TDP; Hemedex, Cambridge, Massachusetts, USA), giving results in absolute units. This probe may be inserted into the brain parenchyma, close to the ICP/PbtO2 probes (cf. multimodality concept). It can be either tunnelled from the surgical area or directly bolted (stable fixation of the probe through a skull bolt to avoid catheter dislodgement). Similar to PbtO2, the probe tip provides a quantitative measurement only in the spherical volume of tissue surrounding the sensor. The TDP technology was first successfully validated by comparing the rCBF measurements with the xenonCT [142]. Insertion of the probe 2.5 cm below the dura in the white matter is checked using a CTscan. Otherwise, for the rCBF assessment, the TDP remains dependent on a stable patient temperature trend. Severe hyperthermia and the patient's temperature instability significantly affect the rCBF numerical value.

In brain injured patients (subarachnoid haemorrhage, trauma, etc.), the TDP combined withPbtO2 seems very relevant for optimising CPP management [143] [144]. The results suggest that rCBF-guided MAP/CPP increase could efficiently replace the classical "triple-H" therapy. The main problem remains to define the most judicious site of insertion of the electrode [145]-[147]. Placed at a good site, rCBF allows the assessment of cerebrovascular reactivity to PaCO2 variations, which is greatly useful for driving moderate hyperventilation, particularly in patients with at least partially altered cerebral autoregulation [148] [149].

Less advanced than PbtO2 technology in its systematic integration into multimodal neuro-monitoring, rCBF could progressively take a part after, of course, the confirmation of its validity and its implementation in a large population of neurological patients.

10.2. Local CBF

For the continuous measurement of CBF at the patient's bedside, Laser Doppler Flowmetry (LDF)represents an old but efficient alternative. The Oxylab LDF system(Oxford Optronix, Abingdon, UK) measures red blood cell movements within the microcirculation only 1cm below the dural surface [150] [151], using several possible local devices (surface angular, needle and micro-needle, and endoscope). The physical principle is to invest a smallvolume of cerebral matter (limited to the cortex), but with the highest possible spatial resolution. This is why the LDF does not qualify as regional CBF monitoring but only as local CBF monitoring and is, till now, mainly used in laboratories for fundamental neuro-investigations in small animals (rats, gerbils, rabbits, or cats), for which it is currently a sort of gold standard. However, the LDF has been investigated for use in neurosurgery for a long time, with satisfactory results regarding the early detection of ischaemia and treatment guidance and adjustment [152]-[155], but a possible significant and beneficial impact on patient outcome was never proved. On the other hand, some authors have considered the mapped multi-insertion of LDF probes as a solution to the problem of the limited volume of investigated cerebral matter, at the main condition to select as judiciously as possible the different probe insertion sites. However, this has never been reported in clinical practice. On the other hand, the LDF has been proved to monitor efficiently local spinal cord blood flow in one animal model [156]. Unfortunately, no consistent comparative data have been published on local CBF monitoring using LDF and rCBF, followed up with TDP. However, in a recent article, LDF seems to be logically more sensitive than TCD in detecting cortical autoregulation disturbance during rising ICP and falling CPP in the area of distribution of the middle cerebral artery [157]. This lack of clinical results makes it quite impossible to have a definitive overview and is a little frustrating.

10.3. TCD, Microvascular Doppler, and Cerebral Tissue Doppler

Today, TCD is a full element of CNS monitoring despite its limited metabolic and functional dimension, being completely indirect. With the constant and even growing interest in this technology, it is regularly upgraded [158]. In fact, except rCBF and local CBF monitoring, TCD provides the only Foods and Drugs Administration-cleared method to continuously and directly monitor change in cerebral haemodynamics, mainly in perioperative and critical care settings, to give clinically valuable and potentially life-saving information [159] [160]. The technology evolution gives the operator the opportunity of more and more substantial morphological information's [161] about the cerebral vasculature. However, the quality of this monitoring is heavily influenced by the training, skill, experience, and practice of the sonographer. Beside TCD, microvascular Doppler ultrasonography [162] is the only dedicated intraoperative to the check of vascular neurosurgery (aneurysm clipping, vascular bypass of giant aneurysm or arteriovenous malformation, etc.) as a potentially powerful alternative to fluorescein angiography, since the Doppler technology is able to give not only qualitative but also quantitative information. Additionally, it is increasing thought that Doppler technology can be used not only to monitor cerebral vessels but also brain parenchyma, where it would probably be very informative about CBF in a less limited area than the two other methods.

To summarise regarding CBF monitoring methods (**Table 8**), TCD has advantages with possible evolutions and improvements, may be completed by the assessment of tissue blood flow by Doppler. This sort of a multimodal Doppler tool could be very valuable and powerful. In the meantime, the more limited (local or regional) methods of monitoring of CBF remain of interest, but what can be done with them and for which types of patients have not been clearly defined.

11. Conclusions

To conclude, I would like to first list some key learning points that form the foundation of efficient neuro-monitoring:

Table 8. The three methodological options regarding cerebral blood flow (CBF) monitoring.

	Regional CBF (rCBF) Thermal Diffusion Probe (TDP)	Local CBF (lCBF) Laser Doppler Flowmetry (LDF)	Transcranial Doppler (TCD)
Basic principle -indicator	Thermal diffusion in a spherical volume around the tip of the probe	Red blood cell movement within the microcirculation beside the probe	Major vascular Doppler effect coupled with two-dimensional ultrasonography
Applicability	Continuous at bedside	Continuous at bedside	Continuous at bedside
Application fields	Intraoperative (to be developed) ICU	Intraoperative (to be re-evaluated and developed) ICU	Intraoperative ICU
Device	Minimally invasive (2 - 2.5 cm below the dura)	Minimally invasive (1cm below the dura)	Non-invasive (main advantage)
Limitations of use	-Measurement and monitoring of rCBF only in the spherical area (1 - 1.5 cm diameter) around the probe tip -Site-dependent measurement	-Measurement and monitoring of lCBF only in the 1 or 2 mm surrounding the probe tip -Site-dependent measurement	-Arterial CBF in medium size vessels (MCA > ACA > PCA) -Not tissue monitoring -Possible instability of the probe
Cost-investment	-Monitoring -Probe (single use)	-Monitoring -Probe (single use)	-Monitoring -Probe (reusable) -Fixation system for probes
Technical expertise, management & nursing	Basic Time-consuming	Basic Time-consuming	Advanced
Specific infrastructure for insertion	Special need (minimally invasive, ICU, or OR) Probe tunneled or bolted	Special need (minimal invasive, ICU or OR) Probe tunnelled or bolted	No need
Ischaemia detection	Local or regional Cortical and subcortical (following the insertion's adequacy)	Local Cortical (following the insertion's adequacy)	Hemispheric or global
CPP correlation	Vasoreactivity and autoregulation	Vasoreactivity and autoregulation	Variable Vasoreactivity and autoregulation
Numeric values	-Normal: 40 - 70 mL$\cdot$100$^{-1}\cdot$min^{-1}	-Normal: 80 mL$\cdot$100$^{-1}\cdot$min^{-1} (temporo-sylvian cortex) and 60 - 65 mL$\cdot$100$^{-1}\cdot$min^{-1} (fronto-latero-dorsal cortex)	-Normal: 30 - 80 mL$\cdot$100$^{-1}\cdot$min^{-1} Following the artery and based on the velocity assessment

MCA: middle cerebral artery; *ACA*: anterior cerebral artery; *PCA*: posterior cerebral artery; *ICU*: intensive care unit; *OR*: operating room; *CPP*: cerebral perfusion pressure.

Table 9. Proposal about the potential multimodal combinations of neuro-parameters of advanced neuro-monitoring in the near future for the intraoperative and/or intensive care unit settings (based on the scientific literature reflecting the actual worldwide practice and on my own practice). For each clinical situation, two to three technologies can be combined. Dark grey indicates validated usual and recommended elements of monitoring. Medium grey indicates parameters with a high level of evidence (equivalent to a recommendation or quite equivalent) In this case; there is consistent scientific literature to support making these parameters probably recommended in the next years. Light grey indicates parameters that require clinical investigations to try to define or to refine the real value. For these, clinical recommendations remain unclear and only potential. Very light grey (regional cerebral blood flow [rCBF] column) is just to point out that rCBF by TDP could be an alternative (or a second choice) to lCBF by LDF that is preferred because of the smallness of the probe.

	EEG‡	EP	MCD	SvjO2	PbtO2	SctO2 (NIRS)	rCBF (TDP)	lCBF (LDF)	TCD
Intraoperative neuromonitoring									
1. Neurosurgery									
Invasive spine or spinal cord surgery		SEP/MEP							
Deep or intermediate hypothermia for brain vascular neurosurgery		SEP/VEP AEP							
Normothermic brain vascular neurosurgery		SEP/VEP AEP							
Cortical brain tumour resection (meningioma and astrocytoma)									
Posterior fossa surgery*		SEP/AEP							
Epilepsy surgery**									
Awake surgery***									
Optic nerve, hypothalamic, pituitary gland, and diaphragma sellae surgery****		VEP							
Surgical peripheral nerve release		SEP/MEP							
2. Cardiac & vascular surgery									
Normothermic thoracic and thoracoabdominal aortic surgery		SEP/MEP							
Normothermic cardiac or vascular surgery									
Intermediate hypothermia for cardiac or vascular surgery		SEP/VEP							
Deep hypothermia for cardiac or vascular surgery§		SEP/VEP							
Carotid endarterectomy		SEP/VEP							
Intensive care unit									
Post-anoxic coma		SEP/VEP SEP/AEP							
Hypothermic coma		SEP/VEP SEP/AEP							
Intoxication and poisoning		SEP/VEP SEP/AEP							
Brain death		SEP/VEP SEP/AEP							
Non-epileptic seizures		SEP/VEP							
Status epilepticus		SEP/VEP							
Subarachnoid haemorrhage		SEP/VEP SEP/AEP							
Stroke (acute phase)		SEP/VEP SEP/AEP							
Trauma brain injury		SEP/VEP SEP/AEP							
Trauma spinal cord injury		SEP/MEP							

‡including quantitative EEG (QEEG) but not necessarily simplified forehead EEG-derived technologies; *including intra- and extracranial surgery of the auditory and/or facial nerves; **including surgical lobectomies and other resections, electrocorticography and stereo-EEG electrodes insertion, and intraoperative cortical stimulation; ***including fully awake procedures and asleep-awake-asleep procedures; ****including open and/or endonasal approaches; §including therapeutic and deliberate cardiac arrest; *rCBF*: regional cerebral blood flow; *TDP*: thermal diffusion probe; *lCBF*: local cerebral blood flow; *LDF*: laser Doppler flowmetry; *EEG*: electroencephalogram; *EP*: evoked potentials; *MCD*: microdialysis; *SvjO2*: jugular venous oxygen saturation; *PbtO2*: brain tissue oxygen tension; *SctO2*: Cerebral oximetry using near infrared spectrometry; *TCD*: transcranial Doppler.

1) The variability of CNS metabolism and function is typical of the different anesthetic phases and in comatose patients. Influenced by physiological and pathophysiological factors, one of our main challenges is to impact it as efficiently as possible.

2) Regarding CNS metabolism and function monitoring, a minimal subdivision has to be respected: the cerebral cortex and deeper structures as interdependent entities, each with a high level of differentiation and complexity.

3) The different cerebral cortical areas are dedicated to different functions and their pharmacological and pathophysiological sensitivity is not similar orhomogeneous. This underlies the concept of topographical investigations for mapping.

4) Regarding not only the electrical signals of the CNS but also the other specialized neuro-monitoring modalities, they potentially have dual dimensions: basic spontaneous activities and advanced evoked responses.

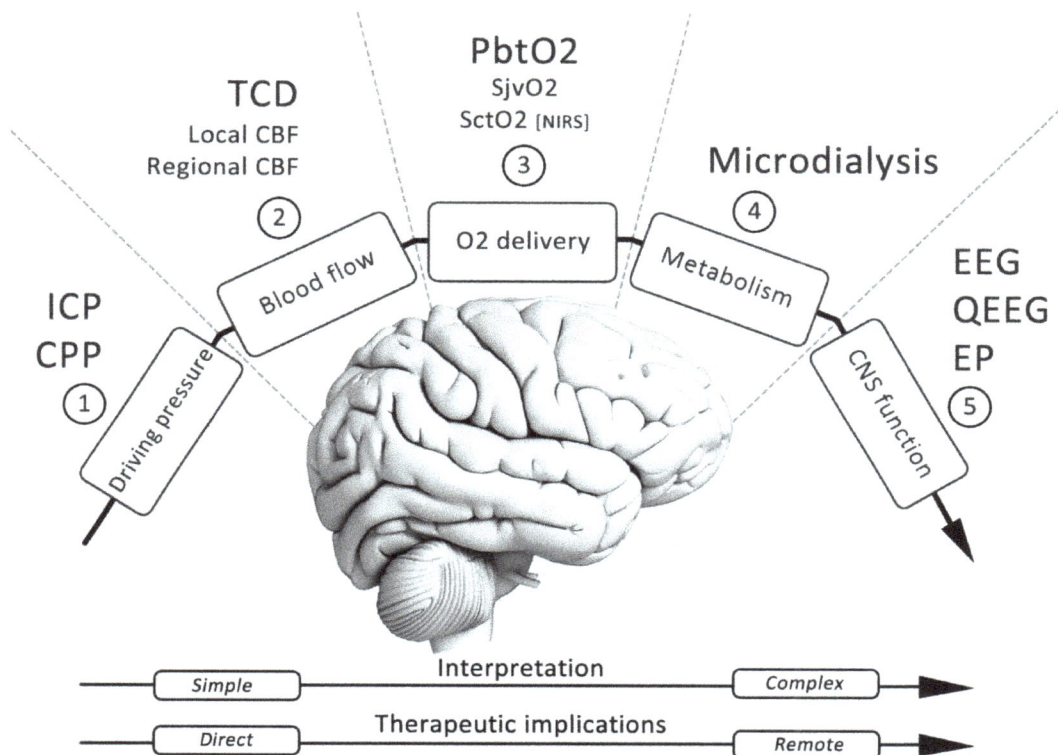

Figure 1. Do we need a more advanced brain and spinal cord monitoring to follow metabolism and function? To make more concrete the multimodal approach, it is possible to put in accordance the different possible modalities of CNS monitoring to the respective level in the phenomenological chain leading to the highest complexity: the CNS function and neurons functioning, on right. First, the driving pressure method is based on the usual and continuous monitoring of the ICP and CPP. Second, about CBF assessment, the TCD remains the reference technique even if local CBF (lCBF) or regional CBF (rCBF) would deserve to be considered a new time. Third, to follow the 02 delivery, the PbtO2 has progressively supplanted the classical SjvO2, without to be really competed with the cerebral oximetry, remaining an O2 cerebral diffusion indicator rather than a really metabolic parameter. Fourth, the metabolism is essentially related by the microdialysis technique for which an increased glutamate, a high lactate/pyruvate ratio with a low glucose in the brain relate a CNS cellular hypoxia. Finally, in point 5, the electrophysiology is alone able to give an idea of the CNS function and neurons functioning. About the phenomenological chain from point 1 to point 5, each item is required for the further factors downstream as in a sort of cascade. The corresponding monitoring items progress from the most basic (on left) with the simplest interpretation to the most advanced (on right) with more complex results sometime difficult to put in perspective with the patient situation. Similarly, the impact on the patients' treatment varies from direct to remote or indirect. However, the level of the accuracy of the information's given by the successive monitoring's is progressively growing up, counterbalancing the apparent awkwardness of use. The investment of time to know how to use the different modalities of this monitoring would be always very productive and beneficial either for the clinicians or particularly for the patients.

5) Multimodality, which is more and more recommended in practice, has to try to define the most judicious combination of parameters from different origins (electrical, oxygen consumption and supply, and blood perfusion and supply) to give the best possible answer for the specific patient's situation.

6) Electrophysiology (EEG, QEEG, and evoked potentials) represents a cornerstone but remains underused because of the absolute need for education.

7) Regarding brain oxygen monitoring, PbtO2 has now supplanted SjvO2 and represents the reference technology. As for SctO2 by NIRS, it is still controversial and we have to wait some more years for definite and strict recommendations for use.

8) Regarding cerebral perfusion, rCBF is interesting but is, unfortunately, too site-dependent to be sufficient. LDF has to be re-evaluated in clinical practice to refine its real interest, specificity and sensitivity. This is the only one with a specific potential interest about spinal cord blood flow monitoring owing to the smallness of its probe.

Finally, regarding brain and spinal cord metabolism and function, continual developments in monitoring methods provide more and more valuable information and more and more accurate answers to questions about potential problems. As to what is called "multimodality" and within the available technologies listed in this article, someone's, older, are more investigated and evaluated in clinical practice and others, more recent are still waiting to find their respective position in the neuro-monitoring arsenal. Far from excluding any technology, the best remains to learn and to know as much as possible what they are and what we can expect of them, to limit the risk of misuse and misevaluation. The development of a real effective neuro-monitoring, combining one monitoring modality of each family (electrophysiology, microdialysis, brain oxygen, and CBF) could be the final solution (**Table 9**). To make more concrete this sort of methodic approach, it is also possible to classify the different modalities according the level in the phenomenological chain leading to the highest step of complexity: the brain or spinal cord function (**Figure 1**). For now, this idea remains only conceptual but this is our role for the next years, to drive investigations to have the opportunity to justify the usefulness of this second generation neuro-monitoring.

References

[1] Sebel, P. and Fitch, W. (1994) Monitoring the Central Nervous System. Blackwell Science, London, 479.

[2] Grundy, B.L. (1982) Monitoring of Sensory Evoked Potentials during Neurosurgical Operations: Methods and Applications. *Neurosurgery*, **11**, 556-575. http://dx.doi.org/10.1227/00006123-198210000-00020

[3] Grundy, B.L. (1983) Intraoperative Monitoring of Sensory-Evoked Potentials *Anesthesiology*, **58**, 72-87. http://dx.doi.org/10.1097/00000542-198301000-00011

[4] Grundy, B.L. (1984) Evoked Potentials in the Operating Rooms. *Mount Sinai Journal of Medicine*, **51**, 585-591.

[5] Thornton, C., Catley, D.M., Jordan, C., Lehane, J.R., Royston, D. and Jones, J.G. (1983) Enflurane Anaesthesia Causes Graded Changes in the Brainstem and the Early Cortical Auditory Evoked Response in Man. *British Journal of Anaesthesia*, **55**, 479-486. http://dx.doi.org/10.1093/bja/55.6.479

[6] Thornton, C., Heneghan, C.P., James, M.F. and Jones, J.G. (1984) Effects of Halothane or Enflurane with Controlled Ventilation on Auditory Evoked Potentials. *British Journal of Anaesthesia*, **56**, 315-323. http://dx.doi.org/10.1093/bja/56.4.315

[7] Lee, S.H. and Dan, Y. (2012) Neuromodulation of Brain States. *Neuron*, **76**, 209-222. http://dx.doi.org/10.1016/j.neuron.2012.09.012

[8] Pandin, P. and Dewitte, O. (2007) Open Low-Field Intraoperative MRI for Transsphenoidal Pituitary Surgery. *Anesthesia & Analgesia*, **105**, 886. http://dx.doi.org/10.1213/01.ane.0000268558.02855.73

[9] Vespa, P. (2005) Continuous EEG Monitoring for the Detection of Seizures in Traumatic Brain Injury, Infarction, and Intracerebral Hemorrhage: "To Detect and Protect". *Journal of Clinical Neurophysiology*, **22**, 99-106. http://dx.doi.org/10.1097/01.WNP.0000154919.54202.E0

[10] Vespa, P. (2005) Multimodality Monitoring and Telemonitoring in Neurocritical Care: From Microdialysis to Robotic Telepresence. *Current Opinion in Critical Care*, **11**, 133-138. http://dx.doi.org/10.1097/01.ccx.0000155353.01489.58

[11] Guérit, J.M., Amantini, A., Amodio, P., Andersen, K.V., Butler, S., de Weerd, A., *et al.* (2009) Consensus on the Use of Neurophysiological Tests in the Intensive Care Unit (ICU): Electroencephalogram (EEG), Evoked Potentials (EP), and Electroneuromyography (ENMG). *Clinical Neurophysiology*, **39**, 71-83. http://dx.doi.org/10.1016/j.neucli.2009.03.002

[12] Kurtz, P., Hanafy, K.A. and Claassen, J. (2009) Continuous EEG Monitoring: Is It Ready for Prime Time? *Current*

Opinion in Critical Care, **15**, 99-109. http://dx.doi.org/10.1097/MCC.0b013e3283294947

[13] Tamaki, T. and Kubota, S. (2007) History of the Development of Intraoperative Spinal Cord Monitoring. *European Spine Journal*, **16**, S140-S146. http://dx.doi.org/10.1007/s00586-007-0416-9

[14] Nash Jr., C.L., Lorig, R.A., Schatzinger, L.A. and Brown, R.H. (1977) Spinal Cord Monitoring during Operative Treatment of the Spine. *Clinical Orthopaedics and Related Research*, **126**, 100-105.

[15] Coles, J.G., Wilson, G.J., Sima, A.F., Klement, P. and Tait, G.A. (1982) Intraoperative Detection of Spinal Cord Ischemia Using Somatosensory Cortical Evoked Potentials during Thoracic Aortic Occlusion. *The Annals of Thoracic Surgery*, **34**, 299-306. http://dx.doi.org/10.1016/S0003-4975(10)62499-X

[16] Oddo, M., Villa, F. and Citerio, G. (2012) Brain Multimodality Monitoring: An Update. *Current Opinion in Critical Care*, **18**, 111-118. http://dx.doi.org/10.1016/S0003-4975(10)62499-X

[17] Grocott, H.P., Davie, S. and Fedorow, C. (2010) Monitoring of Brain Function in Anesthesia and Intensive Care. *Current Opinion in Anaesthesiology*, **23**, 759-764. http://dx.doi.org/10.1097/ACO.0b013e3283404641

[18] John, E.R. (2002) The Neurophysics of Consciousness. *Brain Research Reviews*, **39**, 1-28. http://dx.doi.org/10.1016/S0165-0173(02)00142-X

[19] John, E.R. and Prichep, L.S. (2005) The Anesthetic Cascade: A Theory of How Anesthesia Suppresses Consciousness. *Anesthesiology*, **102**, 447-471. http://dx.doi.org/10.1097/00000542-200502000-00030

[20] John, E.R. and Prichep, L.S. (2006) The Relevance of QEEG to the Evaluation of Behavioral Disorders and Pharmacological Interventions. *Clinical EEG and Neuroscience*, **37**, 135-143. http://dx.doi.org/10.1177/155005940603700210

[21] Nuwer, M.R. (1994) Electroencephalograms and Evoked Potentials. Monitoring Cerebral Function in the Neurosurgical intensive Care Unit. *Neurosurgery Clinics of North America*, **5**, 647-659.

[22] Nuwer, M. (1997) Assessment of Digital EEG, Quantitative EEG, and EEG Brain Mapping: Report of the American Academy of Neurology and the American Clinical Neurophysiology Society. *Neurology*, **49**, 277-292. http://dx.doi.org/10.1212/WNL.49.1.277

[23] Nuwer, M.R. (2007) ICU EEG Monitoring: Nonconvulsive Seizures, Nomenclature, and Pathophysiology. *Clinical Neurophysiology*, **118**, 1653-1654. http://dx.doi.org/10.1016/j.clinph.2007.01.026

[24] Kochs, E., Bischoff, P., Pichlmeier, U. and Esch, S.J. (1994) Surgical Stimulation Induces Changes in Brain Electrical Activity during Isoflurane/Nitrous Oxide Anesthesia. A Topographic Electroencephalographic Analysis. *Anesthesiology*, **80**, 1026-1034. http://dx.doi.org/10.1097/00000542-199405000-00012

[25] Pandin, P., Van Cutsem, N., Tuna, T. and D'hollander, A. (2006) Bispectral Index Is a Topographically Dependent Variable in Patients Receiving Propofol Anaesthesia. *British Journal of Anaesthesia*, **97**, 676-680. http://dx.doi.org/10.1093/bja/ael235

[26] Rampil, I. (1998) A Primer for EEG Signal Processing in Anesthesia. *Anesthesiology*, **89**, 980-1002. http://dx.doi.org/10.1097/00000542-199810000-00023

[27] Jameson, L.C. and Sloan, T.B. (2006) Using EEG to Monitor Anesthesia Drug Effects during Surgery. *Journal of Clinical Monitoring and Computing*, **20**, 445-472. http://dx.doi.org/10.1007/s10877-006-9044-x

[28] Jameson, L.C. and Sloan, T.B. (2012) Neurophysiologic Monitoring in Neurosurgery. *Anesthesiology Clinics*, **30**, 311-331. http://dx.doi.org/10.1016/j.anclin.2012.05.005

[29] Jäntti, V. and Yli-Hankala, A. (2000) Neurophysiology of Anaesthesia. *Supplements to Clinical Neurophysiology*, **53**, 84-88. http://dx.doi.org/10.1016/S1567-424X(09)70142-4

[30] Guérit, J.M. (2000) The Usefulness of EEG, Exogeneous Evoked Potentials and Cognitive Evoked Potentials in the Acute Stage of Post-Anoxic and Post-Traumatic Coma. *Acta Neurologica Belgica*, **100**, 229-236.

[31] Sloan, T.B. (1995) Electrophysiologic Monitoring in Head Injury. *New Horizons*, **3**, 431-438.

[32] Vato, A., Bonzano, L., Chiappalone, M., Cicero, S., Morabito, F., Novellino, A., *et al.* (2004) Spike Manager: A New Tool for Spontaneous and Evoked Neuronal Networks Activity Characterization. *Neurocomputing*, **58-60**, 1153-1161. http://dx.doi.org/10.1016/j.neucom.2004.01.180

[33] Pasternak, J.J. and Lanier, W.L. (2012) Neuroanesthesiology Update. *Journal of Neurosurgical Anesthesiology*, **24**, 85-112. http://dx.doi.org/10.1097/ANA.0b013e31824a8152

[34] Bratton, S.L., Chestnut, R.M., Ghajar, J., Hammond, F.F.M., Harris, O.A., Hartl, R., *et al.* (2007) Guidelines for the Management of Severe Traumatic Brain Injury. VI. Indications for Intracranial Pressure Monitoring. *Journal of Neurotrauma*, **24**, S37-S44. http://dx.doi.org/10.1089/neu.2007.9990

[35] Andrews, P.J. and Citerio, G. (2004) Intracranial Pressure. Part One: Historical Overview and Basic Concepts. *Intensive Care Medicine*, **30**, 1730-1733.

[36] Citerio, G. and Andrews, P.J. (2004) Intracranial Pressure. Part Two: Clinical Applications and Technology. *Intensive*

Care Medicine, **30**, 1882-1885. http://dx.doi.org/10.1007/s00134-004-2377-3

[37] Mokri, B. (2001) The Monro-Kellie Hypothesis. *Neurology*, **56**, 1746-1748. http://dx.doi.org/10.1212/WNL.56.12.1746

[38] Treggiari, M.M., Schutz, N., Yanez, N.D. and Romand, J.A. (2007) Role of Intracranial Pressure Values and Patterns in Predicting Outcome in Traumatic Brain Injury: A Systematic Review. *Neurocritical Care*, **6**, 104-112. http://dx.doi.org/10.1007/s12028-007-0012-1

[39] Kirkman, M.A. and Smith, M. (2014) Intracranial Pressure Monitoring, Cerebral Perfusion Pressure Estimation, and ICP/CPP-Guided Therapy: A Standard of Care or Optional Extra after Brain Injury? *British Journal of Anaesthesia*, **112**, 35-46. http://dx.doi.org/10.1093/bja/aet418

[40] Chesnut, R.M., Tembin, N., Carney, N., Dikmen, S., Rondina, C., Videtta, W., *et al.* (2012) A Trial of Intracranial-Pressure Monitoring in Traumatic Brain Injury. *The New England Journal of Medicine*, **367**, 2471-2481. http://dx.doi.org/10.1056/NEJMoa1207363

[41] Kristiansson, H., Nissborg, E., Bartek, J., Andresen, M., Reinstrup, P. and Romner, B. (2013) Measuring Elevated Intracranial Pressure through Noninvasive Methods: A Review of the Literature. *Journal of Neurosurgical Anesthesiology*, **25**, 372-385. http://dx.doi.org/10.1097/ANA.0b013e31829795ce

[42] Manwaring, P.K., Moodie, K.L., Hartov, A., Manwaring, K.H. and Halter, R.J. (2013) Intracranial Electrical Impedance Tomography: A Method of Continuous Monitoring in an Animal Model of Head Trauma. *Anesthesia & Analgesi*, **117**, 866-875. http://dx.doi.org/10.1213/ANE.0b013e318290c7b7

[43] Bouzat, P., Francony, G., Fauvage, B. and Payen, J.F. (2010) Transcranial Doppler Pulsatility Index for Initial Management of Brain-Injured Patients. *Neurosurgery*, **67**, E1863-E1864. http://dx.doi.org/10.1227/NEU.0b013e3181f932e7

[44] Rajajee, V., Vanaman, M., Fletcher, J.J. and Jacobs, T.L. (2011) Optic Nerve Ultrasound for the Detection of Raised Intracranial Pressure. *Neurocritical Care*, **15**, 506-515. http://dx.doi.org/10.1007/s12028-011-9606-8

[45] Dubost, C., Le Gouez, A., Jouffroy, V., Roger-Christoph, S., Benhamou, D., Mercier, F.J., *et al.* (2012) Optic Nerve Sheath Diameter Used as Ultrasonographic Assessment of the Incidence of Raised Intracranial Pressure in Preeclampsia: A Pilot Study. *Anesthesiology*, **116**, 1066-1071. http://dx.doi.org/10.1097/ALN.0b013e318246ea1a

[46] Voss, S.E., Horton, N.J., Tabucchi, T.H., Folowosele, F.O. and Shera, C.A. (2006) Posture-Indiced Changes in Distorsion-Product Otoacoustic Emissions and the Potential for Noninvasive Monitoring of Intracranial Pressure. *Neurocritical Care*, **4**, 251-257. http://dx.doi.org/10.1385/NCC:4:3:251

[47] Lin, A.P., Liao, H.J., Merugumala, S.K., Prabhu, S.P., Meehan, W.P. and Ross, B.D. (2012) Metabolic Imaging of Mild Traumatic Brain Injury. *Brain Imaging and Behavior*, **6**, 208-223. http://dx.doi.org/10.1007/s11682-012-9181-4

[48] Stam, C.J. and van Straaten, E.C. (2012) The Organization of Physiological Brain Networks. *Clinical Neurophysiology*, **123**, 1067-1087. http://dx.doi.org/10.1016/j.clinph.2012.01.011

[49] Pandin P. (2004) The Neuro-Anaesthesiology Assisted by the Electroencephalogram. *Annales Françaises d'Anesthésie et de Réanimation*, **23**, 395-403. http://dx.doi.org/10.1016/j.annfar.2004.01.006

[50] Abend, N.S., Dlugos, D.J., Hahn, C.D., Hirsch, L.J. and Herman, S.T. (2010) Use of EEG Monitoring and Management of Nonconvulsive Seizures in Critically Ill Patients: A Survey of Neurologists. *Neurocritical Care*, **12**, 382-389. http://dx.doi.org/10.1007/s12028-010-9337-2

[51] Rossetti, A.O. and Oddo, M. (2010) The Neuro-ICU Patient and Electroencephalography Paroxysms: If and When to Treat. *Current Opinion in Critical Care*, **16**, 105-109. http://dx.doi.org/10.1097/MCC.0b013e3283374b5b

[52] Vespa, P.M., Miller, C., McArthur, D., Eliseo, M., Etchepare, M., Hirt, D., *et al.* (2007) Nonconvulsive Electrographic Seizures after Traumatic Brain Injury Result in a Delayed, Prolonged Increase in Intracranial Pressure and Metabolic Crisis. *Critical Care Medicine*, **35**, 2830-2836. http://dx.doi.org/10.1097/01.CCM.0000295667.66853.BC

[53] Vespa, P.M., McArthur, D.L., Xu, Y., Eliseo, M., Etchepare, M., Dinov, I., *et al.* (2010) Nonconvulsive Seizures after Traumatic Brain Injury ARE Associated with Hippocampal Atrophy. *Neurology*, **75**, 792-798. http://dx.doi.org/10.1212/WNL.0b013e3181f07334

[54] Friedman, D., Claassen, J. and Hirsch, L.J. (2009) Continuous Electroencephalogram Monitoring in the Intensive Care Unit. *Anesthesia & Analgesia*, **109**, 506-523. http://dx.doi.org/10.1213/ane.0b013e3181a9d8b5

[55] Olivecrona, M., Zetterlund, B., Rodling-Wahlström, M., Naredi, S. and Koskinen, L.O.D. (2009) Absence of Electroencephalographic Seizure Activity in Patients Treated for Head Injury with an Intracranial Pressure-Targeted Therapy. *Journal of Neurosurgery*, **110**, 300-305. http://dx.doi.org/10.3171/2008.4.17538

[56] Naidech, A.M., Garg, R.K., Liebling, S., Levasseur, K., Macken, M.P., Schuele, S.U., *et al.* (2009) Anticonvulsant Use and Outcomes after Intracerebral Hemorrhage. *Stroke*, **40**, 3810-3815. http://dx.doi.org/10.1161/STROKEAHA.109.559948

[57] Claassen, J., Hirsch, L.J., Kreiter, K.T., Du, E.Y., Connolly, E.S., Emerson, R.G., *et al.* (2004) Quantitative Conti-

nuous EEG for Detecting Delayed Cerebral Ischemia in patients with Poor-Grade Subarachnoid Hemorrhage. *Clinical Neurophysiology*, **115**, 2699-2710. http://dx.doi.org/10.1016/j.clinph.2004.06.017

[58] Rathakrishnan, R., Gotman, J., Dubeau, F. and Angle, M. (2011) Using Continuous Electroencephalography in the Management of Delayed Cerebral Ischemia Following Subarachnoid Hemorrhage. *Neurocritical Care*, **14**, 152-161. http://dx.doi.org/10.1007/s12028-010-9495-2

[59] Diedler, J., Sykora, M., Bast, T., Poli, S., Veltkamp, R., Mellado, P., *et al.* (2009) Quantitative EEG Correlates of Low Cerebral Perfusion in Severe Stroke. *Neurocritical Care*, **11**, 210-216. http://dx.doi.org/10.1007/s12028-009-9236-6

[60] Bosco, E., Marton, E., Feletti, A., Scarpa, B., Longatti, P., Zanatta, P., *et al.* (2011) Dynamic Monitors of Brain Function: A New Target in Neurointensive Care Unit. *Critical Care*, **15**, R170. http://dx.doi.org/10.1186/cc10315

[61] Rossetti, A.O., Oddo, M., Logroscino, G. and Kaplan, P.W. (2010) Prognostication after Cardiac Arrest and Hypothermia: A Prospective Study. *Annals of Neurology*, **67**, 301-307.

[62] Rossetti, A.O., Urbano, L.A., Delodder, F., Kaplan, P.W. and Oddo, M. (2010) Prognostic Value of Continuous EEG Monitoring during Therapeutic Hypothermia after Cardiac Arrest. *Critical Care*, **14**, R173. http://dx.doi.org/10.1186/cc9276

[63] Rundgren, M., Westhall, E., Cronberg, T., Rosén, I. and Friberg, H. (2010) Continuous Amplitude-Integrated Electro encephalogram Predicts Outcome in Hypothermia-Treated Cardiac Arrest Patients. *Critical Care Medicine*, **38**, 1838-1844. http://dx.doi.org/10.1097/CCM.0b013e3181eaa1e7

[64] Coates, S., Clarke, A., Davison, G. and Patterson, V. (2012) Tele-EEG in the UK: A Report of over 1,000 Patients. *Journal of Telemedicine and Telecare*, **18**, 243-246. http://dx.doi.org/10.1258/jtt.2012.111003

[65] Palendeng, M.E., Zhang, Q., Pang, L. and Li, Y. (2012) EEG Data Compression to Monitor DoA in Telemedicine. *Studies in Health Technology and Informatics*, **178**, 163-168.

[66] D'Arcy, R.C., Hajra, S.G., Liu, C., Sculthorpe, L.D. and Weaver, D.F. (2011) Towards Brain First-Aid: A Diagnostic Device for Conscious Awareness. *IEEE Transactions on Biomedical Engineering*, **58**, 750-754. http://dx.doi.org/10.1109/TBME.2010.2090880

[67] Lasierra, N., Alesanco, A., Campos, C., Caudevilla, E., Fernández, J. and García, J. (2009) Experience of a Real-Time Tele-EEG Service. *Annual International Conference of the IEEE Engineering in Medicine and Biology Society*, **2009**, 5211-5214.

[68] Campos, C., Caudevilla, E., Alesanco, A., Lasierra, N., Martinez, O., Fernández, J., *et al.* (2012) Setting up a Telemedicine Service for Remote Real-Time Video-EEG Consultation in La Rioja (Spain). *International Journal of Medical Informatics*, **81**, 404-414. http://dx.doi.org/10.1016/j.ijmedinf.2012.01.006

[69] Toleikis, J.R. (2005) Intraoperative Monitoring Using Somatosensory Evoked Potentials. A Position Statement by the American Society of Neurophysiological Monitoring. *Journal of Clinical Monitoring and Computing*, **19**, 241-258. http://dx.doi.org/10.1007/s10877-005-4397-0

[70] American Electroencephalographic Society (1994) Guidelines for Intraoperative Monitoring of Sensory Evoked Potentials. *Journal of Clinical Neurophysiology*, **11**, 77-87. http://dx.doi.org/10.1097/00004691-199401000-00012

[71] American Electroencephalographic Society (1987) Guidelines for Intraoperative Monitoring of Sensory Evoked Potentials. *Journal of Clinical Neurophysiology*, **4**, 397-416. http://dx.doi.org/10.1097/00004691-198710000-00005

[72] Guerit, J.M. (1999) EEG and Evoked Potentials in the Intensive Care Unit. *Neurophysiologie Clinique*, **29**, 301-317. http://dx.doi.org/10.1016/S0987-7053(99)90044-8

[73] Sloan, T.B. and Heyer, E.J. (2002) Anesthesia for Intraoperative Neurophysiologic Monitoring of the Spinal Cord. *Journal of Clinical Neurophysiology*, **19**, 430-443. http://dx.doi.org/10.1097/00004691-200210000-00006

[74] Sloan, T. (2002) Anesthetics and the Brain. *Anesthesiology Clinics of North America*, **20**, 265-292.

[75] International Organization of Societies for Electrophysiological Technology (OSET) (1999) Guidelines for Performing EEG and Evoked Potential Monitoring during Surgery. *American Journal Of Electroneurodiagnostic Technology*, **39**, 257-277.

[76] Padberg, A.M., Russo, M.H., Lenke, L.G., Bridwell, K.H. and Komanetsky, R.M. (1996) Validity and Reliability of Spinal Cord Monitoring in Neuromuscular Spinal Deformity Surgery. *Journal of Spinal Disorders*, **9**, 150-158. http://dx.doi.org/10.1097/00002517-199604000-00012

[77] Pelosi, L., Lamb, J., Grevitt, M., Mehdian, S.M.H., Webb, J.K. and Blumhardt, L.D. (2002) Combined Monitoring of Motor and Somatosensory Evoked Potentials in Orthopaedic Spinal Surgery. *Clinical Neurophysiology*, **113**, 1082-1091. http://dx.doi.org/10.1016/S1388-2457(02)00027-5

[78] Guerit, J.M. (2010) Neurophysiological Testing in Neurocritical Care. *Current Opinion in Critical Care*, **16**, 98-104. http://dx.doi.org/10.1097/MCC.0b013e328337541a

[79] Kim, S.M., Kim, S.H., Seo, D.W. and Lee, K.W. (2013) Intraoperative Neurophysiologic Monitoring: Basic Principles

and Recent Update. *Journal of Korean Medical Science*, **28**, 1261-1269.
http://dx.doi.org/10.3346/jkms.2013.28.9.1261

[80] Hillered, L., Vespa, P.M. and Hovda, D.A. (2005) Translational Neurochemical Research in Acute Human Brain Injury: the Current Status and Potential Future for Cerebral Microdialysis. *Journal of Neurotrauma*, **22**, 3-41.
http://dx.doi.org/10.1089/neu.2005.22.3

[81] Sarrafzadeh, A.S., Nagel, A., Czabanka, M., Denecke, T., Vajkoczy, P. and Plotkin, M. (2010) Imaging of Hypoxic-Ischemic Penumbra with (18)F-Fluoromisonidazole PET/CT and Measurement of Related Cerebral Metabolism in Aneurysmal Subarachnoid Hemorrhage. *Journal of Cerebral Blood Flow & Metabolism*, **30**, 36-45.
http://dx.doi.org/10.1038/jcbfm.2009.199

[82] Adamides, A.A., Rosenfeldt, F.L., Winter, C.D., Pratt, N.M., Tippett, N.J., Lewis, P.M., *et al.* (2009) Brain Tissue Lactate Elevations Predict Episodes of Intracranial Hypertension in Patients with Traumatic Brain Injury. *Journal of the American College of Surgeons*, **209**, 531-539. http://dx.doi.org/10.1016/j.jamcollsurg.2009.05.028

[83] Oddo, M., Schmidt, J.M., Carrera, E., Badjatia, N., Connolly, E.S., Presciutti, M., *et al.* (2008) Impact of Tight Glycemic Control on Cerebral Glucose Metabolism after Severe Brain Injury: A Microdialysis Study. *Critical Care Medicine*, **36**, 3233-3238.

[84] Meierhans, R., Béchir, M., Ludwig, S., Sommerfeld, J., Brandi, G., Haberthür, C., *et al.* (2010) Brain Metabolism Is Significantly Impaired at Blood Glucose below 6mM and Brain Glucose Below 1mM in Patients with Severe Traumatic Brain Injury. *Critical Care*, **14**, R13. http://dx.doi.org/10.1186/cc8869

[85] Ko, S.B., Choi, H.A., Parikh, G., Helbok, R., Schmidt, J.M., Lee, K., *et al.* (2011) Multimodality Monitoring for Cerebral Perfusion Pressure Optimization in Comatose Patients with Intracerebral Hemorrhage. *Stroke*, **42**, 3087-3092.
http://dx.doi.org/10.1161/STROKEAHA.111.623165

[86] Schmidt, J.M., Ko, S.B., Helbok, R., Kurtz, P., Stuart, R.M., Presciutti, M., *et al.* (2011) Cerebral Perfusion Pressure Thresholds for Brain Tissue Hypoxia and Metabolic Crisis after Poor-Grade Subarachnoid Hemorrhage. *Stroke*, **42**, 1351-1356. http://dx.doi.org/10.1161/STROKEAHA.110.596874

[87] Oddo, M., Milby, A., Chen, I., Frangos, S., MacMurtrie, E., Maloney-Wilensky, E., *et al.* (2009) Hemoglobin Concentration and Cerebral Metabolism in Patients with Aneurysmal Subarachnoid Hemorrhage. *Stroke*, **40**, 1275-1281.
http://dx.doi.org/10.1161/STROKEAHA.110.596874

[88] Diringer, M.N., Bleck, T.P., Claude Hemphill 3rd, J., Menon, D., Shutter, L., Vespa, P., *et al.* (2011) Critical Care Management of Patients Following Aneurysmal Subarachnoid Hemorrhage: Recommendations from the Neurocritical Care Society's Multidisciplinary Consensus Conference. *Neurocritical Care*, **15**, 211-240.
http://dx.doi.org/10.1007/s12028-011-9605-9

[89] Bellander, B.M., Cantais, E., Enblad, P., Hutchinson, P., Nordström, C.H., Robertson, C., *et al.* (2004) Consensus Meeting on Microdialysis in Neurointensive Care. *Intensive Care Medicine*, **30**, 2166-2169.
http://dx.doi.org/10.1007/s00134-004-2461-8

[90] Andrews, P.J., Citerio, G., Longhi, L., Polderman, K., Sahuquillo, J. and Vajkoczy, P. (2008) NICEM Consensus on Neurological Monitoring in Acute Neurological Disease. *Intensive Care Medicine*, **34**, 1362-1370.
http://dx.doi.org/10.1007/s00134-008-1103-y

[91] Timofeev, I., Carpenter, K.L., Nortje, J., Al-Rawi, P.G., O'Connell, M.T., Czosnyka, M., *et al.* (2011) Cerebral Extracellular Chemistry and Outcome Following Traumatic Brain Injury: A Microdialysis Study of 223 Patients. *Brain*, **134**, 484-494. http://dx.doi.org/10.1093/brain/awq353

[92] Poca, M.A., Sahuquillo, J., Vilalta, A., Rios, J.D.L., Robles, A. and Exposito, L. (2006) Percutaneous Implantation of Cerebral Microdialysis Catheters by Twist-Drill Craniostomy in Neurocritical Patients: Description of the Technique and Results of a Feasibility Study in 97 Patients. *Journal of Neurotrauma*, **23**, 1510-1517.
http://dx.doi.org/10.1089/neu.2006.23.1510

[93] Verweij, B.H., Amelink, G.J. and Muizelaar, J.P. (2007) Current Concepts of Cerebral Oxygen Transport and Energy Metabolism after Severe Traumatic Brain Injury. *Progress in Brain Research*, **161**, 111-124.
http://dx.doi.org/10.1016/S0079-6123(06)61008-X

[94] Feldman, Z. and Robertson, C.S. (1997) Monitoring of Cerebral Hemodynamics with Jugular Bulb Catheters. *Critical Care Clinics*, **13**, 51-77. http://dx.doi.org/10.1016/S0749-0704(05)70296-7

[95] Macmillan, C.S. and Andrews, P.J. (2000) Cerebrovenous Oxygen Saturation Monitoring Considerations and Clinical Relevance. *Intensive Care Medicine*, **26**, 1028-1036. http://dx.doi.org/10.1007/s001340051315

[96] Reilly, P.L. (2001) Brain Injury: The Pathophysiology of the First Hours. "Talk and Die Revisited". *Journal of Clinical Neuroscience*, **8**, 398-403. http://dx.doi.org/10.1054/jocn.2001.0916

[97] Rosenthal, G., Hemphill 3rd, J.C., Sorani, M., Martin, C., Morabito, D., Obrist, W.D., *et al.* (2008) Brain Tissue Oxygen Tension Is More Indicative of Oxygen Diffusion than Oxygen Delivery and Metabolism in Patients with Traumatic

Brain Injury. *Critical Care Medicine*, **36**, 1917-1924. http://dx.doi.org/10.1097/CCM.0b013e3181743d77

[98] Jaeger, M., Dengl, M., Meixensberger, J. and Schuhmann, M.U. (2010) Effects of Cerebrovascular Pressure Reactivity-Guided Optimization of Cerebral Perfusion Pressure on Brain Tissue Oxygenation after Traumatic Brain Injury. *Critical Care Medicine*, **38**, 1343-1347.

[99] Jaeger, M., Schuhmann, M.U., Soehle, M., Nagel, C. and Meixensberger, J. (2007) Continuous Monitoring of Cerebrovascular Autoregulation after Subarachnoid Hemorrhage by Brain Tissue Oxygen Pressure Reactivity and Its Relation to Delayed Cerebral Infarction. *Stroke*, **38**, 981-986. http://dx.doi.org/10.1161/01.STR.0000257964.65743.99

[100] Rangel-Castilla, L., Lara, L.R., Gopinath, S., Swank, P.R., Valadka, A. and Robertson, C. (2010) Cerebral Hemodynamic Effects of Acute Hyperoxia and Hyperventilation after Severe Traumatic Brain Injury. *Journal of Neurotrauma*, **27**, 1853-1863. http://dx.doi.org/10.1089/neu.2010.1339

[101] Oddo, M., Nduom, E., Frangos, S., MacKenzie, L., Chen, I., Maloney-Wilensky, E., *et al.* (2010) Acute Lung Injury Is an Independent Risk Factor for Brain Hypoxia after Severe Traumatic Brain Injury. *Neurosurgery*, **67**, 338-344. http://dx.doi.org/10.1227/01.NEU.0000371979.48809.D9

[102] Le Roux, P.D. (2011) Anemia and Transfusion after Subarachnoid Hemorrhage. *Neurocritical Care*, **15**, 342-353. http://dx.doi.org/10.1007/s12028-011-9582-z

[103] Maloney-Wilensky, E., Gracias, V., Itkin, A., Hoffman, K., Bloom, S., Yang, W., *et al.* (2009) Brain Tissue Oxygen and Outcome after Severe Traumatic Brain Injury: A Systematic Review. *Critical Care Medicine*, **37**, 2057-2063.

[104] Oddo, M., Levine, J.M., Mackenzie, L., Frangos, S., Feihl, F., Kasner, S.E., *et al.* (2011) Brain Hypoxia Is Associated with Short-Term Outcome after Severe Traumatic Brain Injury Independent of Intracranial Hypertension and Low Cerebral Perfusion Pressure. *Neurosurgery*, **69**, 1037-1045.

[105] Bratton, S.L., Chestnut, R.M., Ghajar, J., Hammond, F.M., Harris, O.A., Hartl, R., *et al.* (2007) Guidelines for the Management of Severe Traumatic Brain Injury. X. Brain Oxygen Monitoring and Thresholds. *Journal of Neurotrauma*, **24**, S65-S70. http://dx.doi.org/10.1089/neu.2007.9986

[106] Hänggi, D. (2011) Monitoring and Detection of Vasospasm II: EEG and Invasive Monitoring. *Neurocritical Care*, **15** 318-323. http://dx.doi.org/10.1007/s12028-011-9583-y

[107] Bohman, L.E., Heuer, G.G., Macyszyn, L., Maloney-Wilensky, E., Frangos, S., Le Roux, P.D., *et al.* (2011) Medical Management of Compromised Brain Oxygen in Patients with Severe Traumatic Brain Injury. *Neurocritical Care*, **14**, 361-369. http://dx.doi.org/10.1007/s12028-011-9526-7

[108] Nangunoori, R., Maloney-Wilensky, E., Stiefel, M., Park, S., Kofke, W.A., Levine, J.M., *et al.* (2012) Brain Tissue Oxygenbased Therapy and Outcome after Severe Traumatic Brain Injury: A Systematic Literature Review. *Neurocritical Care*, **17**, 131-138. http://dx.doi.org/10.1007/s12028-011-9621-9

[109] Hoshi, Y. (2007) Functional Near-Infrared Spectroscopy: Current Status and Future Prospects. *Journal of Biomedical Optics*, **12**, Article ID 062106. http://dx.doi.org/10.1117/1.2804911

[110] Rolfe, P. (2000) *In Vivo* Near-Infrared Spectroscopy. *Annual Review of Biomedical Engineering*, **2**, 715-754. http://dx.doi.org/10.1146/annurev.bioeng.2.1.715

[111] Wolf, M., Ferrari, M. and Quaresima, V. (2007) Progress of Near-Infrared Spectroscopy and Topography for Brain and Muscle Clinical Applications. *Journal of Biomedical Optics*, **12**, Article ID: 062104. http://dx.doi.org/10.1117/1.2804899

[112] Ghosh, A., Elwell, C. and Smith, M. (2012) Cerebral Near-Infrared Spectroscopy in Adults: A Work in Progress. *Anesthesia & Analgesia*, **115**, 1373-1383. http://dx.doi.org/10.1213/ANE.0b013e31826dd6a6

[113] Gazzaniga, M.S. (2000) Regional Differences in Cortical Organization. *Science*, **289**, 1887-1888. http://dx.doi.org/10.1126/science.289.5486.1887

[114] Gazzaniga, M.S. (2005) What's on Your Mind? *New Science*, **186**, 48-50.

[115] Ferrari, M., Wilson, D.A., Hanley, D.F., Hartmann, J.F. and Traystman, R.J. (1989) Determination of Cerebral Venous Hemoglobin Saturation by Derivative near Infrared Spectroscopy. *Advances in Experimental Medicine and Biology*, **248**, 47-53. http://dx.doi.org/10.1007/978-1-4684-5643-1_6

[116] Ferrari, M. and Quaresima, V. (2012) A Brief Review on the History of Human Functional Near-Infrared Spectroscopy (fNIRS) Development and Fields of Application. *Neuroimage*, **63**, 921-935. http://dx.doi.org/10.1016/j.neuroimage.2012.03.049

[117] Calderon-Arnulphi, M., Alaraj, A. and Slavin, K.V. (2009) Near Infrared Technology in Neuroscience: Past, Present and Future. *Neurological Research*, **31**, 605-614. http://dx.doi.org/10.1179/174313209X383286

[118] Wallois, F., Mahmoudzadeh, M., Patil, A. and Grebe, R. (2012) Usefulness of Simultaneous EEG-NIRS Recording in Language Studies. *Brain and Language*, **121**, 110-123. http://dx.doi.org/10.1016/j.bandl.2011.03.010

[119] Ito, H., Ibaraki, M., Kanno, I., Fukuda, H. and Miura, S. (2005) Changes in the Arterial Fraction of Human Cerebral

Blood Volume during Hypercapnia and Hypocapnia Measured by Positron Emission Tomography. *Journal of Cerebral Blood Flow & Metabolism*, **25**, 852-857. http://dx.doi.org/10.1038/sj.jcbfm.9600076

[120] Thavasothy, M., Broadhead, M., Elwell, C., Peters, M. and Smith, M. (2002) A Comparison of Cerebral Oxygenation as Measured by the NIRO 300 and the INVOS 5100 Near-Infrared SPECTROPHOTOMETERS. *Anaesthesia*, **57**, 999-1006. http://dx.doi.org/10.1046/j.1365-2044.2002.02826.x

[121] Giustiniano, E., Alfano, A., Battistini, G.M., Gavazzeni, V., Spoto, M.R. and Cancellieri, F. (2010) Cerebral Oximetry during Carotid Clamping: Is Blood Pressure Raising Necessary? *Journal of Cardiovascular Medicine*, **11**, 522-528. http://dx.doi.org/10.2459/JCM.0b013e32833246e7

[122] Picton, P., Chambers, J., Shanks, A. and Dorje, P. (2010) The Influence of Inspired Oxygen Fraction and End-Tidal Carbon Dioxide on Post-Crossclamp Cerebral Oxygenation during Carotid Endarterectomy under General Anesthesia. *Anesthesia & Analgesia*, **110**, 581-587. http://dx.doi.org/10.1213/ANE.0b013e3181c5f160

[123] Stoneham, M.D., Lodi, O., de Beer, T.C. and Sear, J.W. (2008) Increased Oxygen Administration Improves Cerebral Oxygenation in Patients Undergoing Awake Carotid Surgery. *Anesthesia & Analgesia*, **107**, 1670-1675. http://dx.doi.org/10.1213/ane.0b013e318184d6c3

[124] Mauermann, W.J., Crepeau, A.Z., Pulido, J.N., Lynch, J.J., Lobbestael, A., Oderich, G.S., *et al.* (2013) Comparison of Electroencephalography and Cerebral Oximetry to Determine the Need for In-Line Arterial Shunting in Patients Undergoing Carotid Endarteriectomy. *Journal of Cardiothoracic and Vascular Anesthesia*, **27**, 1253-1259. http://dx.doi.org/10.1053/j.jvca.2013.02.013

[125] Pedrini, L., Magnoni, F., Sensi, L., Pisano, E., Ballestrazzi, M.S., Cirelli, M.R., *et al.* (2012) Is Near-Infrared Spectroscopy a Reliable Method to Eveluate Clamping Ischemia during Carotid Surgery? *Stroke Research and Treatment*, **2012**, Article ID 156975.

[126] Uchino, H., Nakamura, T., Kuroda, S., Houkin, K., Murata, J. and Saito, H. (2012) Intraoperative Dual Monitoring during Carotid Endarterectomy Using Motor Evoked Potentials and Near-Infrared Spectroscopy. *World Neurosurgery*, **78**, 651-657. http://dx.doi.org/10.1016/j.wneu.2011.10.039

[127] Vohra, H.A., Modi, A. and Ohri, S.K. (2009) Does Use of Intra-Operative Cerebral Regional Oxygen Saturation Monitoring during Cardiac Surgery Lead to Improved Clinical Outcomes? *Interactive CardioVasc Thoracic Surgery*, **9**, 318-322. http://dx.doi.org/10.1510/icvts.2009.206367

[128] Murkin, J.M. and Arango, M. (2009) Near-Infrared Spectroscopy as an Index of Brain and Tissue Oxygenation. *British Journal of Anaesthesia*, **103**, i3-i13. http://dx.doi.org/10.1093/bja/aep299

[129] Selnes, O.A., Gottesman, R.F., Grega, M.A., Baumgartner, W.A., Zeger, S.L. and McKhann, G.M. (2012) Cognitive and Neurologic Outcomes after Coronary-Artery Bypass Surgery. *The New England Journal of Medicine*, **366**, 250-257. http://dx.doi.org/10.1056/NEJMra1100109

[130] Smith, M. (2011) Shedding Light on the Adult Brain: A Review of the Clinical Applications of Near-Infrared Spectroscopy. *Philosophical Transactions of the Royal Society A*, **369**, 4452-4469. http://dx.doi.org/10.1098/rsta.2011.0242

[131] D'Alessio, J.G., Rosenblum, M., Shea, K.P. and Freitas, D.G. (1995) A Retrospective Comparison of Interscalene Block and General Anesthesia for Ambulatory Surgery Shoulder Arthroscopy. *Regional Anesthesia*, **20**, 62-68.

[132] Friedman, D.J., Parnes, N.Z., Zimmer, Z., Higgins, L.D. and Warner, J.J. (2009) Prevalence of Cerebrovascular Events during Shoulder Surgery and Association with Patient Position. *Orthopedics*, **32**, 256.

[133] Dippmann, C., Winge, S. and Nielsen, H.B. (2010) Severe Cerebral Desaturation during Shoulder Arthroscopy in the Beach-Chair Position. *Arthroscopy*, **26**, S148-S150. http://dx.doi.org/10.1016/j.arthro.2010.03.012

[134] Fischer, G.W., Torrillo, T.M., Weiner, M.M. and Rosenblatt, M.A. (2009) The Use of Cerebral Oximetry as a Monitor of the Adequacy of Cerebral Perfusion in a Patient Undergoing Shoulder Surgery in the Beach Chair Position. *Pain Practice*, **9**, 304-307. http://dx.doi.org/10.1111/j.1533-2500.2009.00282.x

[135] Murphy, G.S., Szokol, J.W., Marymont, J.H., Greenberg, S.B., Avram, M.J., Vender, J., *et al.* (2010) Cerebral Oxygen Desaturation Events Assessed by Near-Infrared Spectroscopy during Shoulder Arthroscopy in the Beach Chair and Lateral Decubitus Positions. *Anesthesia & Analgesia*, **111**, 496-505. http://dx.doi.org/10.1213/ANE.0b013e3181e33bd9

[136] Li, Z., Wang, Y., Li, Y., Wang, Y., Li, J. and Zhang, L. (2010) Wavelet Analysis of Cerebral Oxygenation Signal Measured by Near Infrared Spectroscopy in Subjects with Cerebral Infarction. *Microvascular Research*, **80**, 142-147. http://dx.doi.org/10.1016/j.mvr.2010.02.004

[137] Leal-Noval, S.R., Cayuela, A., Arellano-Orden, V., Marín-Caballos, A., Padilla, V., Ferrándiz-Millón, C., *et al.* (2010) Invasive and Noninvasive Assessment of Cerebral Oxygenation in Patients with Severe Traumatic Brain Injury. *Intensive Care Medicine*, **36**, 1309-1317. http://dx.doi.org/10.1007/s00134-010-1920-7

[138] Debevec, T. and Mekjavic, I.B. (2012) Short Intermittent Hypoxic Exposures Augment Ventilation but Do Not Alter Regional Cerebral and Muscle Oxygenation during Hypoxic Exercise. *Respiratory Physiology & Neurobiology*, **181**,

132-142. http://dx.doi.org/10.1016/j.resp.2012.02.008

[139] Ferrari, M., Muthalib, M. and Quaresima, V. (2011) The Use of Near-Infrared Spectroscopy in Understanding Skeletal Muscle Physiology: Recent Developments. *Philosophical Transactions of the Royal Society A*, **28**, 4577-4590. http://dx.doi.org/10.1098/rsta.2011.0230

[140] Tax, N., Urlesberger, B., Binder, C., Pocivalnik, M., Morris, N. and Pichle, G. (2013) The Influence of Perinatal Asphyxia on Peripheral Oxygenation and Perfusion in Neonates. *Early Human Development*, **89**, 483-486. http://dx.doi.org/10.1016/j.earlhumdev.2013.03.011

[141] Mittnacht, A.J. (2010) Near Infrared Spectroscopy in Children at High Risk of Low Perfusion. *Current Opinion in Anaesthesiology*, **23**, 342-347. http://dx.doi.org/10.1097/ACO.0b013e3283393936

[142] Vajkoczy, P., Roth, H., Horn, P., Lucke, T., Thomé, C., Hubner, U., *et al.* (2000) Continuous Monitoring of Regional Cerebral Blood Flow: Experimental and Clinical Validation of a Novel Thermal Diffusion Microprobe. *Journal of Neurosurgery*, **93**, 265-274. http://dx.doi.org/10.3171/jns.2000.93.2.0265

[143] Muench, E., Horn, P., Bauhuf, C., Roth, H., Philipps, M., Hermann, P., *et al.* (2007) Effects of Hypervolemia and Hypertension on Regional Cerebral Blood Flow, Intracranial Pressure, and Brain Tissue Oxygenation after Subarachnoid Hemorrhage. *Critical Care Medicine*, **35**, 1844-1851.

[144] Rosenthal, G., Sanchez-Mejia, R.O., Phan, N., Hemphill 3rd, J.C., Martin, C. and Manley, G.T. (2011) Incorporating a Parenchymal Thermal Diffusion Cerebral Blood Flow Probe in Bedside Assessment of Cerebral Autoregulation and Vasoreactivity in Patients with Severe Traumatic Brain Injury. *Journal of Neurosurgery*, **114**, 62-70. http://dx.doi.org/10.3171/2010.6.JNS091360

[145] Ponce, L.L., Pillai, S., Cruz, J., Li, X., Julia, H., Gopinath, S., *et al.* (2012) Position of the Probe Determines Prognostic Information of Brain Tissue PO2 in Severe Traumatic Brain Injury. *Neurosurgery*, **70**, 1492-1502. http://dx.doi.org/10.1227/NEU.0b013e31824ce933

[146] Helbok, R., Madineni, R.C., Schimedt, M.J., Kurtz, P., Fernandez, L., Ko, S.B., *et al.* (2011) Intracerebral Monitoring of Silent Infarcts after Subarachnoid Hemorrhage. *Neurocritical Care*, **14**, 162-167. http://dx.doi.org/10.1007/s12028-010-9472-9

[147] Maloney-Wilensky, E. and Le Roux, P. (2010) The Physiology Behind Direct Brain Oxygen Monitors and Practical Aspects of Their Use. *Child's Nervous System*, **26**, 419-430. http://dx.doi.org/10.1007/s00381-009-1037-x

[148] Green, J.A., Pellegrini, D.C., Vanderkolk, W.E., Figueroa, B.E. and Eriksson, E.A. (2013) Goal Directed Brain Tissue Oxygen Monitoring versus Conventional Management in Truamtic Brain Injury: An Analysis of in Hospital Recovery. *Neurocritical Care*, **18**, 20-25. http://dx.doi.org/10.1007/s12028-012-9797-7

[149] Bouzat, P., Sala, N., Payen, J.F. and Oddo, M. (2013) Beyond Intracranial Pressure: Optimization of Cerebral Blood Flow, Oxygen, and Substrate Delivery after Traumatic Brain Injury. *Annals of Intensive Care*, **10**, 3-23.

[150] Salerud, E.G. and Nilsson, G.E. (1986) Integrating Probe for Tissue Laser Doppler Flowmeters. *Medical and Biological Engineering and Computing*, **24**, 415-419. http://dx.doi.org/10.1007/BF02442697

[151] Salerud, E.G. and Öberg, P.Å. (1987) Single-Fiber Laser Doppler Flowmetry. *Medical and Biological Engineering and Computing*, **25**, 329-334. http://dx.doi.org/10.1007/BF02447433

[152] Arbit, E., DiResta, G.R., Bedford, R.F., Shah, N.K. and Galicich, J.H. (1989) Intraoperative Measurement of Cerebral and Tumor Blood Flow with Laser-Doppler Flowmetry. *Neurosurgery*, **24**, 166-170. http://dx.doi.org/10.1227/00006123-198902000-00003

[153] Iadecola, C. and Reis, D.J. (1990) Continuous Monitoring of Cerebrocortical Blood Flow during Stimulation of the Cerebellar Fastigial Nucleus. *Journal of Cerebral Blood Flow & Metabolism*, **10**, 608-617. http://dx.doi.org/10.1038/jcbfm.1990.112

[154] Haberl, R.L., Heizer, M.L., Marmarou, A. and Ellis, E.F. (1989) Laser-Doppler Assessment of Brain Microcirculation: Effect of Systemic Alterations. *American Journal of Physiology, Heart and Circulatory*, **256**, H1247-H1254.

[155] Haberl, R.L., Heizer, M.L. and Ellis, E.F. (1989) Laser-Doppler Assessment of Brain Microcirculation: Effect of Local Alterations. *American Journal of Physiology, Heart and Circulatory*, **256**, H1255-H1260.

[156] Lindsberg, P.J., O'Neill, J.T., Paakkari, I.A., Hallenbeck, J.M. and Feuerstein, G. (1989) Validation of Laser-Doppler Flowmetry in Measurement of Spinal Cord Blood Flow. *American Journal of Physiology, Heart and Circulatory*, **257**, H674-H680.

[157] Zweifel, C., Czonyka, M., Lavinio, A., Castellani, G., Kim, D.J., Carrera, E., *et al.* (2010) A Comparison Study of Cerebral Autoregulation Assessed with Transcranial Doppler and Cortical Laser Doppler Flowmetry. *Neurological Research*, **32**, 425-428. http://dx.doi.org/10.1179/174313209X459165

[158] Topcuoglu, M.A. (2012) Transcranial Doppler Ultrasound in Neurovascular Diseases: Diagnostic and Therapeutic Aspects. *Journal of Neurochemistry*, **123**, 39-51. http://dx.doi.org/10.1111/j.1471-4159.2012.07942.x

[159] Edmonds Jr., H.L., Isley, M.R., Sloan, T.B., Alexandrov, A.V. and Razumovsky, A.Y. (2011) American Society of Neurophysiologic Monitoring and American Society of Neuroimaging Joint Guidelines for Transcranial Doppler Ultrasonic Monitoring. *Journal of Neuroimaging*, **21**, 177-183. http://dx.doi.org/10.1111/j.1552-6569.2010.00471.x

[160] Kassah, M.Y., Majid, A., Farooq, M.U., Azhary, H., Hershey, L.A., Bednarczyk, E.M., *et al.* (2007) Transcranial Doppler: An Introduction for Primary Care Physicians. *Journal of the American Board of Family Medicine*, **20**, 65-71. http://dx.doi.org/10.3122/jabfm.2007.01.060128

[161] Greke, C., Neulen, A., Kantelhardt, S.R., Birkenmayer, A., Vollmer, F.C., Thiemann, I., *et al.* (2013) Image-Guided Transcranial Doppler Sonography for Monitoring of Defined Segments of Intracranial Arteries. *Journal of Neurosurgical Anesthesiology*, **25**, 55-61. http://dx.Doi.org/10.1097/ANA.0b013e31826b3d55

[162] Stendel, R., Pietilä, T., Al Hassan, A.A., Schillingb, A. and Brock, M. (2000) Intraoperative Microvascular Doppler Ultrasonography in Cerebral Aneurysm Surgery. *Journal of Neurology, Neurosurgery, and Psychiatry*, **68**, 29-35. http://dx.doi.org/10.1136/jnnp.68.1.29

6

Long Lasting Effects of Breastfeeding on Metabolism in Women with Prior Gestational Diabetes

Luca Mattei*, Antonietta Colatrella, Olimpia Bitterman, Paola Bianchi, Chiara Giuliani, Giona Roma, Camilla Festa, Gianluca Merola, Vincenzo Toscano, Angela Napoli

Faculty of Medicine and Psychology, Sapienza University of Rome, Rome, Italy
Email: *mluca982@hotmail.it

Abstract

Background & Aims: Breastfeeding improves glucose tolerance in the early postpartum period of women with prior gestational diabetes GDM, but it is unclear whether future risk of metabolic alterations, like type 2 diabetes, is reduced. The aim of this study was to investigate the effect of lactation, three years after pregnancy, on glucose and lipid metabolism in women with prior gestational diabetes. Materials & Methods: A population of women with prior gestational diabetes (Carpenter and Coustan Criteria) was evaluated with comparison of results for "lactating" [BF] versus "nonlactating women" [non BF]. Breast feeding was defined [BF] if lasting? 4 weeks. In each woman a 75-g oral glucose tolerance test (OGTT) was performed to analyze the glucose tolerance, insulin sensitivity/resistance and b-cell function. Fasting serum was used to study their lipid profile (total cholesterol, high-density lipoprotein [HDL] cholesterol, low-density lipoprotein [LDL] cholesterol, and triglycerides), apolipoprotein B, apolipoprotein A1, homocysteine, fibrinogen, hs-CRP, uric acid, microalbuminuria. Statistics: Paired and Un-paired t-test, Mann-Whitney and χ^2 tests were used, as appropriate. Results: A total of 81 women were evaluated (62 [BF] and 19 [non BF]). Maternal age (37.1 ± 4.6 vs 37.4 ± 4.9 years), body mass index (26.3 ± 5.6 vs 26.4 ± 5.3 kg/m^2), parity (1.9 ± 0.8 vs 1.7 ± 0.8) and length of follow-up (32.2 ± 20.2 vs 32.1 ± 20,0) were not different between the two groups. No effect was visible on glucose tolerance, HOMA-IR and other b-cell function indexes as well as hs-CRP (not significantly lower in non BF), uric acid, total cholesterol, HDL and LDL cholesterol. Levels of significance were only reached for "HOMA-IS" [BF] 1.0 ± 0.7 vs [non BF] 0.6 ± 0.4, p = 0.04) and triglycerides [BF] 83.8 ± 46.7 vs [non BF] 123.2 ± 94.0 mg/dl, p = 0.02). Conclusions: Breastfeeding does not improve the glucose tolerance of our women with prior GDM three years after delivery, even though lower levels of triglycerides and improved insulin sensitivity are still visible.

*Corresponding author.

Keywords

Breastfeeding, Gestational Diabetes, Metabolism

1. Background

Gestational diabetes mellitus (GDM) is common and transient glucose intolerance, first diagnosed during pregnancy and often resolving at delivery. However, women with GDM have an increased risk for postpartum abnormalities in insulin secretion and insulin action, as well as type 2 diabetes [1].

In these women, a deficit in insulin secretion/action may be observed even if post-partum glucose tolerance is normal, as well as different levels of insulin resistance [2].

Therefore, a "healthy" lifestyle and/or the presence of other risk factors after pregnancy can influence the chance of developing diabetes later in life [3].

Breastfeeding is recommended by many health agencies as the best method to feed infants for at least one year after birth, because of its multiple immediate and long-term benefits for both child and mother (infectious diseases, obesity, immune-related diseases; breast cancer) [4].

Breastfeeding confers health benefits to women with a history of GDM in terms of glucose tolerance in the early postpartum period [5], but it's unclear whether future risk of type 2 diabetes is reduced [6] [7].

A 2001 study found that within a matched population of women with a history of GDM, three months of breastfeeding was associated to improved pancreatic beta-cell function, but not to any significant difference in glucose tolerance, adipose tissue mass, or adipose distribution [8].

The primary aim of this study was to investigate the effect of breastfeeding on glucose metabolism as well as on beta cell function in women with prior GDM, three years after pregnancy.

The secondary aim was to evaluate in these women lipid and inflammatory profile and the prevalence of metabolic syndrome (M.S.).

2. Patients and Methods

Women were successively recruited from January 2007 to December 2009 in our 'Diabetes in Pregnancy" outpatient's office, at S. Andrea Hospital of "Sapienza" University, Rome.

A cohort of 81 women, three years after a pregnancy complicated by GDM (diagnosed through Carpenter & Coustan Criteria) [9], with negative anti GAD antibodies at diagnosis, was evaluated according to their breastfeeding habits. Also patients with just one altered value in the OGTT [defined OAV ("one abnormal value")] had been considered [10].

None of the women was treated with medications and/or substances potentially conditioning metabolism at the moment of follow up.

Arbitrarily, we defined breastfeeding only if lactation duration was longer than four weeks.

Other parameters evaluated at follow up visit were: age, follow up length (measured as months after delivery), BMI (kg/m^2), waist circumference (cm), systolic and diastolic blood pressure, conventionally measured (mmHg) and familiarity for type 2 diabetes.

Laboratory parameters studied were: total, LDL and HDL-cholesterol, triglycerides, Apo lipoprotein B, Apo lipoprotein A1, homocysteine, fibrinogen, hs-CRP, uric acid, TSH, micro albuminuria.

At follow up visit, in the morning, after an overnight fasting period of at least eight hours, all patients performed a 75 g OGTT for glycaemia and insulin (samples at 0', 30' 60', 90' and 120'). All blood samples were analysed in the same laboratory in our university hospital. Plasma glucose levels were determined with a Beckman Glucose Analyzer 2 by glucose oxidase method, and plasma insulin concentration was measured by radioimmunoassay.

Women were defined normal, IFG (impaired fasting glucose), IGT (impaired glucose tolerance) or diabetic, through basal glucose measurements ± OGTT according to ADA diagnostic criteria [11].

Insulin sensitivity and secretion indexes were obtained using plasma glucose and insulin values in the OGTT; insulin sensitivity was estimated using HOMA and HOMA calculator [12] and ISI as proposed by Matsuda *et al.* [13]. To evaluate β-cell secretion, we considered an insulinogenic index expressed as Ins30'/Glic30', a surrogate of the first phase of insulin secretion, and the areas under glucose and insulin curves (AUC), calculated by a trapezoidal method [14]. Disposition index was used as β-cell function index [15].

Metabolic syndrome and hypertension were defined by ATP III 2004 criteria [16].

All the biochemical tests were performed in Sant' Andrea university hospital laboratory, in Rome.

2.1. Statistic

We used Paired & Un-Paired t-test, Mann-Whitney & χ^2 tests. Data concerning glucose profile are expected to follow a normal distribution and are expressed in terms of their mean and standard deviation.

2.2. Informed Consent

According to our usual practice, a written informed consent was obtained by all the women attending our out-patient's office at the first visit in pregnancy, later confirmed after delivery and at the moment of the last clinical and metabolic evaluation.

3. Results

3.1. General Characteristics

A cohort of 81 women was followed up about three years after delivery (32.2 ± 20.2 months after delivery). According to our definition of breastfeeding habit, 62 women were classified as breastfeeding only [BF] and 19 as not-breastfeeding [non-BF]. At the follow up visit none of the women was still lactating.

The two groups were similar in terms of follow up length, age, parity, number of children, smoking habit, type 2 diabetes familiarity in first-degree relatives. On average, women breastfed for 25.5 ± 19.2 weeks (range 4 - 96 weeks). Regarding anthropometric parameters, there were no differences in BMI and waist circumference (**Table 1**).

3.2. Glycaemic Homeostasis

According to the number of glucose alteration in the OGTT performed in pregnancy, BF group included 46 GDM and 16 OAV, while non-BF group included 14 GDM and 5 OAV. Moreover, 63% BF and 78% non-BF women (χ^2, ns) required insulin treatment.

At follow up, no difference was found in glucose and insulin levels at each time point in the OGTT. Among non-BF women, 13 (68.4%) were normal, 4 (21.0%) were IFG, 1 (5.3%) was diabetic and 1 was IGT/IFG (5.3%); among BF women 44 (71.0%) were normal, 5 was IFG (8.0%), 6 were IGT (9.7%), and 7 were diabetic (11.3%) (χ^2, ns). These two groups were similar in terms of insulin resistance indexes, except for HOMA-IS (BF 1.0 ± 0.7 vs non-BF 0.6 ± 0.4, p = 0.04). No differences were found in insulinogenic index and disposition index (**Table 2**).

Table 1. General characteristics.

	BF n = 62/81	non-BF n = 19/81	p
Follow up length (months)	32.2 ± 20.2	32.1 ± 20.0	0.86
Age (y)	37.1 ± 4.6	37.2 ± 5.1	0.89
Parity (n)	2.3 ± 1.1	2.1 ± 1.0	0.39
Number of child (n)	1.9 ± 0.89	1.68 ± 0.88	0.31
Smoking habit (%)	15	25	0.85
DMT2 familiarity (%)	53.3	47.1	0.64
BMI (kg/m^2)	26.3 ± 5.6	26.4 ± 5.3	0.86
Waist circumference (cm)	87.5 ± 10.4	83.5 ± 10.3	0.20

Table 2. Glycaemic homeostasis.

	BF n = 62/81	non-BF n = 19/81	p
OGTT 0	90.1 ± 16.4	92.2 ± 8.9	0.61
OGTT 30	142.5 ± 34.3	140.1 ± 40.1	0.82
OGTT 60	140.7 ± 42.4	124.0 ± 33.0	0.16
OGTT 90	113.6 ± 36.8	107.0 ± 32.1	0.54
OGTT 120	101.5 ± 28.1	101.2 ± 26.9	0.97
OGTT alteration (%) DM/IFG/IGT (n°)	29 7 DM, 5 IFG, 6 IGT	31.6 1 DM, 4 IFG, 1 IFG/IGT	0.34
Homa-IR	2.2 ± 3.9	2.7 ± 2.7	0.64
ISI	8.1 ± 4.2	6.8 ± 3.6	0.34
Homa-IS	1.0 ± 0.7	0.6 ± 0.4	0.04
Insulinogenic index	14.1 ± 14.0	11.7 ± 29.9	0.68
AUCIRI/AUCBG	0.3 ± 0.2	0.4 ± 0.2	0.80
Disposition index	2.5 ± 1.08	1.96 ± 0.62	0.78
Cholesterol (mg/dl)	191.9 ± 37.7	203.4 ± 40	0.31
HDL (mg/dl)	55.9 ± 14.7	55.7 ± 15.4;	0.95
LDL (mg/dl)	116.3 ± 40.7	120.3 ± 29.6	0.76
Triglycerides (mg/dl)	83.8 ± 46.7	123.2 ± 94.0	0.03 Mann-Whitney
ApoA1 (mg/dl)	147.6 ± 22.9	150 ± 37.9	0.79
ApoB (mg/dl)	93.13 ± 25.8	106.8 ± 23.6	0.13
ApoB/ApoA1	0.65 ± 0.23	0.73 ± 0.16	0.31
hs-CRP (mg/L)	0.5 ± 0.7	2.3 ± 6.2	0.08
Homocysteine (μmoli/L)	8.6 ± 3.2	7.9 ± 2.3	0.52
Systolic (mmHg)	112.17 ± 15.7	110 ± 11.9	0.66
Diastolic (mmHg)	71.6 ± 10.6	72.6 ± 9.2	0.73
MS/ATPIII (%)	50.0	27.7	0.67

3.3. Lipidic Profile

There were no differences in total cholesterol, HDL and LDL levels between the two groups. Significant lower triglycerides values were observed in BF women (BF 83.8 ± 46.7 vs non-BF 123.2 ± 94.0 mg/dl; p = 0.03, Mann Whitney) (**Table 2**).

3.4. Inflammatory Markers

There were no differences in inflammatory markers: hs-CRP, homocysteine. We did not find any difference in ApoA1 and ApoB values and ApoB/ApoA1 ratio (**Table 2**).

3.5. Blood Pressure and Metabolic Syndrome

We did not found significant differences either in systolic or diastolic blood pressure values.

No difference was observed in prevalence of MS (**Table 2**).

4. Discussion

According to our results, breastfeeding has no long term impact on glucose tolerance in women with prior GDM. Three years after delivery, OGTT glycaemic levels were similar at each time point in the two groups, as well as insulin resistance and secretion indexes. These results are partially explained by the fact that more than 60% of the studied population needed insulin treatment. An improvement in metabolic profile is observed in breast-feeding women with mild GDM [5].

However, HOMA-IS index still suggests a protective role of breastfeeding on insulin sensitivity; while the other insulin sensitivity indexes show a similar trend, without reaching the level of significance.

Many studies investigated the role of breast-feeding early after delivery. McManus et al. demonstrated a greater beta-cell compensation to insulin resistance, associated to lower OGTT glycaemic levels, in women with recent GDM still BF, three months after delivery. The same authors did not find any significant difference in adipose tissue mass or distribution through CT [8]. These results are likely to be due to a higher glucose consumption for milk production through a non insulin-related pathway. Therefore, a reduction in glucose stimulation on beta-cells could potentially prevent progression towards type 2 diabetes, as observed by Kjos, who showed a lower diabetes prevalence in BF women (4.2% BF vs 9.4% non-BF). Moreover, despite diabetes was more frequent in women who needed insulin therapy during pregnancy, breast feeding was still a protective factor at follow up, so that in insulin treated group 12.6% of "BF" resulted affected from diabetes compared to 22% of "non-BF" [5].

Recently, the "Atlantic DIP Study" confirmed the protective role of breastfeeding 12 weeks after delivery in a cohort of women from five Irish regions, 300 with previous GDM and 220 with normal glucose tolerance in pregnancy. In the OGTT performed after pregnancy, 19% of the women with previous GDM vs 2.7% of controls had an impaired glucose tolerance, with 8.2% reduction of "persistent hyperglycaemia" in BF vs non-BF. Risk factors were non-European ethnic group, type diabetes family history, higher BMI and insulin therapy in pregnancy, while breastfeeding had a protective role [17].

There are few follow-up studies investigating if the protective effect of lactation on late development of insulin resistance and insulin secretion defects persists after weaning. Diniz did not observe any association between breastfeeding duration and insulin sensitivity in 67 women from health population evaluated 12 and 18 months after delivery [18]. Chouinard-Castonguay showed that a total breastfeeding period of at least ten months leads to improved glucose tolerance as well as improved insulin sensitivity and insulin secretion [19].

The "Nurses Health Study", a prospective observational cohort study on 83,585 parous women, and the "Nurses Health Study II", a retrospective observational cohort study on 73,418 parous women, showed that long lasting breastfeeding, particularly if exclusive, is associated to a fifteen percent decrease of type 2 diabetes risk, for each additional year. However, the same studies failed to find any protective effect of breastfeeding on diabetes risk, in women with a history of gestational diabetes [20].

Two studies on Latin American women with previous GDM, showed that diabetes diagnosis were halved in breastfeeding patient 4 - 12 weeks after delivery, but not after 11 - 26 months [21] [22].

Ziegler and colleagues prospectively investigated the impact of breastfeeding on diabetes outcome in women with prior GDM up to 19 years after delivery and observed a >40% long term risk reduction. Diabetes risk was related to treatment received during pregnancy (insulin vs diet), BMI, and presence/absence of islet autoantibodies. Among islet autoantibody-negative women, breastfeeding was associated to a median period to diabetes diagnosis of 12.3 years compared to 2.3 years in women who did not breastfeed. The lowest postpartum diabetes risk was observed in women who breastfed for 3 months [23].

Recently, a systematic review shows a 9% reduction in relative risk for developing T2DM for each 12-month increase in lifetime duration of breastfeeding and this inverse association appears to be independent of other important risk factors for type 2 diabetes, including BMI, smoking, alcohol, physical activity, education, income, parity and family history of diabetes [24].

In our study, breastfeeding was not correlated either to type 2 diabetes or any alteration of glucose tolerance (IGT and/or IFG and/or Diabetes), as well as to BMI and the other investigated risk factors.

Several studies demonstrated that lipid panel can be modified by breastfeeding [5]. Kjos et al. found higher HDL cholesterol levels in BF women with previous GDM, 4 - 12 weeks after delivery. In our study lower triglycerides levels were found in "BF women", with no difference in total, HDL and LDL cholesterol.

Gunderson et al. noted an inverse association between breastfeeding and metabolic syndrome incidence in women with previous GDM; in particular, the incidence rate of metabolic syndrome was 6 fold lower when women breastfed at least nine months [25]. Our results do not confirm the protective role of breastfeeding on metabolic syndrome, by contrast of what observed by the "CARDIA Study", 20 years after delivery.

Two-thirds of our population is breastfed exclusively. Recently, Matias *et al.* demonstrated that maternal obesity, insulin treatment, and suboptimal in-hospital breastfeeding were essential risk factors for delayed lactogenesis onset [26].

Finally, as ours is a retrospective study, we do not have data about some of the many variables affecting metabolic syndrome risk, such as physical activity and food habits, during follow-up. However, all the women had received general recommendations about lifestyle to prevent metabolic diseases.

5. Conclusions

Breastfeeding protective role on metabolic profile in women with previous GDM is still evident in a long-term follow up study.

All the available resources should be used already in pregnancy to implement education programs [27].

References

[1]   Bellamy, L., Casas, J.P., Hingorani, A.D. and Williams, D. (2009) Type 2 Diabetes Mellitus after Gestational Diabetes: A Systematic Review and Meta-Analysis. *Lancet*, **373**, 1773-1779. http://dx.doi.org/10.1016/S0140-6736(09)60731-5

[2]   Retnakaran, R., Qi, Y., Sermer, M., Connelly, P.W. and Hanley, A.J.G. and Zinman, B. (2010) β-Cell Function Declines within the First Year Postpartum in Women with Recent Glucose Intolerance in Pregnancy. *Diabetes Care*, **33**, 1798-1804. http://dx.doi.org/10.2337/dc10-0351

[3]   Schack-Nielsen, L. and Michaelsen, K.F. (2006) Breast Feeding and Future Health. *Current Opinion in Clinical Nutrition and Metabolic Care*, **9**, 289-296. http://dx.doi.org/10.1097/01.mco.0000222114.84159.79

[4]   American Dietetic Association (1997) Position of the American Dietetic Association: Promotion of Breastfeeding. *Journal of the American Dietetic Association*, **97**, 662-666. http://dx.doi.org/10.1016/S0002-8223(97)00167-3

[5]   Kjos, S.L., Henry, O., Lee, R.M., Buchanan, T.A. and Mishell Jr., D.R. (1993) The Effect of Lactation on Glucose and Lipid Metabolism in Women with Recent Gestational Diabetes. *Obstetrics Gynecology*, **82**, 451-455.

[6]   Gunderson, E.P. (2007) Breastfeeding after Gestational Diabetes Pregnancy. *Diabetes Care*, **30**, S161-S168. http://dx.doi.org/10.2337/dc07-s210

[7]   Aune, D., Norat, T., Romundstad, P. and Vatten, L.J. (2014) Breastfeeding and the Maternal Risk of Type 2 Diabetes: A Systematic Review and Dose-Response Meta-Analysis of Cohort Studies. *Nutrition, Metabolism Cardiovascular Diseases*, **24**, 107-115. http://dx.doi.org/10.1016/j.numecd.2013.10.028

[8]   McManus, R.M., Cunningham, I., Watson, A., Harker, L. and Finegood, D.T. (2001) Beta-Cell Function and Visceral Fat in Lactating Women with a History of Gestational Diabetes. *Metabolism—Clinical and Experimental*, **50**, 715-719. http://dx.doi.org/10.1053/meta.2001.23304

[9]   Carpenter, M.W. and Coustan, D.R. (1982) Criteria for Screening Test for Gestational Diabetes. *American Journal of Obstetrics Gynecology*, **144**, 768-773.

[10]   Langer, O., Brustman, L., Anyaegbunam, A. and Mazze, R. (1987) The Significance of One Abnormal Glucose Tolerance Test Value on Adverse Outcome in Pregnancy. *American Journal of Obstetrics Gynecology*, **157**, 758-763. http://dx.doi.org/10.1016/S0002-9378(87)80045-5

[11]   American Diabetes Association (2014) Diagnosis and Classification of Diabetes Mellitus. *Diabetes Care*, **37**, S81-S90. http://dx.doi.org/10.2337/dc14-S081

[12]   Matthews, D.R., Hosker, J.P., Rudenski, A.S., Naylor, B.A., Treacher, D.F. and Turner, R.C. (1985) Homeostasis Model Assessment: Insulin Resistance and β-Cell Function from Fasting Plasma Glucose and Insulin Concentrations in Man. *Diabetologia*, **28**, 412-419. http://dx.doi.org/10.1007/BF00280883

[13]   Matsuda, M. and DeFronzo, R. (1999) Insulin Sensitivity Indices Obtained from Oral Glucose Tolerance Testing. Comparison with the Euglycemic Insulin Clamp. *Diabetes Care*, **22**, 1462-1470. http://dx.doi.org/10.2337/diacare.22.9.1462

[14]   Stumvoll, M., Mitralou, A., Pimenta, W., Jenssen, T., Yki-Jarvinen, H., Van Haeften, T., Renn, W. and Gerich, J. (2000) Use of the Oral Glucose Tolerance Test to Assess Insulin Release and Insulin Sensitivity. *Diabetes Care*, **23**, 295-301. http://dx.doi.org/10.2337/diacare.23.3.295

[15]   Utzschneider, K.M., Prigeon, R.L., Faulenbach, M.V., Tong, J., Carr, D.B., Boyko, E.J., Leonetti, D.L., McNeely, M.J., Fujimoto, W.Y. and Kahn, S.E. (2009) Oral Disposition Index Predicts the Development of Future Diabetes Above and Beyond Fasting and 2-h Glucose Levels. *Diabetes Care*, **32**, 335-341. http://dx.doi.org/10.2337/dc08-1478

[16] Grundy, S.M., Brewer Jr., H.B., Cleeman, J.I., Smith Jr., S.C. and Lenfant, C. (2004) Definition of Metabolic Syndrome: Report of the National Heart, Lung, and Blood Institute/American Heart Association Conference on Scientific Issues Related to Definition. *Circulation*, **109**, 433-438. http://dx.doi.org/10.1161/01.CIR.0000111245.75752.C6

[17] O'Reilly, M.W., Avalos, G., Dennedy, M.C., O'Sullivan, E.P. and Dunne, F. (2011) Atlantic DIP: High Prevalence of Abnormal Glucose Tolerance Postpartum Is Reduced by Breast-Feeding in Women with Prior Gestational Diabetes Mellitus. *European Journal of Endocrinology*, **165**, 953-959. http://dx.doi.org/10.1530/EJE-11-0663

[18] Diniz, J.M. and Da Costa, T.H. (2004) Independent of Body Adiposity, Breastfeeding Has a Protective Effect on Glucose Metabolism in Young Adult Women. *British Journal of Nutrition*, **92**, 905-912. http://dx.doi.org/10.1079/BJN20041288

[19] Chouinard-Castonguay, S., Weisnagel, S.J., Tchernof, A. and Robitaille, J. (2013) Relationship between Lactation Duration and Insulin and Glucose Response among Women with Prior Gestational Diabetes. *European Journal of Endocrinology*, **168**, 515-523. http://dx.doi.org/10.1530/EJE-12-0939

[20] Stuebe, A.M., Rich-Edwards, J.W., Willett, W.C., Manson, J.E. and Michels, K.B. (2005) Duration of Lactation and Incidence of Type 2 Diabetes. *JAMA*, **294**, 2601-2610. http://dx.doi.org/10.1001/jama.294.20.2601

[21] Kjos, S.L., Peters, R.K., Xiang, A., Henry, O.A., Montoro, M. and Buchanan, T.A. (1995) Predicting Future Diabetes in Latino Women with Gestational Diabetes: Utility of Early Postpartum Glucose Tolerance Testing. *Diabetes*, **44**, 586-591. http://dx.doi.org/10.2337/diab.44.5.586

[22] Buchanan, T.A., Xiang, A.H., Kjos, S.L., Trigo, E., Lee, W.P. and Peters, R.K. (1999) Antepartum Predictors of the Development of Type 2 Diabetes in Latino Women 11-26 Months after Pregnancies Complicated by Gestational Diabetes. *Diabetes*, **48**, 2430-2436. http://dx.doi.org/10.2337/diabetes.48.12.2430

[23] Ziegler, A.G., Wallner, M., Kaiser, I., Rossbauer, M., Harsunen, M.H., Lachmann, L., Maier, J., Winkler, C. and Hummel, S. (2012) Long-Term Protective Effect of Lactation on the Development of Type 2 Diabetes in Women with Recent Gestational Diabetes Mellitus. *Diabetes*, **61**, 3167-3171. http://dx.doi.org/10.2337/db12-0393

[24] Aune, D., Norat, T., Romundstad, P. and Vatten, L.J. (2014) Breastfeeding and the Maternal Risk of Type 2 Diabetes: A Systematic Review and Dose Response Meta-Analysis of Cohort Studies. *Nutrition, Metabolism and Cardiovascular Diseases*, **24**, 107-115. http://dx.doi.org/10.1016/j.numecd.2013.10.028

[25] Gunderson, E.P., Jacobs Jr., D.R., Chiang, V., Lewis, C.E., Feng, J., Quesenberry Jr., C.P. and Sidney, S. (2010) Duration of Lactation and Incidence of the Metabolic Syndrome in Women of Reproductive Age According to Gestational Diabetes Mellitus Status: A 20-Year Prospective Study in CARDIA (Coronary Artery Risk Development in Young Adults). *Diabetes*, **59**, 495-504. http://dx.doi.org/10.2337/db09-1197

[26] Matias, S.L., Dewey, K.G., Quesenberry Jr., C.P. and Gunderson, E.P. (2014) Maternal Prepregnancy Obesity and Insulin Treatment during Pregnancy Are Independently Associated with Delayed Lactogenesis in Women with Recent Gestational Diabetes Mellitus. *American Journal of Clinical Nutrition*, **99**, 115-121. http://dx.doi.org/10.3945/ajcn.113.073049

[27] World Health Organization (2013) Health Topics, Nutrition Topics, 10 Facts on Breastfeeding. http://www.who.int/features/factfiles/breastfeeding/facts/en/index.html

7

The Mitochondrial Pyruvate Carrier and Metabolic Regulation

Bor Luen Tang

Department of Biochemistry, Yong Loo Lin School of Medicine, National University of Singapore, Singapore
Email: bchtbl@nus.edu.sg

Abstract

Pyruvate is a key intermediate at the branchpoint of anaerobic and aerobic energy metabolism. Its transport into the mitochondrial matrix is necessary prior to its decarboxylation into acetyl-CoA, which feeds the reducing equivalent-generating tricarboxylic acid (TCA) cycle. Although the existence of specific carrier transport of cytosolic pyruvate into the mitochondria has been inferred from a myriad of studies, the identities of the mitochondrial pyruvate carrier (MPC) were only confirmed very recently. Identification of the MPC facilitated several other recent advances. These include the finding of MPC's inhibition by the insulin-sensitizing drug family thiazolidinediones, how cells respond flexibly to a reduction in MPC functionality, as well as insights into how changes in MPC levels affect oncogenic potential of cancer cells. These new findings, discussed here in this brief review, have important implications in therapeutic approaches towards metabolic disorders and cancer.

Keywords

Cancer, Energy Metabolism, Mitochodrial Pyruvate Carrier (MPC), Pyruvate, Warburg Effect

1. Introduction

The 3-carbon monocarboxylate pyruvate is a product of cytosolic glycolysis, and is a key meeting point of the principal metabolic pathways of sugars, fatty acids and amino acids. In anaerobic glycolysis, pyruvate could be fermented to lactate in the cytosol by lactate dehydrogenase (LDH). In aerobic respiration, pyruvate needs to enter the mitochondria and be decarboxylated into the 2-carbon acetyl-CoA that feeds into the TCA cycle in the mitochondrial matrix. Pyruvate could be converted back to glucose by the process of gluconeogenesis and deaminated to form the amino acid alanine. In the mitochondria, it could also be carboxylated into the 4-carbon oxaloacetate (OAA), which could enter the TCA cycle or participate in anabolic pathways of glucose, amino acid and fatty acid synthesis (**Figure 1**).

While the need for cytosolic pyruvate to be transported into the mitochondrial matrixin aerobic respiration is basic textbook knowledge, how exactly pyruvate is transported was somewhat controversial. The outer mitochondrial membrane (OMM) is rather permeable to small molecules, but pyruvate in its ionized form is unlikely to negotiate the inner mitochondrial membrane (IMM) by passive diffusion. Although there was some early evidence for a significant degree of pyruvate free diffusion across artificial membranes, subsequent studies using purified mitochondria demonstrated saturation kinetics [1], thus suggesting the existence of a specific carrier(s). This notion is supported by the discovery of an inhibitor, the cinnamate α-cyano-4-hydroxycinnamate (CHC) [2], which inhibited pyruvate oxidation in intact but not disrupted mitochondria [3]. The cinnamate derivativealpha-cyano-beta-(1-phenylindol-3-yl)acrylate] (UK5099) was shown to diminish labelling by [^{3}H]N-phenylmaleimide (a thiol-blocking agent which inhibits pyruvate transport) of a 15 kDa protein in heart and liver mitochondria [4]. The molecular size of this unidentified protein actually coincided well with those MPC components eventually found (which are small proteins of 14 - 16 kDa in size) [5]. The exact molecular identity of the MPC has, however, remained elusive for some time. Its recent identification shall be described in more detail below.

As a key metabolic node, enzymes directly involved in pyruvate metabolism are tightly regulated [6] [7]. Likewise, pyruvate influx into the mitochondria is also likely regulated by multiple inputs from connecting pathways, and these regulatory mechanisms could be defective in disease conditions. Importantly, dysregulation of pyruvate mitochondrial influx could tip the balance between aerobic respiration and anaerobic glycolysis. A prominent example of such an imbalance is the Warburg effect [8]. As was observed and documented by Nobelist Otto Warburg in 1927 [9], tumor cells preferentially produce energy by heightened glycolysis and pyruvate-lactate fermentation rather than oxidation of pyruvate in mitochondria. Although the effect could be exaggerated

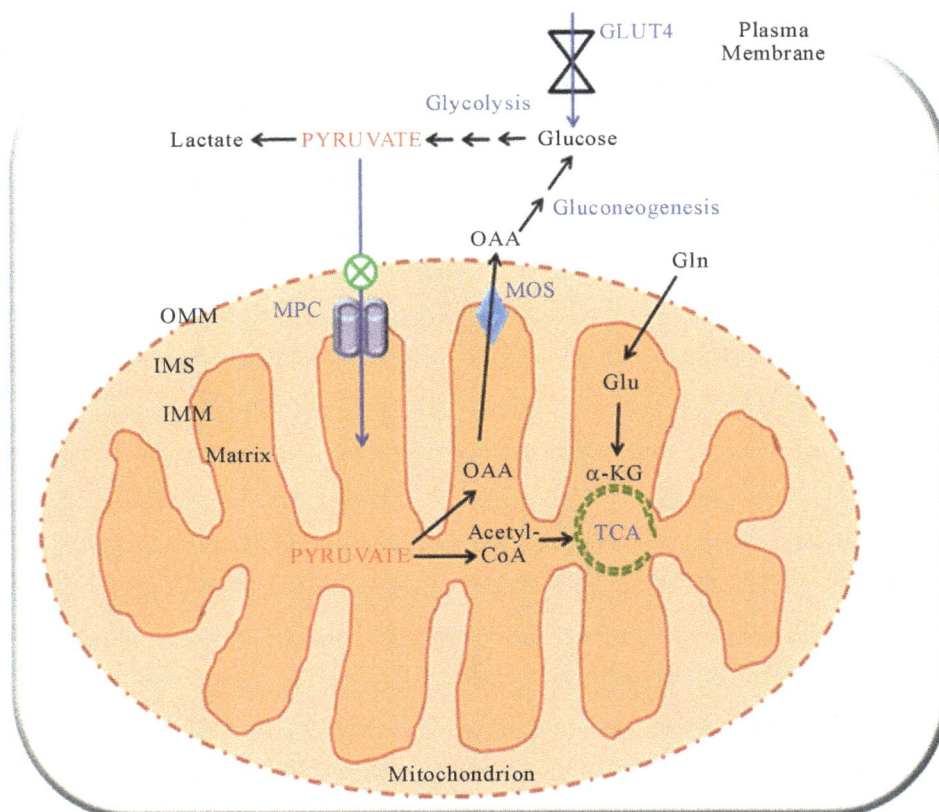

Figure 1. Schematic diagram of a mitochondrion illustrating the cellular components associated with pyruvate transport and metabolism. MPC—mitochondrial pyruvate carrier; MOS—Malate-OAA shuttle; OMM—outer mitochondrial membrane; IMS—intermembrane space; IMM—inner mitochondrial membrane; OAA—oxaloacetate; α-KG—α-ketoglutarate; TCA—tricarboxylic acid cycle.

by an increased intumor-specific pyruvate kinase isozyme M2 (PKM2) [10] and LDH, or a general mitochondrial dysfunction in cancer cells, defects in pyruvate influx is also a possibility. Pyruvate uptake by isolated mitochondria is a relatively slow process and evidence suggests that mitochondrial pyruvate transport might be rate limiting for mitochondrial pyruvate oxidation [11] [12].

With the molecular identification of MPC [13] [14], investigations into its role in metabolic regulation in normal can cancer cells are now feasible. In this brief review, I shall provide an update of some recent findings associated with the MPC.

2. Identification of the Mitochondrial Pyruvate Carrier (MPC) Complex

Identification of CHC as an inhibitor of pyruvate transport activity facilitated early attempts at partial purification and cell-free functional constitution of MPC [15]-[17]. Attempts were also made with affinity chromatography on immobilized CHC [18]. These attempts did not lead to any definitive identification of polypeptides that correspond to a functional MPC. A possible breakthrough came in 2003 when Halestrap's laboratory identified a possible MPC candidate in the yeast *S. cerevisiae* by a genetics approach. The authors measured UK5099-sensitive pyruvate uptake into mitochondria from 18 mitochondrial carrier family (MCF) deletion mutants. Only one mutant, *YIL006W*, exhibited no inhibitor-sensitive pyruvate transport, and the gene encodes a MCF family protein with likely mammalian homologues [19]. However, *YIL006W* was later shown by cloning and liposomal functional reconstitution assays to be one of two isoforms of the yeast NAD^+ transporters (Ndt1p) [20]. The highly anticipated molecular identification of MPC had to wait for almost another 10 years.

Rutter's laboratory was examining groups of mitochondrial proteins that are evolutionarily conserved, and noted the homologous *YGL080W*, *YHR162W*, and *YGR243W* genes which encode yeast *Mpc1*, *Mpc2* and *Mpc3*, respectively [13]. The authors localized the gene products of these, which encode small polypeptides of 14 - 16 kDa, to the mitochondrial inner membrane. *Mpc1* and *Mpc2* were found to form a multimeric complex of ~150 kD. *mpc1Δ* and *mpc2Δ* cells (but not *mpc3Δ*) displayed mild growth defects on nonfermentable carbon sources, and *Drosophila* or human *MPC1* orthologs, could both rescue the *mpc1Δ* phenotype. The *Drosophila dMPC1* mutants have defective carbohydrate metabolism as they are sensitive to a diet consisting of only carbohydrates. Metabolomic analyses revealed that d*MPC1* mutants on a sugar diet had high levels of pyruvate but a significant depletion of TCA cycle intermediates. A corresponding elevation/reduction profile of amino acids and other intermediates that could be derived from either cytosolic pyruvate or mitochondrial acetyl-CoA was also observed. Clear functional evidence that these genes encode MPC components came from a combination of biochemical and genetic experiments. Mitochondria of yeast *mpc1Δ* mutant exhibited no ^{14}C-pyruvate uptake, a defect that could be effectively rescued by transgenic *MPC1* in a MPC inhibitor UK5099-sensitive manner. The authors have also identified a yeast *MPC1* mutation, Asp118 → Gly, which confers resistance to the MPC inhibitor UK-5099. A very clinically relevant and significant finding of the Rutter's group is the identification of *BRP44L* (human *MCP1*) mutations in families with impaired basal and uncoupling agent FCCP-stimulated pyruvate oxidation. Transgenic expression of wild type human *MPC1* in cells derived from patients rescued the pyruvate oxidation defect, while mutant forms of human *MPC1*s have diminished or no rescue effect of the yeast deletion.

The Martinou group discovered MPC components while investigating defects in the synthesis of lipoic acid, a co-factor of several multi-subunit dehydrogenase complexes in the mitochondrial matrix [14]. The authors have previously identified Brp44L (human *MPC1*) in a proteomics analysis [21] and noted its homology with the yeast *YGL080W*, *YHR162W*, and *YGR243W* genes. They also found that the *mpc1Δ* and *mpc2Δ mpc3Δ* deletion mutants grew more slowly in amino acid-free medium, a phenotype that was relieved by addition of the amino acids valine or leucine, but not other amino acids. ^{14}C tracer analysis showed that *mpc1Δ* cells have drastically reduced $^{14}CO_2$ release that corresponded with decreased dehydrogenase activities and their lipoylation, and lipoic acid production. The authors traced these defects to an upstream event of acetyl-CoA production and mitochondrial uptake of ^{14}C pyruvate, and like the Rutter group, found that mammalian (mouse) *MPC1* could rescue the yeast defects. A key additional functional test performed by the Martinou group was the expression of *mMPC1* and *mMPC2*, alone and in combination, in the bacteria *Lactococcus lactis*, a naïve system. Expression of both MPC proteins resulted in pyruvate uptake that was sensitive to UK5099, and with similar properties to mitochondrial pyruvate transport.

The genetic conservation and compelling biochemical and functional evidence for the MPCs discovered in the works described above provided strong evidence that the real MPC has now been identified. The polypeptides

Mpc1 and *Mpc2* form functional multimeric complexes at the IMM to mediate pyruvate translocation. It would appear that *Mpc3*, which is highly homologous to *Mpc2*, may have functional redundancy with the latter. Some caveats to this notion have been pointed out by Halestrap [22], and pyruvate transport by the purified protein(s) functionally reconstitution of into liposomes have not yet been demonstrated. We now await the structural analysis of these proteins in anticipation of the functional insights that shall be obtained. Interestingly, another recent report implicated an *Arabidopsis thaliana* gene, *NRGA1*, which is homologous to *MPC2* and when co-expressed with *AtMPC1*, complemented the yeast *mpc2Δ/mpc3Δ* mutation [23]. *NRGA1* negatively regulates abscisic acid-induced signaling in *Arabdopsis* guard cells in response to drought, but how this is connected to pyruvate transport is unclear at the moment.

3. Aspects of Metabolic Regulation Unveiled by MPC Inhibition

Several recent studies have been aided by the molecular identification of MPC. Murphy and colleagues found that the anti-diabetic drug family of thiazolidinediones (TZDs), better known as peroxisome proliferator-activated receptor gamma (PPARγ) inhibitors [24], also inhibits MPC at clinically relevant concentrations [25]. The authors showed that low dosages of TZD acted like UK5099 and specifically inhibited pyruvate and not glutamate of succinate oxidation in several cell types. The IMM-permeable methyl pyruvate rescued both the TZD and UK5099 inhibition, as it did the respiratory defects in cells with *MPC1* or *MPC2* silenced by lentiviral-shRNA. Importantly, MPC inhibition by TZD underlies its stimulation of glucose uptake, degrees of which in myotubes and myocytes were directly proportional to the level of respiratory inhibition by TZDs or UK5099. TZD activation of the energy status-sensing, catabolism driver AMP-activated protein kinase (AMPK) [26], is also mimicked by UK5099. In another report, MCP1 and MCP2 were identified as mitochondrial proteins that could be chemically crosslinked to TZD [27] in a manner that could be blocked by UK5099. These authors also showed that TZDs altered the incorporation of ^{13}C-labeled carbon from glucose into acetyl CoA. These findings thus connect mitochondrial pyruvate uptake to acute responses in glucose sensing and uptake, which could be therapeutically useful.

Another recent finding further suggests that MPC activity affects glucose sensing and insulin sensitivity. In mice, loss of *Mpc2* is embryonically lethal, but Vigueira *et al.* generated a viable *MPC2* hypomorphic mouse line harboring an N-terminally truncated protein and exhibiting reduced capacity for mitochondrial pyruvate oxidation [28]. These mice have elevated blood glucose and lactate when subjected to an intraperitoneal pyruvate bolus. The mice are insulin-sensitive, but had reduced plasma insulin. Glucose intolerance in this strain was attributed to impaired glucose-stimulated pancreatic insulin secretion, which could be corrected by sulfonylurea treatment. This rather specific insulin secretion defect in a *MPC2* hypomorph is interesting, and attested again to a connection between mitochondrial pyruvate uptake and glucose sensing.

What exactly would the consequences of MPC inhibition be on the core metabolic pathways such as the TCA cycle? A recent study by Vacanti *et al.* using ^{13}C metabolic flux analysis of cells after genetic or pharmacological ablation of MPC activity revealed a surprising degree of cellular metabolic flexibility and adaptation [29]. In MPC-deficient cells, both glucose and pyruvate oxidation were suppressed. However, the authors found that cell growth, oxygen consumption, and the TCA cycle functionality were surprisingly maintained by enhanced oxidative glutaminolysis. Also, MPC silencing increased fatty acid β-oxidation and branched-chain amino acid oxidation. This response is therefore unlike those observed during inhibition of the electron transport chain complex I or PDH, and cells could apparently reprogram to adapt to a reduction in mitochondrial pyruvate transport by channeling in products of amino acids and fatty acid metabolism to feed the TCA cycle.

The findings of Vacanti *et al.* are mirrored by another report. Yang *et al.* have previously found that glucose deprivation in c-Myc transformed cancer cells prompted acetyl-CoA generation via glutamine, which isconverted into glutamate by glutaminase and subsequently α-ketoglutarate by elevated glutamate dehydrogenase (GDH) activity [30]. With tracer experiments, the authors now found that glucose and pyruvate transport into mitochondria suppresses GDH and acetyl-CoA formation from glutamine [31]. Impairment of pyruvate transport into mitochondria by UK5099 inhibition of MPC conversely induces glutamine-dependent acetyl-CoA formation. While UK5099 and glutaminase or GDH inhibitors only moderately suppressed cell proliferation and did not cause significant cell death, a combination UK5099 with inhibition of either glutaminase or GDH synergistically increased growth suppression and cell death. Interestingly, a combination of MPC and GDH inhibitors also impaired tumor growth in mouse xenografts. Other than uncovering aspects of metabolic flexibility, these results also suggest that pyruvate transport may be considered as a potential target in cancer therapeutics.

4. MPC, Mitochondrial Pyruvate Transport and Cancer

Cancer cells have profound metabolic alterations compared to noncancerous cells [32]. One prominent feature, termed the Warburg effect [8], is highlighted by the fact that many cancer cells tend to generate lactate from pyruvate and have reduced aerobic oxidation, even under normoxic and aerobic conditions. This has been attributed to mitochondrial damage and impaired aerobic respiration. However, many cancer cells with an intact TCA cycle nonetheless exhibit the Warburg effect. Alternative explanations for the effect include decrease pyruvate production by PKM2, upregulated LDH and increase expression of PDH kinase PDK1. Rutter's group now showed that impaired mitochondrial transport due to *MPC1* deletion or diminished expression could also explain the Warburg effect [33]. The authors found that while the gene locus of *MPC2* is not frequently loss or altered in cancer, the *MPC1* locus is within the most frequently deleted region across all cancer samples investigated. *MPC1* expression is also reduced in all cancer types examined, with its reduced expression correlating with poor disease prognosis. Re-expressing of *MPC1* and *MPC2* in cells increased mitochondrial pyruvate oxidation, and interestingly impaired anchorage-independent growth and xenograft growth of these cells. The cancers cells therefore appeared to lose oncogenic potential, but did not suffer impaired health or viability.

How exactly does expression of MPC reverse the cancer phenotype? The authors noted that the enzyme aldehyde dehydrogenase (ALDH), a cancer stem cell marker [34] [35], was significantly decreased in the MPC-expressing tumors. Further examination revealed other stem cell markers such as LGR5 [36], LIN28A [37] and NANOG [38] were decreased in cells upon MPC expression. The mitochondrial pyruvate transport, or indeed the carrier itself, could have profound effects on the oncogenic expression profile of cancer cells beyond the superficially perceived alteration in metabolic profile.

5. Concluding Remarks

In the paragraphs above, recent advances in the molecular cloning and identification of the mitochondrial transport carrier were outlined, and some recent intriguing findings that have been facilitated by the discovery of MPC were discussed. Much remains to be learned about the MPC-mediated pyruvate transport process itself, such as the mechanism of transport and its regulation. Manipulations of MPC-dependent pyruvate transport into the mitochondria through MPCs have already revealed some surprising findings pertaining to metabolic flexibility of cells, and we could expect more revelations along this line in the near future. That MPC levels or function affect expression profiles of cancer stem cell markers is unexpected and exciting. We could look forward to the resolution of the underlying mechanism, and anticipate how this might become applicable in terms of cancer therapeutics.

Acknowledgements

The author declares no conflict of interest.

References

[1]   Papa, S., Francavilla, A., Paradies, G. and Meduri, B. (1971) The Transport of Pyruvate in Rat Liver Mitochondria. *FEBS Letters*, **12**, 285-288. http://dx.doi.org/10.1016/0014-5793(71)80200-4

[2]   Halestrap, A.P. and Denton, R.M. (1974) Specific Inhibition of Pyruvate Transport in Rat Liver Mitochondria and Human Erythrocytes by alpha-Cyano-4-hydroxycinnamate. *Biochemical Journal*, **138**, 313-316.

[3]   Halestrap, A.P. and Denton, R.M. (1975) The Specificity and Metabolic Implications of the Inhibition of Pyruvate Transport in Isolated Mitochondria and Intact Tissue Preparations by alpha-Cyano-4-hydroxycinnamate and Related Compounds. *Biochemical Journal*, **148**, 97-106.

[4]   Thomas, A.P. and Halestrap, A.P. (1981) Identification of the Protein Responsible for Pyruvate Transport into Rat Liver and Heart Mitochondria by Specific Labelling with [3H]N-Phenylmaleimide. *Biochemical Journal*, **196**, 471-479.

[5]   Schell, J.C. and Rutter, J. (2013) The Long and Winding Road to the Mitochondrial Pyruvate Carrier. *Cancer & Metabolism*, **1**, 6.

[6]   Gray, L.R., Tompkins, S.C. and Taylor, E.B. (2014) Regulation of Pyruvate Metabolism and Human Disease. *Cellular*

and Molecular Life Sciences, **71**, 2577-2604. http://dx.doi.org/10.1007/s00018-013-1539-2

[7] Jeoung, N.H., Harris, C.R. and Harris, R.A. (2014) Regulation of Pyruvate Metabolism in Metabolic-Related Diseases. *Reviews in Endocrine & Metabolic Disorders*, **15**, 99-110. http://dx.doi.org/10.1007/s11154-013-9284-2

[8] Palsson-McDermott, E.M. and O'Neill, L.A.J. (2013) The Warburg Effect Then and Now: From Cancer to Inflammatory Diseases. *Bioessays*, **35**, 965-973. http://dx.doi.org/10.1002/bies.201300084

[9] Warburg, O., Wind, F. and Negelein, E. (1927) The Metabolism of Tumors in the Body. *The Journal of General Physiology*, **8**, 519-530. http://dx.doi.org/10.1085/jgp.8.6.519

[10] Iqbal, M.A., Gupta, V., Gopinath, P., Mazurek, S. and Bamezai, R.N.K. (2014) Pyruvate Kinase M2 and Cancer: An Updated Assessment. *FEBS Letters*, **588**, 2685-2692. http://dx.doi.org/10.1016/j.febslet.2014.04.011

[11] Pande, S.V. and Parvin, R. (1978) Pyruvate and Acetoacetate Transport in Mitochondria. A Reappraisal. *Journal of Biological Chemistry*, **253**, 1565-1573.

[12] Shearman, M.S. and Halestrap, A.P. (1984) The Concentration of the Mitochondrial Pyruvate Carrier in Rat Liver and Heart Mitochondria Determined with Alpha-Cyano-Beta-(1-phenylindol-3-yl)acrylate. *Biochemical Journal*, **223**, 673-676.

[13] Bricker, D.K., Taylor, E.B., Schell, J.C., Orsak, T., Boutron, A., Chen, Y.C., Cox, J.E., Cardon, C.M., Van Vranken, J.G., Dephoure, N., Redin, C., Boudina, S., Gygi, S.P., Brivet, M., Thummel, C.S. and Rutter, J. (2012) A Mitochondrial Pyruvate Carrier Required for Pyruvate Uptake in Yeast, *Drosophila*, and Humans. *Science*, **337**, 96-100. http://dx.doi.org/10.1126/science.1218099

[14] Herzig, S., Raemy, E., Montessuit, S., Veuthey, J.L., Zamboni, N., Westermann, B., Kunji, E.R.S. and Martinou, J.C. (2012) Identification and Functional Expression of the Mitochondrial Pyruvate Carrier. *Science*, **337**, 93-96. http://dx.doi.org/10.1126/science.1218530

[15] Brailsford, M.A., Thompson, A.G., Kaderbhai, N. and Beechey, R.B. (1986) The Extraction and Reconstitution of the Alpha-Cyanocinnamate-Sensitive Pyruvate Transporter from Castor Bean Mitochondria. *Biochemical and Biophysical Research Communications*, **140**, 1036-1042. http://dx.doi.org/10.1016/0006-291X(86)90739-4

[16] Nałecz, M.J., Nałecz, K.A., Broger, C., Bolli, R., Wojtczak, L. and Azzi, A. (1986) Extraction, Partial Purification and Functional Reconstitution of Two Mitochondrial Carriers Transporting Keto Acids: 2-Oxoglutarate and Pyruvate. *FEBS Letters*, **196**, 331-336. http://dx.doi.org/10.1016/0014-5793(86)80273-3

[17] Capuano, F., Di Paola, M., Azzi, A. and Papa, S. (1990) The Monocarboxylate Carrier from Rat Liver Mitochondria. Purification and Kinetic Characterization in a Reconstituted System. *FEBS Letters*, **261**, 39-42. http://dx.doi.org/10.1016/0014-5793(90)80631-R

[18] Nałecz, M.J., Nałecz, K.A. and Azzi, A. (1991) Purification and Functional Characterisation of the Pyruvate (Monocarboxylate) Carrier from Baker's Yeast Mitochondria (*Saccharomyces cerevisiae*). *Biochimica et Biophysica Acta*, **1079**, 87-95. http://dx.doi.org/10.1016/0167-4838(91)90028-X

[19] Hildyard, J.C.W. and Halestrap, A.P. (2003) Identification of the Mitochondrial Pyruvate Carrier in *Saccharomyces cerevisiae*. *Biochemical Journal*, **374**, 607-611. http://dx.doi.org/10.1042/BJ20030995

[20] Todisco, S., Agrimi, G., Castegna, A. and Palmieri, F. (2006) Identification of the Mitochondrial NAD$^+$ Transporter in *Saccharomyces cerevisiae*. *Journal of Biological Chemistry*, **281**, 1524-1531. http://dx.doi.org/10.1074/jbc.M510425200

[21] Da Cruz, S., Xenarios, I., Langridge, J., Vilbois, F., Parone, P.A. and Martinou, J.C. (2003) Proteomic Analysis of the Mouse Liver Mitochondrial Inner Membrane. *Journal of Biological Chemistry*, **278**, 41566-41571. http://dx.doi.org/10.1074/jbc.M304940200

[22] Halestrap, A.P. (2012) The Mitochondrial Pyruvate Carrier: Has It Been Unearthed at Last? *Cell Metabolism*, **16**, 141-143. http://dx.doi.org/10.1016/j.cmet.2012.07.013

[23] Li, C.L., Wang, M., Ma, X.Y. and Zhang, W. (2014) NRGA1, a Putative Mitochondrial Pyruvate Carrier, Mediates ABA Regulation of Guard Cell Ion Channels and Drought Stress Responses in *Arabidopsis*. *Molecular Plant*, **7**, 1508-1521. http://dx.doi.org/10.1093/mp/ssu061

[24] Lehmann, J.M., Moore, L.B., Smith-Oliver, T.A., Wilkison, W.O., Willson, T.M. and Kliewer, S.A. (1995) An Antidiabetic Thiazolidinedione Is a High Affinity Ligand for Peroxisome Proliferator-Activated Receptor γ (PPARγ). *Journal of Biological Chemistry*, **270**, 12953-12956. http://dx.doi.org/10.1074/jbc.270.22.12953

[25] Divakaruni, A.S., Wiley, S.E., Rogers, G.W., Andreyev, A.Y., Petrosyan, S., Loviscach, M., Wall, E.A., Yadava, N., Heuck, A.P., Ferrick, D.A., Henry, R.R., McDonald, W.G., Colca, J.R., Simon, M.I., Ciaraldi, T.P. and Murphy, A.N. (2013) Thiazolidinediones Are Acute, Specific Inhibitors of the Mitochondrial Pyruvate Carrier. *Proceedings of the National Academy of Sciences of the United States of America*, **110**, 5422-5427. http://dx.doi.org/10.1073/pnas.1303360110

[26] Hardie, D.G. (2014) AMPK: Positive and Negative Regulation, and Its Role in Whole-Body Energy Homeostasis. *Current Opinion in Cell Biology*, **33C**, 1-7.

[27] Colca, J.R., McDonald, W.G., Cavey, G.S., Cole, S.L., Holewa, D.D., Brightwell-Conrad, A.S., Wolfe, C.L., Wheeler, J.S., Coulter, K.R., Kilkuskie, P.M., Gracheva, E., Korshunova, Y., Trusgnich, M., Karr, R., Wiley, S.E., Divakaruni, A.S., Murphy, A.N., Vigueira, P.A., Finck, B.N. and Kletzien, R.F. (2013) Identification of a Mitochondrial Target of Thiazolidinedione Insulin Sensitizers (mTOT)—Relationship to Newly Identified Mitochondrial Pyruvate Carrier Proteins. *PLoS ONE*, **8**, e61551. http://dx.doi.org/10.1371/journal.pone.0061551

[28] Vigueira, P.A., McCommis, K.S., Schweitzer, G.G., Remedi, M.S., Chambers, K.T., Fu, X., McDonald, W.G., Cole, S.L., Colca, J.R., Kletzien, R.F., Burgess, S.C. and Finck, B.N. (2014) Mitochondrial Pyruvate Carrier 2 Hypomorphism in Mice Leads to Defects in Glucose-Stimulated Insulin Secretion. *Cell Reports*, **7**, 2042-2053. http://dx.doi.org/10.1016/j.celrep.2014.05.017

[29] Vacanti, N.M., Divakaruni, A.S., Green, C.R., Parker, S.J., Henry, R.R., Ciaraldi, T.P., Murphy, A.N. and Metallo, C.M. (2014) Regulation of Substrate Utilization by the Mitochondrial Pyruvate Carrier. *Molecular Cell*, **56**, 425-435. http://dx.doi.org/10.1016/j.molcel.2014.09.024

[30] Yang, C., Sudderth, J., Dang, T., Bachoo, R.M., Bachoo, R.G., McDonald, J.G. and DeBerardinis, R.J. (2009) Glioblastoma Cells Require Glutamate Dehydrogenase to Survive Impairments of Glucose Metabolism or Akt Signaling. *Cancer Research*, **69**, 7986-7993. http://dx.doi.org/10.1158/0008-5472.CAN-09-2266

[31] Yang, C., Ko, B., Hensley, C.T., Jiang, L., Wasti, A.T., Kim, J., Sudderth, J., Calvaruso, M.A., Lumata, L., Mitsche, M., Rutter, J., Merritt, M.E. and DeBerardinis, R.J. (2014) Glutamine Oxidation Maintains the TCA Cycle and Cell Survival during Impaired Mitochondrial Pyruvate Transport. *Molecular Cell*, **56**, 414-424. http://dx.doi.org/10.1016/j.molcel.2014.09.025

[32] Cairns, R.A., Harris, I.S. and Mak, T.W. (2011) Regulation of Cancer Cell Metabolism. *Nature Reviews Cancer*, **11**, 85-95. http://dx.doi.org/10.1038/nrc2981

[33] Schell, J.C., Olson, K.A., Jiang, L., Hawkins, A.J., Van Vranken, J.G., Xie, J., Egnatchik, R.A., Earl, E.G., DeBerardinis, R.J. and Rutter, J. (2014) A Role for the Mitochondrial Pyruvate Carrier as a Repressor of the Warburg Effect and Colon Cancer Cell Growth. *Molecular Cell*, **56**, 400-413. http://dx.doi.org/10.1016/j.molcel.2014.09.026

[34] Moreb, J.S. (2008) Aldehyde Dehydrogenase as a Marker for Stem Cells. *Current Stem Cell Research & Therapy*, **3**, 237-246. http://dx.doi.org/10.2174/157488808786734006

[35] Tirino, V., Desiderio, V., Paino, F., De Rosa, A., Papaccio, F., La Noce, M., Laino, L., De Francesco, F. and Papaccio, G. (2013) Cancer Stem Cells in Solid Tumors: An Overview and New Approaches for Their Isolation and Characterization. *FASEB Journal*, **27**, 13-24. http://dx.doi.org/10.1096/fj.12-218222

[36] Leushacke, M. and Barker, N. (2012) Lgr5 and Lgr6 as Markers to Study Adult Stem Cell Roles in Self-Renewal and Cancer. *Oncogene*, **31**, 3009-3022. http://dx.doi.org/10.1038/onc.2011.479

[37] Zhou, J., Ng, S.B. and Chng, W.J. (2013) LIN28/LIN28B: An Emerging Oncogenic Driver in Cancer Stem Cells. *International Journal of Biochemistry & Cell Biology*, **45**, 973-978. http://dx.doi.org/10.1016/j.biocel.2013.02.006

[38] Iv Santaliz-Ruiz, L.E., Xie, X., Old, M., Teknos, T.N. and Pan, Q. (2014) Emerging Role of Nanog in Tumorigenesis and Cancer Stem Cells. *International Journal of Cancer*, **135**, 2741-2748. http://dx.doi.org/10.1002/ijc.28690

8

Prevalence of Hypogonadotropic Hypogonadism in Type 2 Diabetes Male Patients

Mozhgan Afkhamizadeh[1], Seyed Bahman Ghaderian[2]*, Reza Rajabian[1], Armaghan Moravej Aleali[1]

[1]Endocrine Research Center, Ghaem Hospital, Mashhad University of Medical Sciences, Mashhad, Iran
[2]Health Research Institute, Diabetes Research Center, Ahvaz Jundishapur University of Medical Science, Ahvaz, Iran
Email: *bahmanint@yahoo.com

Abstract

Background: Erectile dysfunction is common in patients with diabetes mellitus. In addition, reduced testosterone itself is considered as a risk factor for diabetes; therefore hypogonadism was studied in diabetes. Objective: This study was done to determine the prevalence of hypo- and hypergonadotropic hypogonadism in the type 2 diabetes male patients in Mashhad in north-east of Iran. Methods: This study was done on type 2 diabetic men aged 40 - 60 years in the endocrine clinic, Endocrinology Research Center, Mashhad University of Medical Sciences, Iran. Fasting blood samples were collected at 8 am for measurement of fasting blood sugar (FBS), HbA1C, total serum testosterone, FSH, Sex Hormone Binding Globulin (SHBG), LH, prolactin, thyroxin-stimulating hormone (TSH), and immediately was sent to laboratory. Results: Out of total 96 type 2 diabetic males (mean age of 51.4 ± 11.26 years, range of 40 - 60 years), 11 (12.94%) patients were excluded because of inadequate samples, insufficient information and fulfillment of the exclusion criteria of the study. Hypogonadism based on Testosterone, Calculated free testosterone (CFT), and boiavailable testosterone (BT) were observed in 10 (11.8%), 31 (36.6%), and 30 (35.3%) of the patients, respectively. Libido was decreased in 55 (64.7%) of the patients. Based on the obtained SHBG values there were 7 (8.2%), 52 (61.2%), and 26 (30.6%) cases of low, normal and high values, respectively. According to TSH observed values there were 6 (7.1%) patients and 1 case of sub-clinical hypothyroidism and hyperthyroidism, respectively, and the rest 78 (91.8%) cases were euthyroid. Prolactin level was normal in all cases. Conclusion: Hypogonadotropic hypogonadism is common in type 2 diabetic men, and whether its treatment is useful for erectile dysfunction or not, needed additional investigation.

*Corresponding author.

Keywords

Type 2 Diabetes, Testosterone, Hypogonadism, Hypogonadotropic

1. Background

Diabetes is a common endocrine disease, which causes many complications in other organs in the body. One of these complications is erectile dysfunction (ED). Erectile dysfunction and reverse ejaculation are common in patients with diabetes mellitus and may be one of the first symptoms of diabetic neuropathy. Erectile dysfunction prevalence increases with increasing age and duration of diabetes, and may occur in the absence of other signs of diabetic autonomic neuropathy [1]. If hypogonadism has a significant role in the development of erectile dysfunction in diabetics, administration of testosterone could be useful in treatment of ED. Therefore hypogonadism is studied in diabetics. But in various studies, the prevalence of hypogonadism in diabetes has been reported differently [2]-[9]. Also hypogonadism, increases lipid mass, reduces muscle mass, accelerates bone loss and consequently increases bone fractures, decreases libido and makes erectile dysfunction. On the other hand, testosterone has anti-inflammatory and anti-atherosclerosis properties which might be involved in causing other complications of diabetes [10]. In addition, reduced testosterone itself is considered as a risk factor for diabetes and may lead to worsening glycemic control [11]. So study on hypogonadism in diabetes is useful.

2. Objective

This study was conducted due to conflicting and limited information about the presence or absence of hypo- and hypergonadotropic hypogonadism in type 2 diabetes male patients and its prevalence especially in Iran.

3. Patients and Methods

This study was done on patients with type 2 diabetic men aged 40 - 60 years in the endocrine clinic, Endocrinology Research Center, Mashhad University of Medical Sciences, Iran from October 2006 to April 2008. This study was approved by the medical ethics committee of Mashhad University of Medical Science.

Inclusion criteria: Type 2 diabetic males aged 40 - 60 years.

Exclusion criteria: Known cases of hypo- or hypergonadotropic hypogonadism were excluded. Other exclusion criteria were chronic debilitating diseases such as cirrhosis and HIV and also addiction.

Measurements and data collection: Questionnaires were prepared for patients and information about age, duration of diabetes, family history of diabetes, drugs, history of renal disease, thyroid, cardiovascular disease, hypertension, hyperlipidemia and libido were collected. Height (cm) and weight (kg) were measured using mechanic scales for the patients with their clothed in underwear, and body mass index (BMI) was calculated according to the standard formula [BMI = Weight (kg)/Height^2 $(meter)$]. Fasting blood samples were collected at 8 am for measurement of fasting blood sugar (FBS), HbA1C, total serum testosterone, FSH, Sex Hormone Binding Globulin (SHBG), LH, prolactin, Thyroxin-Stimulating Hormone (TSH), and immediately was sent to laboratory. Total serum testosterone was measured by RIA; SHBG, TSH, prolactin, LH and FSH were measured by IRMA. Calculated free testosterone (CFT) was calculated using Vermelune method by software at website: www.issam.ch/Free testo.htm based on testosterone and SHBG (Fier from Belgium. Bioavailable testosterone (BT) was calculated by Dr. Fier formula.

4. Statistical Methods

Data were analyzed using SPSS 13.0 software. Mann Whitney test was used for comparing nonparametric data, and t test was used to compare parametric data. χ^2 test was also used to compare qualitative variables. Spearman correlation (for nonparametricdata) or Pearson correlation (for parametric data) was used to establish correlations. P value less than 0.05 was considered significant.

5. Results

Out of total 96 type 2 diabetic males (mean age of 51.4 ± 11.26 years, range of 40 - 60 years), 11 (12.94%) patients were excluded because of inadequate samples, insufficient information and fulfillment of the exclusion criteria of the study. The mean and standard deviation of weight, height, BMI, Testosterone, FBS, HbA1C1, systolic and diastolic blood pressure and duration of diabetes has been shown in **Table 1**. The mean LH and FSH values were not elevated, and all the cases were hypogonadotropic hypogonadism (**Table 1**).

The family history of diabetes has been observed in 60 (70.6%) of the patients. Out of 85 patients, 14 (16.5%) cases had a history of cardiovascular disease, 26 (30.6%) subjects had a history of hypertension, and none of the cases had a history of renal and thyroid diseases (**Table 2**). The libido was decreased in 55 (64.7%) of the patients. Hypogonadism based on Testosterone, CFT, and BT were observed in 10 (11.8%), 31 (36.6%), and 30 (35.3%) of the patients, respectively (**Table 2**). According to TSH observed values there were 6 (7.1%) patients and 1 case of sub-clinical hypothyroidism and hyperthyroidism, respectively, and the rest 78 (91.8%) cases were euthyroid (**Table 2**). Based on the obtained SHBG values there were 7 (8.2%), 52 (61.2%), and 26 (30.6%) cases of low, normal and high values, respectively (**Table 2**). The prolactin level was normal in all cases. In case of anti-diabetic drugs 62 (72.9%), 66 (77.6%), and 7 (8.2%) cases used metformin, glibenclamide, and insulin, respectively (**Table 2**).

There was a significant correlation in duration of diabetes between two study groups (**Table 3**). There were no significant correlations in term of mean age, BMI, FBS, HbA1C, SHBG, TT, CFT, and BT between two study groups (**Table 3**). Also between mean of SBP, DBP, TSH, prolactin, LH and FSH, there were no significant differences among study groups (**Table 3**). The TT showed significant positive correlations with SHBG and prolactin, negative correlation with BMI, FBS and HbA1C, and no significant correlation with FSH, TSH, LH, duration of diabetes and DBP (**Table 3**). The age showed significant positive correlations with TT and SHBG,

Table 1. The mean and standard deviation of variables of interest.

Variable	Mean ± SD	Range
Weigh (kg)	75.85 ± 12.6	123.5 - 56
Height (cm)	168.3 ± 5.1	182 - 152
BMI (kg/m²)	26.6 ± 3.6	20.2 - 38.5
FPG (mg/dl)	197.7 ± 74.5	79 - 511
HbA1c (%)	8.81 ± 2.1	4.5 - 15
Duration of diabetes (year)	8.3 ± 5.85	0.6 - 30
Systolic Blood Pressure (mmhg)	129.23 ± 20.5	80 - 200
Diastolic Blood Pressure (mmhg)	77.4 ± 12.5	40 - 120
Testosterone (ng/dl)	460.3 ± 136.6	190 - 810
CFT (ng/dl)	7.5 ± 2.34	3.66 - 13.2
BT (ng/dl)	172.8 ± 62.2	13 - 310
LH (mIu/ml)	5.56 ± 3.8	1 - 19
FSH (mIu/ml)	10.15 ± 9.7	2 - 20
TSH (mIu/ml)	1.73 ± 3.1	0.2 - 29
SHBG (nmol/L)	51.7 ± 29.5	10 - 150
Prolactine (ng/ml)	9.15 ± 8.8	2 - 19
Anti-diabetic drugs		
Metformin (mg)	1076 ± 499	---------
Glibenclamide (mg)	8.5 ± 4.59	-------------
Insulin (U)	33 ± 12.7	-----------

FPG: Fasting Plasma Glucose; **BMI:** Body Mass Index.

Table 2. The history of a disease among the patients of interest.

Variables	Number	Percentage
Family history of diabetes	60	70.6%
History of renal disease	0	0%
History of thyroid disease	0	0%
History of cardiovascular disease	14	16.5%
History of hypertension	26	60.6%
Decreased libido	55	64.7%
Hypogonadism based on		
Testosterone values (<300 ng/dL)	10	11.8%
CFT values (<6.48 ng/dL)	31	36.6%
BT values (<150 ng/dL)	30	35.3%
Thyroid disorder based on the TSH values		
Sub-clinical hyperthyroidism	6	7.1%
Hypothyroidism	1	1.2%
Euthyroidism	78	91.8%
SHBG condition		
Low	7	8.2%
Normal	52	61.2%
High	26	30.6%
Anti-diabetic drug		
Metformin	62	72.9%
Glibenclamide	66	77.6%
Insulin	7	8.2%

Table 3. The mean and standard deviation of variables in patients with normal and low free testosterone.

	Low free testosterone group	Normal free testosterone group
Number of patients	32	53
Age (y)	52.5 ± 4.8	50.7 ± 6.4
Diabetes duration (y)	9.4 ± 5.5	7.6 ± 5.8
TSH (mIu/L)	1.5 ± 1.03	1.85 ± 3.97
Prolactin (ng/ml)	7.12 ± 3.07	10.2 ± 10.9
LH (mIu/ml)	6.06 ± 4.7	5.3 ± 3.17
FSH (mIu/ml)	13.4 ± 4.3	8.1 ± 4.3
SHBG (nmol/L)	69.6 ± 31.5	40.5 ± 21.8
TT (ng/dl)	281.4 ± 38.4	465.3 ± 121.4
FBS (mg/dl)	200.7 ± 74.8	196 ± 74.1
HbA1C (%)	9.08 ± 2.28	8.76 ± 2.06

negative correlation with BMI, and, and no significant correlation with FSH, TSH, LH, FBS, HbA1C, prolactin and DBP (**Table 3**). The BT has no significant correlations with FSH, TSH, LH, FBS, HbA1C, BMI, DBP, duration of diabetes and prolactin, which only showed significant positive correlations with SHBG (**Table 3**). The

CFT has no significant correlations with FSH, TSH, LH, FBS, HbA1C, BMI, DBP, duration of diabetes and prolactin, which only showed significant positive correlations with SHBG and negative correlation with age (**Table 3**). LH level showed significant positive correlations with DBP and FSH, and no significant correlation with FSH, TSH, LH, BMI, SBP and prolactin (**Table 3**). FSH level showed significant positive correlations with DBP and FBS, and no significant correlation with TSH, LH, BMI, SBP and prolactin (**Table 3**). Prolactin showed no significant correlation with all other variables (**Table 3**).

6. Discussion

The present study, regardless of the glycemic control, duration of the disease and complications of diabetes or obesity, typically revealed that hypogonadotropic hypogonadism is common in type 2 diabetes. The prevalence of hypogonadism based on age criteria was higher than of what is expected. Age naturally is associated with the 0.5% to 2% decrease in the level of testosterone. The decrease in testosterone is gradual and stable, and begins in early life stages, probably after the third decade [12]. In our study, we limited the age into the range of 40 to 60-year in order to minimize the changes in testosterone according to the age.

In a study that has been conducted on the old men of Massachusetts the testosterone had decreased by the rate of 1.6% per year, and SHBG increased with the rate of 1.2% per year [13]. In the BLSA study, one of the most studies of age-related decrease in the expression of testosterone, the mean decrease of this hormone was 0.11 nmol/L in year. In this study, 3661 sample was analyzed for testosterone and SHBG. 16% were diabetic and there was no relationship between testosterone levels and diabetes [14], but in the present study this correlation was observed. The reason may be that diabetes was diagnosed by glucose tolerance test in all volunteers in BLSA study, which probably those cases were mild diabetics or in the early stages of disease compared with the present study. Inspire of measuring the prevalence of hypogonadism using the same criteria that have been used by BLSA, in the present study hypogonadism were more common (10% vs. 16.4%, respectively). We also compared the BT levels in our study with non-diabetic population study from Muller and colleagues [15]. They measured testosterone and SHBG in 400 male volunteers (mean age of 60.2 years, range of 40 - 80 years). In the present study, we reached the conclusion that diabetic people have lower BT levels compared to their non-diabetic subjects (172.8 ng/dL vs. 262 ng/dL). Tsay et al. [16] measured the BT, CFT, SHBG, testosterone Levels in 221 non-diabetic men with mean age 57 years and BMI of 29 kg/m^2, and reported the mean CFT of 0.32 nmol/L (9.2 ng/dL), BT of 7.9 nmol/L (227.5 ng/dL), testosterone of 18 nmol/L (518.4 ng/dL) and SHBG of 42.2 nmol/L. While, in the present study on diabetic patients with a mean age of 51.4 years and BMI of 26.6 kg/m^2, the mean CFT, BT, testosterone and SHBG were 7.5 ng/dL, 172 ng/dL, 460.3 ng/dL and 51.7 nmol/L, respectively. CFT, BT, testosterone were lower in our patients compared to nondiabetic men in their study.

Although, techniques for measuring testosterone and SHBG is fixed and almost same, but cannot deny this fact that there are changes in these two tests in different laboratories with different kit, so we also have compared the testosterone levels in our study with two studies that conducted the CALDIA [7] and Kalndvnyay (an island in France) using same method of measurement of testosterone. In this study, Dfay and colleagues compared the testosterone levels in 16 diabetic male patients with 16 controls in the same population with similar age in both groups (mean age: 46.9 years). People with diabetes had higher BMI (32.8 kg/m^2 in diabetics vs. 25.11 kg/m^2 in the controls), 1.8 years as the mean duration of diabetes, the mean testosterone level in diabetics subjects was 13.8 nmol/L (397 ng/dL) compared to the 20.73 nmol/L (596 ng/dL) in the control group, while, the average mean testosterone level in our study was slightly higher (460.3 ng/dL).

The frequency of hypogonadism was lower in the present study compared to a study that was performed in the New York on 103 men with type 2 diabetes [16] (11.8% vs. 24.6%), which the reason may be less BMI and more SHBG levels. It is not clear that age-related decrease in testosterone whether is due to presence of the chronic disease which increased related to the age or not. Some studies have identified age-related decrease in testosterone levels in healthy individuals [15]. Some chronic diseases coexist with the decrease in the testosterone levels such as infection, malignancy and HIV [17]. Although, both hyper- and hypogonadism have been reported in the chronic diseases previously, but the etiology of hypogonadism in these diseases is complex [17]. In the study of BLSA, the age related presence of the malignant only was associated greater reductions in testosterone levels [18].

Studies have shown that levels of LH and FSH slightly increased according to the age [18] [19]. Increase in LH is not proportional to reduction in testosterone, which shows the change in the mechanism of feedback occurs related to the age [19] [20]. The prolactin level remains constant, or slightly increases or decrease with the increase in the age [13] [18]. In the study of New York the levels of prolactin among different hypogonadal and eugonadal groups had no role and relationship with age, and levels of prolactin was comparable with normal individuals [12]. In our study, FSH, LH had not been increase in hypogonadal people, which revealed that the gonadal effect may not be the reason. Despite previous studies, in our study there was no significant correlation between the age-related changes in FSH, LH and prolactin. Hypothalamic disorders that lead to hypogonadotropic hypogonadism in type 2 diabetes is associated with insulin resistance [21]. Metabolic syndrome, insulin resistance and obesity, are associated with lower level of SHBG and testosterone in men [22] [23]. Tsay and colleagues found that in non-diabetics male, CFT and BT levels had negative correlation with local fat, total fat and insulin resistance [16]. However, CFT and BT levels correlation with the insulin resistance regardless of local and total fats is not remarkable.

In the New York study, testosterone was inversely correlated to BMI values that we also observed in the present study, so BMI and SHBG, both were predictors of testosterone [12], herein, it seems that in diabetes, BMI non-dependent to SHBG levels affect testosterone. It is believed that low testosterone in obesity is due to the low level of SHBG. Zimov and colleagues [24] conducted a study on 48 healthy males (mean age of 32.2 years), with a BMI range between 21 - 95 kg/m^2, and showed that both FT and BT are inversely related with BMI. The researchers reported that increasing in the plasma levels of FT is caused by pre-inflammatory cytokines such as TNFα, IL6 and CRP [24] [25], and has been shown that TNFα and IL$_{1B}$, decrease secretion of LH in the hypothalamus of animal in vitro [26] [27]. But in our study there was no significant correlation between changes in BT and CFT with BMI. In addition, there were no significant correlation between changes of BT and CFT with LH and FSH. However, because there was no clear difference between the present and previous studies, perhaps lower BMI in our study makes this difference. Although in many studies on the frequency of hypogonadism only testosterone is measured, some believe that the presence of hypogonadism should be determined based on clinical syndrome associated with low levels of testosterone and FT. Furthermore, practical test to determine the activity of testosterone is not yet available. In addition, various androgen-dependent physiological functions require different levels of testosterone [28]. Serum testosterone levels could be to establish in the lower range of normal sexual function. In our study, there were no significant relationship between decreased sexual desire levels with TT, CFT, and BT. Muscle strength, muscle size and lean body mass increase due to circulating testosterone dose-dependently, even in the normal range [29] [30]. Hypogonadism increases fat mass, reduces muscle mass, accelerates bone loss and is associated with decrease in libido, which testosterone treatment improved these parameters [31].

High prevalence of hypogonadism in type 2 diabetes, illustrate this fact that diabetes can affect sexual desire, erectile function, muscle mass, abdominal fat, bone density, mood and individual recognition. Recently indicated that testosterone has anti-inflammatory properties and anti-atherosclerosis in animals and humans, which show the importance of testosterone replacement [10]. In the New York study, there were no relationship between TT and CFT with FBS and HbA1C [12], but in the present study there was an inverse significant correlation between TT and FBS and HbA1C. While, between BT and CFT with FBS and HbA1C any relationship did not exist, which the presence of such significant inverse correlation between FBS and SHBG in the present study compared to New York study may be due to the effect of high FBS on testosterone.

7. Conclusion

Hypogonadotropic hypogonadism is common in type 2 diabetic men, and whether its treatment is useful for erectile dysfunction or not, needs additional investigation.

Acknowledgements

The results described in this paper were part of a MD student thesis proposal. The authors would like to thanks to Ghaem hospital laboratory for measuring hormones.

Sources of Funding

Research deputy, Mashhad University of Medical Sciences, Mashhad, Iran.

References

[1]   Martin, J.B., Kasper, D.L., *et al.* (2011) Harrisonns Principles of Internal Medicine. 18th Edition, McGrow Hill, New York.

[2]   Barrett-Conner, E. (1992) Lower Endogenous Androgen Levels and Dyslipidemia in Men with Non-Insulin Dependent Diabetes Mellitus. *Annals of Internal Medicine*, **117**, 807-811. http://dx.doi.org/10.7326/0003-4819-117-10-807

[3]   Barrett-Conner, E., Khow, Kt and Yen, S.S. (1990) Endogenous Sex Hormone Levels in Older Adult Men with Diabetes Mellitus. *American Journal of Epidemiology*, **132**, 895-901.

[4]   Goodman-Gruen, D. and Barrett-Conner, E. (2000) Sex Differences in the Association of Endogenous Sex Hormone Levels and Glucose Tolerance Status in Older Men and Women. *Diabetes Care*, **23**, 912-918. http://dx.doi.org/10.2337/diacare.23.7.912

[5]   Chang, T.C., Tung, C.C. and Hsiao, Y.L. (1994) Hormonal Changes in Elderly Men with Non-Insulin Dependent Diabetes Mellitus and the Hormonal Relationships to Abdominal Obesity. *Gerontology*, **40**, 260-267. http://dx.doi.org/10.1159/000213594

[6]   Ando, S., Rubens, R. and Rottiers, R. (1984) Androgen Plasma Levels in Male Diabetics. *Journal of Endocrinological Investigation*, **7**, 21-24. http://dx.doi.org/10.1007/BF03348370

[7]   Defay, R., Papoz, L., Barney, S., Bonnot-Lours, S., Caces, E. and Simon, D. (1998) Hormonal Status and NIDDM in the European and Melanesian Populations of New Caledonia: A Case-Control Study. The Caledonia Diabetes Mellitus (CALDIA) Study Group. *International Journal of Obesity and Related Metabolic Disorders*, **22**, 927-934. http://dx.doi.org/10.1038/sj.ijo.0800697

[8]   Anderson, B., Marin, P., Lissner, L., Vermeulen, A. and Bjorntorp, P. (1994) Tesosterone Concentration in Women and Men with NIDDM. *Diabetes Care*, **17**, 405-411. http://dx.doi.org/10.2337/diacare.17.5.405

[9]   Betancourt-Albrecht, M. and Cunningham, Gr. (2003) Hypogonadism and Diabetes. *International Journal of Impotence Research*, **15**, 514-520.

[10]   Malkin, C.J., Pugh, P.G., Jones, R.D., Jones, T.H. and Channer, K.S. (2003) Testosterone as a Protective Factor against Atherosclerosis: Immunomodulation and Influence upon Plaque Development and Stability. *Journal of Endocrinology*, **178**, 373-380. http://dx.doi.org/10.1677/joe.0.1780373

[11]   Rauscher, M. (2007) Low Testosterone a Possible Risk Factor for Diabetes in Men. *Diabetes Care*, **30**, 234-238.

[12]   Dhindsa, S., Prabhkar, S., Sethi, M., Bandyopdhyay, A., Chaudhuri, A. and Dahdona, P. (2004) Frequent Occurrence of Hypogonadotropic Hypogonadism in Type 2 Diabetes. *Journal of Clinical Endocrinology & Metabolism*, **89**, 5462-5468. http://dx.doi.org/10.1210/jc.2004-0804

[13]   Vermeulen, A. and Koufman, J.M. (2002) Diagnosis of Hypogonadism in the Aging Male. *Aging Male*, **5**, 170-176. http://dx.doi.org/10.1080/tam.5.3.170.176

[14]   Harman, S.M., Metter, E.J., Tobin, J.D., Pearson, J. and Blackman, M.R. (2001) Longitudinal Effects of Aging on Serum Total and Free Testosterone Levels in Healthy Men: Baltimore Longitudinal Study of Aging. *Journal of Clinical Endocrinology & Metabolism*, **86**, 724-731. http://dx.doi.org/10.1210/jcem.86.2.7219

[15]   Gray, A., Feldman, H.A., McKinlay, J.B. and Longcope, C. (1991) Age, Disease, and Changing Sex Hormone Levels in Middle-Aged Men: Results of the Massachusetts Male Aging Study. *Journal of Clinical Endocrinology & Metabolism*, **73**, 1016-1025. http://dx.doi.org/10.1210/jcem-73-5-1016

[16]   Tsai, E.C., Matsmoto, A.M., Fujimoto, W.Y. and Boyko, E.J. (2004) Association of Bioavailable, Free and Total Testosterone with Insulin Resistance: Influence of Sex Hormone-Binding Globulin and Body Fat. *Diabetes Care*, **27**, 861-868. http://dx.doi.org/10.2337/diacare.27.4.861

[17]   Muller, M., Den tonkelaar, I., Thijssen, J., Grobbeee, D.E. and Van der Schouw, Y.T. (2003) Endogenous Sex Hormones in Men Aged 40 - 80 Years. *European Journal of Endocrinology*, **149**, 583-589. http://dx.doi.org/10.1530/eje.0.1490583

[18]   Bhasin, S. and Bremner, W.J. (1997) Emerging Issues in Androgen Replacement Therapy. *Journal of Clinical Endocrinology & Metabolism*, **82**, 3-8.

[19]   Feldman, H.A., Longcope, C., Derby, C.A., Johannes, C.B., Araujo, A.B., Coviello, A.D., *et al.* (2002) Age Trends in the Level of Serum Testosterone and Other Hormones in Middle-Aged Men: Longitudinal Results of Massachusetts Male Aging Study. *Journal of Clinical Endocrinology & Metabolism*, **87**, 589-598. http://dx.doi.org/10.1210/jcem.87.2.8201

[20]   Morley, J.E., Kaiser, F.E., Perry, H.M., Patrick, P., Morley, P.M., Stauber, P.M., *et al.* (1997) Longitudinal Changes in Testosterone, Lueinizing Hormone, and Follicle Stimulating Hormone in Healthy Older Men. *Metabolism*, **46**, 410-413. http://dx.doi.org/10.1016/S0026-0495(97)90057-3

[21] Mulligan, T., Iranmanesh, A., Kerzner, R., Demers, L.W. and Veldhuis, J.D. (1999) Two Week Pulsatile Gonadotropin Releasing Hormone Infusion Unmasks Dual (Hypothalamic and Leydig Cell) Defects in the Healthy Aging Male Gonadotropic Axis. *European Journal of Endocrinology*, **141**, 257-266. http://dx.doi.org/10.1530/eje.0.1410257

[22] Bruning, J.C., Gautman, D., Burks, D.J., Gillette, J., Schubert, M., Orban, P.C., *et al.* (2000) Role of Brain Insulin Receptor in Control of Body Weight and Reproduction. *Science*, **289**, 2122-2125. http://dx.doi.org/10.1126/science.289.5487.2122

[23] Haffner, S.M., Karhapaa, P., Mykkanen, L. and Laak, M. (1994) Insulin Resistance, Body Fat Distribution, and Sex Hormone in Men. *Diabetes*, **43**, 212-219. http://dx.doi.org/10.2337/diab.43.2.212

[24] Zumoff, B., Strain, G.W., Miller, L.K., Rosner, W., Senie, R., Seres, D.S., *et al.* (1990) Plasma Free and Non-Sex-Hormone-Binding-Globulin Bound Testosterone Are Decreased in Obese Men in Proportion to Their Degree of Obesity. *Journal of Clinical Endocrinology & Metabolism*, **71**, 929-931. http://dx.doi.org/10.1210/jcem-71-4-929

[25] Dandona, P., Weinstock, R., Thusu, K., Abel-Rahman, E., Aljada, A. and Wadden, T. (1998) Tumor Necrosis Factor-Alfa in Sera of Obese Patients: Fall with Weight Loss. *Journal of Clinical Endocrinology & Metabolism*, **83**, 2907-2910.

[26] Weisberg, S.P., McCann, D., Desai, M., Rosenbaum, M., Leibel, R.L. and Ferrante Jr., A.W. (2003) Obesity Is Associated with Macrophage Accumulation in Adipose Tissue. *Journal of Clinical Investigation*, **112**, 1796-1808. http://dx.doi.org/10.1172/JCI200319246

[27] Watanobe, H. and Hayakawa, Y. (2003) Hypothalamic Inerlukin-1β and Tumor Necrosis Factor-α, but Not Interlukin-6 Mediate the Endotoxin-Induced Suppression of the Reproductive Axis in Rats. *Endocrinology*, **144**, 4868-4875. http://dx.doi.org/10.1210/en.2003-0644

[28] Russell, S.H., Small, C.J., Stanley, S.A., Franks, S., Ghateri, M.A. and Bloom, S.R. (2001) The *in Vitro* Role of Tumor Necrosis Factor-α and Interlukin-6 in the Hypothalamic-Pituitary-Gonadal Axis. *Journal of Neuroendocrinology*, **13**, 296-301. http://dx.doi.org/10.1046/j.1365-2826.2001.00632.x

[29] Bhasin, S. (2000) The Dose-Dependent Effects of Testosterone on Sexual Function and on Muscle Mass Function. *Mayo Clinic Proceedings*, **75**, S70-S75, Discussion S75-S76.

[30] Bhasin, S., Woodhouse, L., Casaburi, R., Singh, A.B., Bhasin, D., Berman, N., *et al.* (2001) Testosterone Dose-Response Relationship in Healthy Young Men. *American Journal of Physiology. Endocrinology and Metabolism*, **281**, E1172-E1181.

[31] Snyder, P.J., Peachey, H., Berlin, J.A., Hannoush, P., Haddad, G., Dlewati, A., *et al.* (2000) Effect of Testosterone Replacement in Hypogonadal Men. *Journal of Clinical Endocrinology & Metabolism*, **85**, 2670-2677.

9

Insulin Resistance in Pregnancy Is Correlated with Decreased Insulin Receptor Gene Expression in Omental Adipose: Insulin Sensitivity and Adipose Tissue Gene Expression in Normal Pregnancy

Arnold M. Mahesan[1]*, Dotun Ogunyemi[2], Eric Kim[3], Anthea B. M. Paul[2], Y.-D. Ida Chen[3]

[1]Jones Institute for Reproductive Medicine, Eastern Virginia Medical School, Norfolk, VA, USA
[2]Department of Obstetrics and Gynecology, Oakland University William Beaumont School of Medicine; Royal Oak, MI, USA
[3]LA Biomedical Research Center, Harbor-UCLA Medical Center, Torrance, CA, USA
Email: *am.mahesan@gmail.com

Abstract

Aims: To determine correlations of insulin sensitivity to gene expression in omental and subcutaneous adipose tissue of non-obese, non-diabetic pregnant women. Methods: Microarray gene profiling was performed on subcutaneous and omental adipose tissue from 14 patients and obtained while fasting during non-laboring Cesarean section, using Illumina HumanHT-12 V4 Expression BeadChips. Findings were validated by real-time PCR. Matusda-Insulin sensitivity index (IS) and homeostasis model assessment of insulin resistance (HOMA-IR) were calculated from glucose and insulin levels obtained from a frequently sampled oral glucose tolerance test, and correlated with gene expression. Results: Of genes differentially expressed in omental vs. subcutaneous adipose, in omentum 12 genes were expressed toward insulin resistance, whereas only 5 genes were expressed toward insulin sensitivity. In particular, expression of the insulin receptor gene (INSR), which initiates the insulin signaling cascade, is strongly positively correlated with IS and negatively with HOMA-IR in omental tissue (r = 0.84). Conclusion: Differential gene expression in omentum relative to subcutaneous adipose showed a pro-insulin resistance profile in omentum. A clinical importance of omental adipose is observed here, as downregulation of insulin receptor in omentum is correlated with increased systemic insulin resistance.

---

*Corresponding author.

Keywords

DEG, Insulin Resistance, Insulin Sensitivity, Insulin Signaling Pathway, Adipose Tissue in Pregnancy, Carbohydrate Metabolism, Diabetic Pathways

1. Introduction

Various metabolic pathways are involved in glucose homeostasis and in the development of insulin resistance. The insulin signaling pathway is initiated when insulin binds to its receptor resulting in the tyrosine phosphorylation of insulin receptor substrates (IRS) by the insulin receptor tyrosine kinase (INSR). Tyrosine phosphorylated IRS in turn activates phosphoinositide 3-kinase (PI3K), which further activates Akt. Activated Akt induces glycogen synthesis by inhibiting glycogen synthase kinase 3 (GSK-3), and facilitates mTOR-mediated activation of protein synthesis and cell survival. The PI3k/Akt pathway further stimulates the translocation of GLUT4 vesicles to the plasma membrane and allows the uptake of glucose into muscle and adipose cells [1]-[3].

The role of adipose tissue in the pathophysiology of insulin resistance is well recognized [1] [4]. Pregnancy is associated with insulin resistance and increases risks of gestational diabetes mellitus (GDM) and type II diabetes mellitus (T2DM) [5] [6]. In pregnancy, the cellular mechanisms for decreased insulin sensitivity are multifactorial, involving both skeletal muscle and adipose tissue and remain to be completely elucidated [1] [4]. Human pregnancy is characterized by adipose tissue accretion in early gestation, followed by insulin resistance and facilitated lipolysis in late pregnancy [7]-[9]. Additionally, the adipose tissue transcriptome demonstrates the recruitment of metabolic and immune molecular networks by 8 - 12 weeks of gestation, preceding any pregnancy-related physiological changes associated with insulin resistance [9].

Studies investigating insulin-signaling intermediates have demonstrated reduced IRS-1 protein levels, reduced GLUT4 translocation and subsequent glucose uptake in adipose tissue of obese women with GDM, and T2DM in comparison to controls [10]-[14].

These previous reports studied obese women and those with GDM or T2DM, analyzing mainly subcutaneous adipose tissue. There is data demonstrating that visceral adipose tissue accumulation increases the risk for developing obesity-related diseases such as T2DM, and cardiovascular diseases [15] [16]. Consequently, our study focused on the comparative roles of visceral versus subcutaneous adipose tissue. Furthermore, by choosing to include healthy, non-diabetic, non-obese pregnant women in the current analysis, we are able to examine the function of visceral and subcutaneous adipose tissue in pregnancy without confounding factors that may be associated with disease states.

The objectives of our study were two-fold. The first was to characterize in healthy, non-obese pregnant women differentially expressed genes in visceral and subcutaneous adipose tissue with a focus on insulin signaling, carbohydrate metabolism, and diabetic pathways [17]. The second was to determine associations between systemic insulin sensitivity and gene expression in visceral and subcutaneous adipose tissue.

2. Materials and Methods

2.1. Adipose Tissue Collection

Non-obese healthy pregnant women between the ages of 18 to 45 years old were recruited during prenatal care. Women who were scheduled for an elective cesarean delivery and had a normal glucose challenge test were included. After obtaining informed consent and routine prenatal care, during the cesarean delivery, maternal blood, cord blood, subcutaneous adipose tissue samples (from the abdominal wall at the edge of the surgical incision), and omental adipose tissue samples were all obtained. The adipose tissues were flash frozen in liquid nitrogen and stored in a $-80°C$ freezer. The Cedars-Sinai Medical Center Institutional Review Board approved the study.

2.2. RNA Extraction and Labeling

Total RNA was extracted from adipose tissues using RNeasy Lipid Tissue kit from Qiagen following the manufacturer's instructions. Biotin-labeled cRNA synthesis and amplification was performed using Illumina Total Prep RNA Amplification kit (Ambion) following manufacturers protocol.

2.3. Microarray Hybridization, Staining and Scanning

Biotin labeled cRNA (750 ng) was loaded on to Illumina HumanHT-12 V4.0 Expression BeadChip in hybridization buffer with hybridization controls and incubated for 16 hours at 58°C. After hybridization, BeadChips were washed, blocked with blocking buffer, and stained with streptavidin-Cy3 (Amersham Biosciences). Images of stained BeadChips were captured by Illumina BeadArray Reader.

2.4. Microarray Image Processing and Data Analysis

BeadChip images were loaded into Illumina GenomeStudio for quality determination by evaluation of the present call percentages, signal intensities of hybridization control, biotin controls, and negative controls, with quantile normalization. Signal intensities of each gene/probe were exported into Partek Genomic Suite 6.5 and ANOVA model was used to evaluate the impacts of various variables in the study such as different adipose tissues, patient ethnicity, patient-to-patient variability, etc., on the expression data set. Differentially expressed genes of subcutaneous versus omental adipose tissue were defined as a 1.5-fold difference in either direction plus pair-wise t-test. Benjamini & Hochberg procedure was applied with a false discovery rate (FDR) threshold of $p < 0.05$ to adjust for multiple testing. DAVID Bioinformatics Resources 6.7 was used to conduct functional classification and pathway analysis (National Institute of Allergy and Infectious Diseases, NIAID, NIH) [18]-[20].

2.5. Real-Time PCR Validation of Microarray Results

Quantitative RT-PCR was used to verify the differential expression level of several genes. A ratio greater than 1 reflected a greater level of transcript expression within the omental adipose group compared with the subcutaneous adipose group. We selected the genes that had the highest fold change in the analysis (CLDN1, CFB) as well as six genes (IL-6, IL-1B, SLC2A1, HSD11B1, ADIPOQ, IRS1, PLA2G2A) that had well recognized insulin signaling, inflammatory and metabolic function.

RNA was first reverse-transcribed to cDNA using iScript Reverse Transcription Supermix for RT-qPCR (Bio-rad). About 10 ng cDNA were mixed with gene specific primers and Platinum Sybr Green qPCR Super-Mix-UDG (Invitrogen). Real-time PCR was carried out in ABI 7000 Sequence Detector (AppliedBiosystems) for 40 cycles. The expression level of human GAPDH gene was used as an internal control, and fold changes of omental adipose group versus subcutaneous group were calculated using ΔCT method.

2.6. Matusda-Insulin Sensitivity Calculation

On 11 subjects, a frequently Sampled Oral Glucose Tolerance Test (FSOGTT) was performed. Patients had to be on a 300 grams carbohydrate per day diet. After obtaining a fasting blood sample, a 75 gram glucose solution was ingested orally. Blood samples were obtained every 15 minutes for 3 hours. Glucose and insulin levels were determined and recorded. Insulin sensitivity was calculated using Matsuda index. Matusda *et al.* developed an index of whole-body insulin sensitivity using 10,000/(square root of fasting glucose × fasting insulin × mean glucose × mean insulin during OGTT), which is highly correlated with the rate of whole-body glucose disposal during the euglycemic insulin clamp [21]. The homeostasis model assessment of insulin resistance (HOMA-IR) index, the product of basal glucose and insulin levels divided by 22.5 [22], is regarded as a simple, reliable measure of insulin resistance. HOMA-IR was calculating according to the following formula: fasting insulin (μIU/ml) × fasting glucose (mmol/ml)/22.5 [23].

2.7. Gene Mapping

DEGs were mapped to the Kyoto Encyclopedia of Genes and Genomes (KEGG) pathways; a collection of pathway maps representing current knowledge on molecular interaction and reaction networks classified as Global, Metabolism, Genetic Information Processing, Environmental Information Processing, Cellular Processes, Organismal Systems, Human Diseases and Drug Development with each molecular interaction and reaction network including multiple pathways [17]. Utilizing NIH David [19], Gene Card [24], KEGG pathway database [17], and PubMed [25], extensive review was done of known functions of DEGs in regards to gene tendency towards insulin resistance (IR) or insulin sensitivity (IS). In this review, DEGs whose cellular function would cause decreased plasma glucose level or facilitate insulin action were classified as insulin sensitive and genes whose functions would cause increased plasma glucose levels or block insulin action were classified as insulin resistant.

Pearson's correlation test was applied for transcript expression levels and insulin sensitivity scores. Separate analyses were performed for subcutaneous and visceral adipose tissues. Gene transcripts determined to be significantly correlated with both HOMA-IR score and Matsuda index were selected for pathway analysis. A cutoff p-value of <0.01 was used to determine significance.

3. Results

3.1. Demographic and Categorical Factors

The study is based on 14 patients who had an elective Cesarean section performed between 2008 and 2010. Patients were screened for any pre-existing diabetic condition; oral glucose tolerance test results were normal and excluded gestational diabetes. The mean age was 32.1 years (SD = 6.21), the mean BMI was 23.3 (SD = 2.88), the mean gestational age at delivery was 39 + 0/7 weeks (SD = 4.37 days), and the mean birth weight was 3240 grams (SD = 384.7 grams) (**Table 1**).

Categorical factors including fat, BMI, and race were analyzed using ANOVA to gauge each factor's contribution and for allowing the identification of significant sources of variation. Factors having a ratio greater than 1 were considered significant and not attributable to error. Adipose tissue had almost a five-fold effect with an F ratio of 4.77. BMI had a ratio of 2.02, highlighting the impact of BMI. Anticipating this factor, the study was planned to minimize the effect of obesity by excluding from the study any women with a BMI of 30 (classified as obese). Race had a ratio of 1.8. Although the race factor is higher than can be attributed to error, comparing the interaction of race with adipose tissue on differential gene expression using a mixed model ANOVA showed an effect of only 1.25, suggesting minimal impact of race on the differential gene expression of adipose tissue (**Figure 1**).

Table 1. Demographic data of the study population.

	Race	Age	Gestational AGE	Birth weight	Weight at Delivery	BMI*
Patient 1	Afr Am	33	40 + 0	3213	75.8	22.2
Patient 2	Afr Am	28	39 + 0	3950	77.1	25.5
Patient 3	Afr Am	41	39 + 1	3210	88.9	26.3
Patient 4	Asian	30	39 + 5	2760	59.0	20.7
Patient 5	Asian	31	38 + 2	3230	78.9	23.0
Patient 6	Caucasian	20	39 + 0	3400	75.4	20.8
Patient 7	Caucasian	38	39 + 0	3493	89.0	22.3
Patient 8	Caucasian	36	37 + 2	2850	78.4	24.9
Patient 9	Hispanic	37	39 + 0	2769	56.7	18.7
Patient 10	Hispanic	37	39 + 0	3420	58.0	21.0
Patient 11	Hispanic	26	39 + 1	3460	82.6	21.7
Patient 12	Hispanic	38	38 + 5	2630	77.1	23.0
Patient 13	Hispanic	32	39 + 0	3760	84.8	25.8
Patient 14	Hispanic	23	38 + 5	3210	95.3	29.7
Mean		32.1	39 + 0	3240	77.0	23.3
SD		6.21	4.37 days	384.7	12.3	2.88

Gestational Age given in number of weeks + days/7. Birth weight in grams. Age in years. BMI = Pre-pregnancy body mass index; Afr Am = African American.

3.2. Upregulated and Downregulated Genes in KEGG Pathways

In the comparison of omental versus subcutaneous adipose tissue, 920 genes showed significant relative fold change of expression level, of which 332 genes showed decreased expression levels and 588 genes showed increased expression levels.

We focused our analysis on the 17 differentially expressed genes in the insulin signaling (**Figure 2**), diabetic (**Figure 3**) and carbohydrate metabolism KEGG pathways that were associated in the literature with insulin sensitivity or resistance.

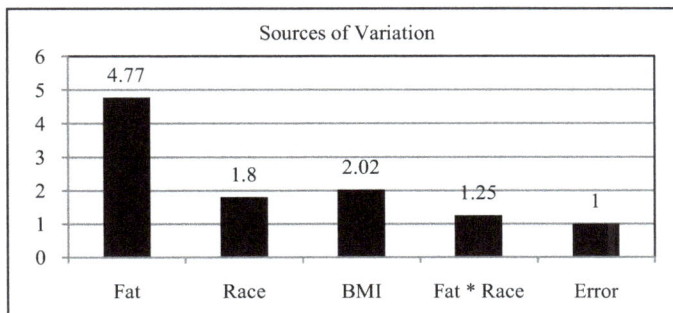

Figure 1. ANOVA model used to evaluate the impacts of the potential confounding variables: fat, race, BMI, fat and race in the differentially expressed genes in the study population. The horizontal column indicates the Mean F Ratio while the various factors analyzed in the multi factor ANOVA are listed horizontally along the x-axis. Any factor that has a Mean F Ratio more than error (1) is considered "significant".

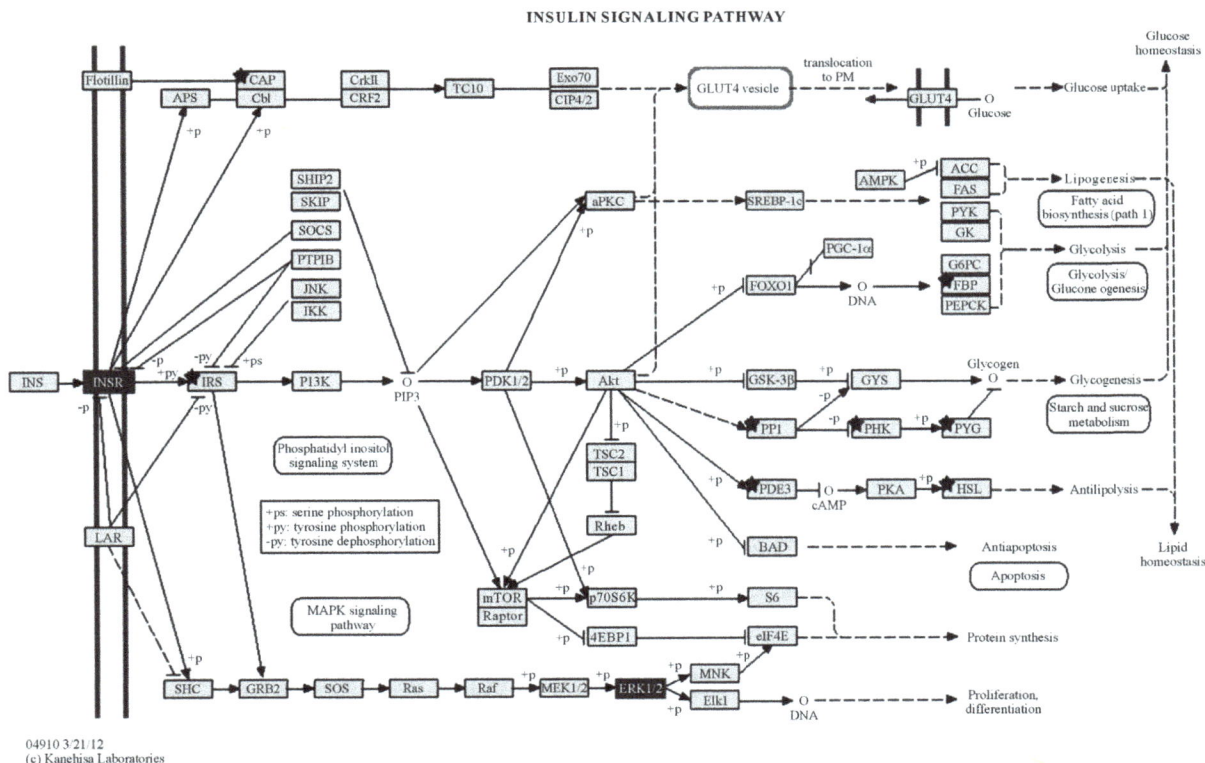

Figure 2. Graphic representation of KEGG insulin signaling pathway. Genes marked with stars are significantly differentially expressed in omental versus subcutaneous adipose tissue.

TYPE II DIABETES MELLITUS

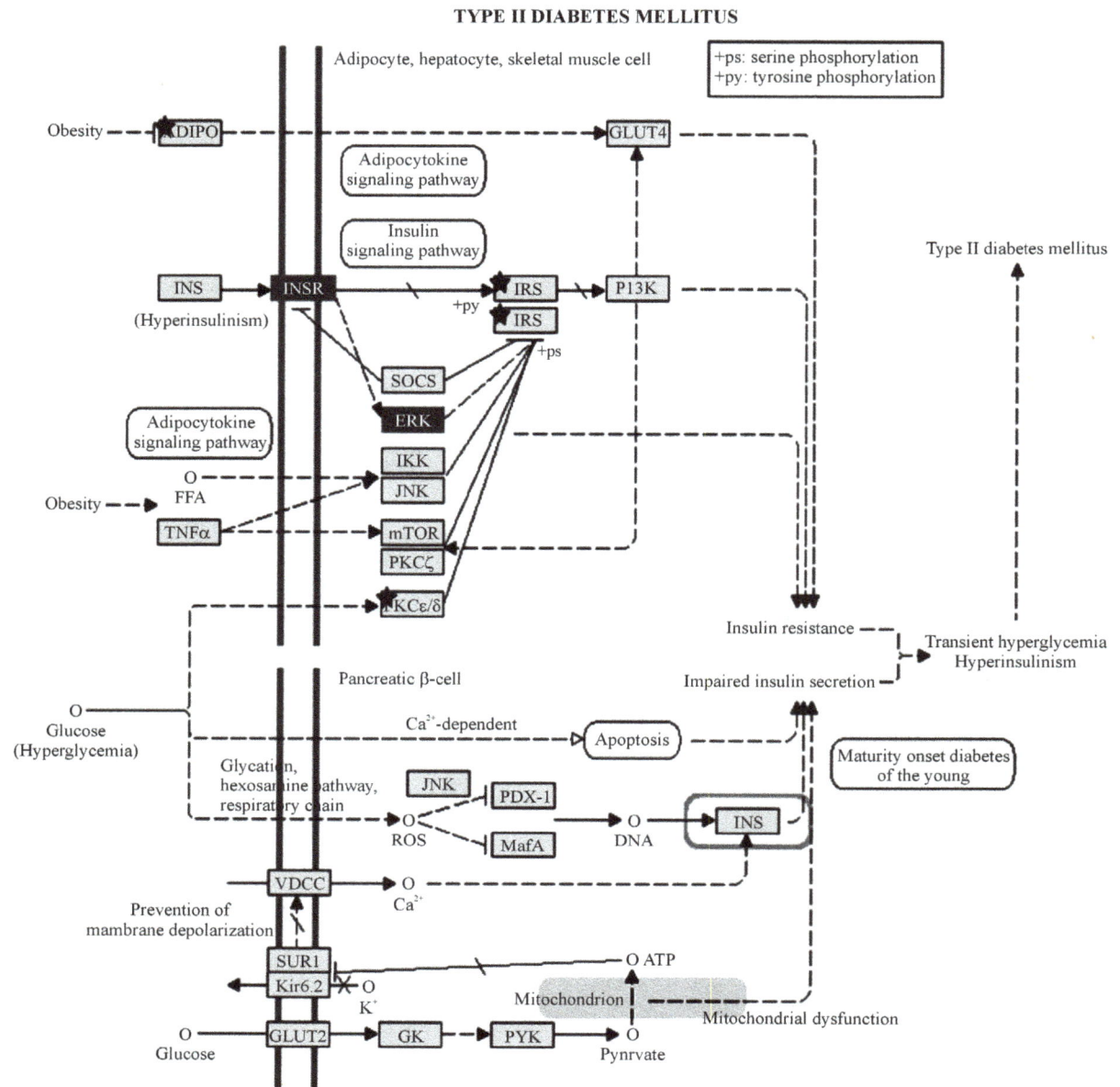

04930 7/2/09
(c) Kanehisa Laboratories

Figure 3. Graphic representation of KEGG Type II diabetes mellitus pathway. Genes marked with stars are significantly differentially expressed in omental versus subcutaneous adipose tissue.

3.3. Genes Differentially Expressed Towards Increased Insulin Sensitivity

2 upregulated genes in omental adipose were associated with increased insulin sensitivity: Protein phosphatase 1, regulatory (inhibitor) subunit 3C (PPP1R3C), and Phosphofructokinase, muscle (PFKM).

3 downregulated genes were associated with increased insulin resistance: Phosphorylase kinase, delta (PHK), Protein kinase C delta (PRKCD), Phosphorylase, glycogen, liver (PYGL) (**Table 2**).

3.4. Genes Differentially Expressed toward Increased Insulin Sensitivity

2 upregulated genes in omental adipose were associated in the literature with increased insulin resistance: FBP1 and GFPT2.

Table 2. Genes differentially expressed towards insulin sensitivity in omental vs. subcutaneous adipose.

Symbol	Gene Name	Gene Function	Microarray Fold Change	p-Value
PHK	Phosphorylasekinase, delta	Catalyzes phosphorylation of serine in substrates. Increases glycogenolysis.	−1.743	6.50E−06
PRKCD	Protein kinase C delta	Functioning as a pro-apoptotic protein during DNA damage-induced apoptosis, may impair insulin secretion due to apoptosis.	−1.63	6.28E−05
PYGL	Phosphorylase, glycogen, liver	Rate-determining enzyme catalyzing glycogen degradation.	−1.50	1.66E−03
PPP1R3C	Protein phosphatase 1, regulatory (inhibitor) subunit 3C	Activates glycogen synthase, reduces glycogen phosphorylase activity and limits glycogen breakdown. Dramatically increases basal and insulin-stimulated glycogen synthesis.	+1.69	1.37E−03
PFKM	Phosphofructokinase, muscle	Catalyzes the phosphorylation of fructose-6-phosphate to fructose-1,6-bisphosphate, prior to its cleavage into glyceraldehyde-3-phosphate which enters the energy generation phase of glycolysis.	+2.27	1.47E−07

10 downregulated DEG associated with increased insulin sensitivity were identified: GBE1, LIPE, SORBS1, IRS1, ADIPOQ, PFKFB3, ME1, IDH1, ACSS2, PFKFB1 (**Table 3**).

3.5. Correlation of Insulin Sensitivity and HOMA-IR with Differentially Expressed Genes

In the second stage of our study, we evaluated the correlation between insulin sensitivity (IS), HOMA-IR, with gene expression in omental and subcutaneous tissue.

In subcutaneous tissue, expression of 22 genes correlated significantly with IS. Of these, 15 had a negative correlation with IS and 7 had a positive correlation with IS. Only 5 genes matched to known genes in NIH David database with none mapping to the insulin signaling, diabetic, or carbohydrate metabolism pathways.

In omental adipose, 509 genes significantly correlated with IS. Of these, 325 matched to known genes in NIH David database. Of these, 2 genes were in the insulin signaling or type 2 diabetic KEGG pathways.

Two genes, insulin receptor (INSR) and mitogen-activated protein kinase 3 (MAPK1), strongly positively correlated with IS (**Table 4**).

3.6. Real-Time PCR Validation of Microarray Results

Table 5 shows the quantitative RT-PCR results for the nine positional candidate genes and confirms the differential expression of all upregulated genes and downregulated genes with the microarray analysis. For example, for the CFB gene the microarray fold change was 10.62 and the RT-PCR fold change was 11.6.

4. Discussion

Pregnancy is associated with a decrease in insulin sensitivity of 50% - 60% by the latter half of pregnancy with a 200% - 250% increase in insulin secretion to maintain euglycemia [26]. Adipose tissue plays a central role in the development of insulin resistance because it is insulin responsive and contributes directly, although quantitatively less than skeletal muscle, to the whole-body glucose disposal [1] [4] [8] [27] [28]. Our results suggest that omental tissue in comparison to subcutaneous adipose tissue may have more metabolic pathways alterations that affect carbohydrate metabolism and insulin function, which may contribute to the decreased insulin sensitivity in pregnancy.

In the insulin-signaling pathway, 4 genes were differentially expressed towards decreased insulin sensitivity in omental vs. subcutaneous adipose. IRS1 is downregulated, and it is a crucial gene in insulin sensitivity because it mediates the various cellular processes of insulin [11] [17] [29] [30]. Also downregulated are sorbin and SH3 domain containing 1 (SORBS1), required for insulin-stimulated glucose transport [31], and Lipase, hormone-sensitive (LIPE), shown to have decreased activity in insulin resistant and obese states [32] [33]. Fructose-1,6-

Table 3. Genes differentially expressed towards insulin resistance in omental vs. subcutaneous adipose.

Symbol	Gene Name	Gene Function	Microarray Fold Change	p-Value
FBP1	fructose-1,6-bisphosphatase 1	Gluconeogenesis regulatory enzyme, catalyzes the hydrolysis of fructose 1,6-bisphosphate to fructose 6-phosphate and inorganic phosphate. upregulation of FBPase in pancreatic islet beta-cells, as occurs in states of lipid oversupply and type 2 diabetes, contributes to insulin secretory dysfunction.	+1.72	2.32E−03
GFPT2	glutamine-fructose-6-phosphate transaminase 2	Controls the flux of glucose into the hexosamine pathway. Regulates availability of precursors for glycosylation of proteins. Increased GFAT activity appears to be associated with insulin resistance, postprandial hyperglycaemia and oxidative stress in T2DM.	+3.47	1.68E−05
GBE1	glucan (1,4-alpha-), branching enzyme 1	Required for sufficient glycogen accumulation. The alpha 1 - 6 branches of glycogen play an important role in increasing the solubility of the molecule and, consequently, in reducing the osmotic pressure within cells.	−4.27	0.000493696
LIPE	Lipase, hormone-sensitive	In adipose tissue, it hydrolyzes stored triglycerides to free fatty acids. Rate-limiting enzyme responsible for triglyceride breakdown. Decreased in IR and obese states	−2.36	7.33E−04
SORBS1	sorbin and SH3 domain containing 1	Required for insulin-stimulated glucose transport.	−2.20	2.34E−04
IRS1	Insulin receptor substrate 1	Mediates cellular processes of insulin. Mutations associated with type II diabetes and insulin resistance.	−1.78	1.46E−05
ADIPOQ	Adiponectin	Important adipokine involved in the control of fat metabolism and insulin sensitivity, with direct anti-diabetic, anti-atherogenic and anti-inflammatory activities. Stimulates AMPK phosphorylation and activation in the liver and the skeletal muscle, enhancing glucose utilization and fatty-acid combustion. Antagonizes TNF-alpha. Inhibits endothelial NF-kappa-B signaling through a cAMP-dependent pathway.	−1.67	3.98E−02
PFKFB3	6-phosphofructo-2-kinase/ fructose-2,6-biphosphatase 3	Catalyzes the synthesis and degradation of fructose 2,6-bisphosphate (F2,6BP), which is a powerful activator of 6-phosphofructo-1-kinase, the rate-limiting enzyme of glycolysis. Induced by insulin in adipose tissue.	−1.67	0.0053397
ME1	Malic enzyme 1, NADP(+)-dependent, cytosolic	Reversible oxidative decarboxylation of malate, links the glycolytic and citric acid cycle.	−1.64	0.00107314
IDH1	Isocitratedehydrogenase 1 (NADP+), soluble	Catalyze the oxidative decarboxylation of isocitrate to 2-oxoglutarate. Significant role in cytoplasmic NADPH production.	−1.63	0.000787487
ACSS2	acyl-CoAsynthetase short-chain family member 2	Catalyzes the activation of acetate for use in lipid synthesis and energy generation.	−1.60	0.000415893
PFKFB1	6-phosphofructo-2-kinase/ fructose-2,6-biphosphatase 1	Activates glycolysis & inhibits gluconeogenesis. Regulate glucose homeostasis.	−1.51	0.0133634

Table 4. Correlations between insulin sensitivity, HOMA-R and microarray differential gene expression mapping to KEGG insulin signaling, type 2 diabetes mellitus and carbohydrate metabolism pathways in omental tissue of healthy non-obese pregnant women.

Gene Name	Gene Symbol	Rho (ISI Matsuda Index)	p-Value (ISI Matsuda Index)	HOMA IR, Rho
Mitogen-activated protein kinase 3	MAPK1 (ERK)	0.78	0.004	-0.52
Insulin receptor	INSR	0.84	0.001	-0.64

Legend: ISI matsuda: Matusda-Insulin sensitivity index; HOMA IR: homeostasis model assessment of insulin resistance; Rho: correlation coefficient.

Table 5. Real-time PCR validation of microarray results.

Gene	Gene Name	Ref_seq	Fold Change	
			Microarray	RT-PCR
IL-6		NM_000600	2.19	1.23
IL-1B		NM_000576	2.00	1.31
CLDN1		NM_021101	18.61	13.89
SLC2A1		NM_006516	1.59	1.93
HSD11B1		NM_181755	2.60	1.95
ADIPOQ		NM_004797	−1.67	−1.58
CFB		NM_001710	10.62	11.60
IRS1		NM_005544	−1.77	−1.48
PLA2G2A		NM_000300	4.48	3.50

Ref_Seq = reference sequence.

bisphosphatase 1 (FBP1) is upregulated, and it is associated with decreased insulin sensitivity because it regulates gluconeogenesis and has been shown to contribute to insulin secretory dysfunction [34].

In the insulin signaling pathway, 3 genes were differentially expressed towards increased insulin sensitivity in omental vs. subcutaneous adipose. Two genes are downregulated: phosphorylase, glycogen, liver (PYGL) which is involved in glycogen degradation [35], and calmodulin 1, phosphorylase kinase, delta (PHK), which increases glycogenolysis [36]. One gene is upregulated: protein phosphatase 1, regulatory (inhibitor) subunit 3C (PPP1R3C), which is associated with insulin sensitivity because it activates glycogen synthase, reduces glycogen phosphorylase activity and limits glycogen breakdown [37].

In the Type-2 diabetic pathway, Adiponectin was downregulated in omental adipose compared with subcutaneous adipose. Adiponectin is an endogenous insulin-sensitizing hormone, which has anti-diabetic, anti-atherogenic and anti-inflammatory roles [30]. Decreased serum levels of adiponectin in early pregnancy have been shown to predict increased risks of GDM [4] [8].

Several genes of carbohydrate metabolism were differentially expressed in omental versus subcutaneous adipose towards insulin resistance. 6-phosphofructo-2-kinase/fructose-2,6-biphosphatase 3 (PFKFB3) [38] [39] was downregulated in omental versus subcutaneous adipose. PFKFB3 is associated with increased insulin sensitivity because it is the rate-limiting enzyme in glycolysis. Glycolysis involves the anaerobic breakdown of glucose to two pyruvates. Pyruvate is converted to acetyl CoA, which enters the TCA cycle. The TCA cycle is used aerobically to generate energy through the oxidization of acetate, derived from carbohydrates, fats and proteins, to carbon dioxide [17] [40]. Other downregulated genes associated with increased insulin sensitivity include other TCA and glycolytic pathway genes (**Table 1**), 1,4-alpha-glucan-branching enzyme 1 (GBE1) which is required for glycogen accumulation [41] [42], and inositol 1,3,4-triphosphate 5/6 kinase (ITPK1) which inhibits TNF alpha induced cell death [43]. Glutamine-fructose-6-phosphate transaminase (GFPT2), associated with insulin resistance and oxidative stress, was upregulated [44]. Further, phosphofructokinase muscle (PFKM), a major insulin glycolytic gene [45] [46], was downregulated, while aldehyde dehydrogenase 3 family, member B1 (ALDH3B1), which converted acetaldehyde to acetate for glycolysis [47] [48], was upregulated in omental vs. subcutaneous adipose.

We identified 5 genes involved in the insulin signaling, diabetic and carbohydrate metabolism pathways in omental adipose that showed significant correlations with IS and HOMA-IR but none in subcutaneous adipose. Insulin sensitivity was strongly positively correlated with insulin receptor (INSR) [49] [50] gene expression in omental adipose (r = 0.84). Insulin receptor binds insulin and is thus a key mediator of the metabolic effects of insulin. MAPK1 [51] [52], which regulates protein synthesis in response to insulin and is associated with cell survival, is also strongly positively correlated (r = 0.78) with insulin sensitivity.

Our findings support and add to previously published studies on adipose tissue. We show a decrease in expression of IRS-1 in omental adipose as compared with subcutaneous adipose, which has been observed in previous studies [10]-[12] [14] [53]. However, we did not find a difference in GLUT4 [13] [14] or in GS activity and GSK-3 expression as in other studies [14] [30]. Notably, previous reports studied diseased states (obesity, GDM and T2DM), and since we investigated only normal non-obese individuals, we would expect the cellular defects to be milder. We further found decreased expressions of adiponectin, glycolysis and TCA genes in omental adipose.

Furthermore, we showed a strong positive correlation between insulin receptor gene expression in omental adipose and systemic insulin sensitivity, with no correlation seen in subcutaneous tissue. This finding suggests the clinical significance of omental adipose of systemic insulin resistance in our study, and calls for further elucidation of the potential role of omental adipose in the pathophysiology of insulin resistance in pregnancy.

Disclosure

None of the authors have a conflict of interest

References

[1] Catalano, P.M. (2010) Obesity, Insulin Resistance, and Pregnancy Outcome. *Reproduction*, **140**, 365-371. http://dx.doi.org/10.1530/REP-10-0088

[2] Ding, A. Insulin Receptor Signaling Pathway. http://www.cellsignal.com/reference/pathway/Insulin_Receptor.html

[3] Kanehisa Laboratories. Insulin Signaling Pathway, KEGG Database. http://www.genome.jp/kegg/pathway/hsa/hsa04910.html

[4] Barbour, L.A., McCurdy, C.E., Hernandez, T.L., Kirwan, J.P., Catalano, P.M. and Friedman, J.E. (2007) Cellular Mechanisms for Insulin Resistance in Normal Pregnancy and Gestational Diabetes. *Diabetes Care*, **30**, S112-S119. http://dx.doi.org/10.2337/dc07-s202

[5] Centers for Disease Control and Prevention (2008) National Diabetes Fact Sheet: General Information and National Estimates on Diabetes in the United States, 2007. U.S. Department of Health and Human Services, Centers for Disease Control and Prevention, Atlanta.

[6] American College of Obstetricians and Gynecologists (2001) Gestational Diabetes. ACOG Practice Bulletin No. 30. *Obstetrics & Gynecology*, **98**, 525-538.

[7] Bergman, R.N., Kim, S.P., Catalano, K.J., *et al.* (2006) Why Visceral Fat Is Bad: Mechanisms of the Metabolic Syndrome. *Obesity*, **14**, 16S-19S. http://dx.doi.org/10.1038/oby.2006.277

[8] Valsamakis, G., Kumar, S., Creatsas, G. and Mastorakos, G. (2010) The Effects of Adipose Tissue and Adipocytokines in Human Pregnancy. *Annals of the New York Academy of Sciences*, **1205**, 76-81. http://dx.doi.org/10.1111/j.1749-6632.2010.05667.x

[9] Resi, V., Basu, S., Haghiac, M., *et al.* (2012) Molecular inflammation and adipose tissue matrix remodeling precede physiological adaptations to pregnancy. *American Journal of Physiology-Endocrinology and Metabolism*, **303**, E832-E840. http://dx.doi.org/10.1152/ajpendo.00002.2012

[10] Friedman, J.E., Ishizuka, T., Shao, J., Huston, L., Highman, T. and Catalano, P. (1999) Impaired Glucose Transport and Insulin Receptor Tyrosine Phosphorylation in Skeletal Muscle from Obese Women with Gestational Diabetes. *Diabetes*, **48**, 1807-1814. http://dx.doi.org/10.2337/diabetes.48.9.1807

[11] Catalano, P.M., Nizielski, S.E., Shao, J., Preston, L., Qiao, L. and Friedman, J.E. (2002) Downregulated IRS-1 and PPAR Gamma in Obese Women with Gestational Diabetes: Relationship to FFA during Pregnancy. *American Journal of Physiology*: Endocrinology and Metabolism, **282**, E522-E533. http://dx.doi.org/10.1152/ajpendo.00124.2001

[12] Tomazic, M., Janez, A., Sketelj, A., Kocijancic, A., Eckel, J. and Sharma, P.M. (2002) Comparison of Alterations in Insulin Signaling Pathway in Adipocytes from Type II Diabetic Pregnant Women with Gestational Diabetes Mellitus. *Diabetologia*, **45**, 502-508. http://dx.doi.org/10.1007/s00125-002-0791-z

[13] Garvey, W.T., Maianu, L., Zhu, J.H., Hancock, J.A. and Golichowski, A.M. (1993) Multiple Defects in the Adipocyte Glucose Transport System Cause Cellular Insulin Resistance in Gestational Diabetes. Heterogeneity in the Number and a Novel Abnormality in Subcellular Localization of GLUT4 Glucose Transporters. *Diabetes*, **42**, 1773-1785. http://dx.doi.org/10.2337/diab.42.12.1773

[14] Colomiere, M., Permezel, M. and Lappas, M. (2010) Diabetes and Obesity during Pregnancy Alter Insulin Signalling and Glucose Transporter Expression in Maternal Skeletal Muscle and Subcutaneous Adipose Tissue. *Journal of Molecular Endocrinology*, **44**, 213-223. http://dx.doi.org/10.1677/JME-09-0091

[15] Linder, K., Arner, P., Flores-Morales, A., Tollet-Egnell, P. and Norstedt, G. (2004) Differentially Expressed Genes in Visceral or Subcutaneous Adipose Tissue of Obese Men and Women. *The Journal of Lipid Research*, **45**, 148-154.

http://dx.doi.org/10.1194/jlr.M300256-JLR200

[16] Lee, Y.H., Nair, S., Rousseau, E., Allison, D.B., Page, G.P., Tataranni, P.A., Bogardus, C. and Permana, P.A. (2005) Microarray Profiling of Isolated Abdominal Subcutaneous Adipocytes from Obese vs Non-Obese Pima Indians: Increased Expression of Inflammation-Related Genes. *Diabetologia*, **48**, 1776-1783. http://dx.doi.org/10.1007/s00125-005-1867-3

[17] Kanehisa Laboratories. KEGG Pathway Database. Accessed 10 December 2013. http://www.genome.jp/kegg/pathway.html

[18] Huang, D.W., Sherman, B.T. and Lempicki, R.A. (2009) Systematic and Integrative Analysis of Large Gene Lists Using DAVID Bioinformatics Resources. *Nature Protocols*, **4**, 44-57. http://dx.doi.org/10.1038/nprot.2008.211

[19] Huang, D.W., Sherman, B.T. and Lempicki, R.A. (2009) Bioinformatics Enrichment Tools: Paths toward the Comprehensive Functional Analysis of Large Gene Lists. *Nucleic Acids Research*, **37**, 1-13. http://dx.doi.org/10.1093/nar/gkn923

[20] National Institute of Allergy and Infectious Diseases (NIAID), NIH. DAVID Bioinformatics Resources 6.7. http://david.abcc.ncifcrf.gov

[21] Matsuda, M. and DeFronzo, R.A. (1999) Insulin Sensitivity Indices Obtained from Oral Glucose Tolerance Testing: Comparison with the Euglycemic Insulin Clamp. *Diabetes Care*, **22**, 1462-1470. http://dx.doi.org/10.2337/diacare.22.9.1462

[22] Matthews, D.R., Hosker, J.P., Rudenski, A.S., Naylor, B.A., Treacher, D.F. and Turner, R.C. (1985) Homeostasis Model Assessment: Insulin Resistance and Beta-Cell Function from Fasting Plasma Glucose and Insulin Concentrations in Man. *Diabetologia*, **28**, 412-419. http://dx.doi.org/10.1007/BF00280883

[23] Song, Y., Manson, J.E., Tinker, L., Howard, B.V., Kuller, L.H., Nathan, L., *et al.* (2007) Insulin Sensitivity and Insulin Secretion Determined by Homeostasis Model Assessment (HOMA) and Risk of Diabetes in a Multiethnic Cohort of Women: The Women's Health Initiative Observational Study. *Diabetes Care*, **30**, 1747-1752. http://dx.doi.org/10.2337/dc07-0358

[24] Crown Human Genome Center, Weizmann Institute of Science. GeneCards. Accessed 5 March 2013. http://www.genecards.org

[25] National Institutes of Health. PubMed. Accessed 5 March 2013. http://www.ncbi.nlm.nih.gov/pubmed

[26] Catalano, P.M., Huston, L., Amini, S.B. and Kalhan, S.C. (1999) Longitudinal Changes in Glucose Metabolism during Pregnancy in Obese Women with Normal Glucose Tolerance and Gestational Diabetes Mellitus. *American Journal of Obstetrics & Gynecology*, **180**, 903-916. http://dx.doi.org/10.1016/S0002-9378(99)70662-9

[27] Hajer, G.R., van Haeften, T.W. and Visseren, F.L.J. (2008) Adipose Tissue Dysfunction in Obesity, Diabetes, and Vascular Diseases. *European Heart Journal*, **29**, 2959-2971. http://dx.doi.org/10.1093/eurheartj/ehn387

[28] Stump, C.S., Henriksen, E.J., Wei, Y. and Sowers, J.R. (2006) The Metabolic Syndrome: Role of Skeletal Muscle Metabolism. *Annals of Medicine*, **38**, 389-402. http://dx.doi.org/10.1080/07853890600888413

[29] Draznin, B. (2006) Molecular Mechanisms of Insulin Resistance: Serine Phosphorylation of Insulin Receptor Substrate-1 and Increased Expression of p85alpha: The Two Sides of a Coin. *Diabetes*, **55**, 2392-2397.

[30] Patel, S., Doble, B.W., MacAulay, K., Sinclair, E.M., Drucker, D.J. and Woodgett, J.R. (2008) Tissue-Specific Role of Glycogen Synthase Kinase 3 Beta in Glucose Homeostasis and Insulin Action. *Molecular and Cellular Biology*, **28**, 6314-6328. http://dx.doi.org/10.1128/MCB.00763-08

[31] Crown Human Genome Center, Weizmann Institute of Science. Sorbin and SH3 Domain Containing 1. Accessed 5 March 2013. http://www.genecards.org/cgi-bin/carddisp.pl?gene=SORBS1

[32] Jocken, J.W., Langin, D., Smit, E., Saris, W.H., Valle, C., Hul, G.B., Holm, C., Arner, P. and Blaak, E.E. (2007) Adipose Triglyceride Lipase and Hormone-Sensitive Lipase Protein Expression Is Decreased in the Obese Insulin-Resistant State. *The Journal of Clinical Endocrinology & Metabolism*, **92**, 2292-2299. http://dx.doi.org/10.1210/jc.2006-1318

[33] Jocken, J.W., Roepstorff, C., Goossens, G.H., van der Baan, P., van Baak, M., Saris, W.H.M., Kiens, B. and Blaak, E.E. (2008) Hormone-Sensitive Lipase Serine Phosphorylation and Glycerol Exchange across Skeletal Muscle in Lean and Obese Subjects: Effect of Beta-Adrenergic Stimulation. *Diabetes*, **57**, 1834-1841. http://dx.doi.org/10.2337/db07-0857

[34] Kebede, M., Favaloro, J., Gunton, J.E., Laybutt, D.R., Shaw, M., Wong, N., Fam, B.C., Aston-Mourney, K., Rantzau, C., Zulli, A., Proietto, J. and Andrikopoulos, S. (2008) Fructose-1,6-bisphosphatase Overexpression in Pancreatic Beta-Cells Results in Reduced Insulin Secretion: A New Mechanism for Fat-Induced Impairment of Beta-Cell Function. *Diabetes*, **57**, 1887-1895. http://dx.doi.org/10.2337/db07-1326

[35] Burwinkel, B., Bakker, H.D., Herschkovitz, E., Moses, S.W., Shin, Y.S. and Kilimann, M.W. (1998) Mutations in the Liver Glycogen Phosphorylase Gene (PYGL) Underlying Glycogenosis Type VI. *The American Journal of Human*

Genetics, **62**, 785-791. http://dx.doi.org/10.1086/301790

[36] Maichele, A.J., Burwinkel, B., Maire, I., Søvik, O. and Kilimann, M.W. (1996) Mutations in the Testis/Liver Isoform of the Phosphorylase Kinase Gamma Subunit (PHKG2) Cause Autosomal Liver Glycogenosis in the *Gsd* Rat and in Humans. *Nature Genetics*, **14**, 337-340. http://dx.doi.org/10.1038/ng1196-337

[37] Crown Human Genome Center, Weizmann Institute of Science. Protein Phosphatase 1, Regulatory Subunit 3C. http://www.genecards.org/cgi-bin/carddisp.pl?gene=PPP1R3C&search=PPP1R3C

[38] Atsumi, T., Nishio, T., Niwa, H., Takeuchi, J., Bando, H., Shimizu, C., Yoshioka, N., Bucala, R. and Koike, T. (2005) Expression of Inducible 6-phosphofructo-2-kinase/fructose-2,6-bisphosphatase/PFKFB3 Isoforms in Adipocytes and Their Potential Role in Glycolytic Regulation. *Diabetes*, **54**, 3349-3357. http://dx.doi.org/10.2337/diabetes.54.12.3349

[39] Huo, Y., Guo, X., Li, H., Xu, H., Halim, V., Zhang, W., *et al.* (2012) Targeted Overexpression of Inducible 6-phosphofructo-2-kinase in Adipose Tissue Increases Fat Deposition but Protects against Diet-Induced Insulin Resistance and Inflammatory Responses. *The Journal of Biological Chemistry*, **287**, 21492-21500. http://dx.doi.org/10.1074/jbc.M112.370379

[40] Kanehisa Laboratories. Type I Diabetes Mellitus—Homo Sapiens, KEGG Database. http://www.genome.jp/kegg/pathway/hsa/hsa04940.html

[41] Kanehisa Laboratories. Citrate Cycle (TCA Cycle). http://www.genome.jp/kegg/pathway/map/map00020.html

[42] Crown Human Genome Center, Weizmann Institute of Science. Glucan (1,4-Alpha-), Branching Enzyme 1. http://www.genecards.org/cgi-bin/carddisp.pl?gene=GBE1&search=GBE1

[43] Sun, Y., Mochizuki, Y. and Majerus, P.W. (2003) Inositol 1,3,4-trisphosphate 5/6-kinase Inhibits Tumor Necrosis Factor-Induced Apoptosis. *The Journal of Biological Chemistry*, **278**, 43645-43653. http://dx.doi.org/10.1074/jbc.M300674200

[44] Srinivasan, V., Sandhya, N., Sampathkumar, R., Farooq, S., Mohan, V. and Balasubramanyam, M. (2007) Glutamine Fructose-6-phosphate Amidotransferase (GFAT) Gene Expression and Activity in Patients with Type 2 Diabetes: Inter-Relationships with Hyperglycaemia and Oxidative Stress. *Clinical Biochemistry*, **40**, 952-957. http://dx.doi.org/10.1016/j.clinbiochem.2007.05.002

[45] Ristow, M., Vorgerd, M., Möhlig, M., Schatz, H. and Pfeiffer, A. (1999) Insulin Resistance and Impaired Insulin Secretion Due to Phosphofructo-1-kinase-deficiency in Humans. *Journal of Molecular Medicine*, **77**, 96-103. http://dx.doi.org/10.1007/s001090050311

[46] García, M., Pujol, A., Ruzo, A., Riu, E., Ruberte, J., Arbós, A., Serafín, A., Albella, B., Felíu, J.E. and Bosch, F. (2009) Phosphofructo-1-kinase Deficiency Leads to a Severe Cardiac and Hematological Disorder in Addition to Skeletal Muscle Glycogenosis. *PLoS Genetics*, **5**, e1000615. http://dx.doi.org/10.1371/journal.pgen.1000615

[47] Wang, Y., Ng, M.C., Lee, S.C., So, W.-Y., Tong, P.C.Y., Cockram, C.S., Critchley, J.A.J.H. and Chan, J.C.N. (2003) Phenotypic Heterogeneity and Associations of Two Aldose Reductase Gene Polymorphisms with Nephropathy and Retinopathy in Type 2 Diabetes. *Diabetes Care*, **26**, 2410-2415. http://dx.doi.org/10.2337/diacare.26.8.2410

[48] Neamat-Allah, M., Feeney, S.A., Savage, D.A., Maxwell, A.P., Hanson, R.L., Knowler, W.C., El Nahas, A.M., Plater, M.E., Shaw, J., Boulton, A.J.M., Duff, G.W. and Cox, A. (2001) Analysis of the Association between Diabetic Nephropathy and Polymorphisms in the Aldose Reductase Gene in Type 1 and Type 2 Diabetes Mellitus. *Diabetic Medicine*, **18**, 906-914. http://dx.doi.org/10.1046/j.0742-3071.2001.00598.x

[49] Jiang, S., Fang, Q., Zhang, F., Wan, H., Zhang, R., Wang, C., *et al.* (2011) Functional Characterization of Insulin Receptor Gene Mutations Contributing to Rabson-Mendenhall Syndrome—Phenotypic Heterogeneity of Insulin Receptor Gene Mutations. *Endocrine Journal*, **58**, 931-940. http://dx.doi.org/10.1507/endocrj.EJ11-0032

[50] Crown Human Genome Center, Weizmann Institute of Science. Insulin Receptor. http://www.genecards.org/cgi-bin/carddisp.pl?gene=INSR

[51] Sale, E.M., Atkinson, P.P., Arnott, C.H., Chad, J.E. and Sale, G.J. (1999) Role of ERK1/ERK2 and p70S6K Pathway in Insulin Signalling of Protein Synthesis. *FEBS Letters*, **446**, 122-126. http://dx.doi.org/10.1016/S0014-5793(99)00193-3

[52] Finlay, D., Healy, V., Furlong, F., O'Connell, F.C., Keon, N.K. and Martin, F. (2000) MAP Kinase Pathway Signaling Is Essential for Extracellular Matrix Determined Mammary Epithelial Cell Survival. *Cell Death & Differentiation*, **7**, 302-313. http://dx.doi.org/10.1038/sj.cdd.4400652

[53] Ogunyemi, D., Xu, J., Mahesan, A., Rad, S., Kim, E., Yano, J., Alexander, C., Rotter, J.I. and Ida Chen, Y.-D. (2013) Differentially Expressed Genes in Adipocytokine Signaling Pathway of Adipose Tissue in Pregnancy. *Journal of Diabetes Mellitus*, **3**, 86-95. http://dx.doi.org/10.4236/jdm.2013.32013

10

Correlation between Dietary Intake and Inflammatory Biomarkers in a Tunisian Obese Group

Manel Ayoub[1], Chedia Zouaoui[2], Nedra Grira[1], Radhia Kochkar[3], Nejla Stambouli[1], Chaker Bouguerra[4], Borni Zidi[2], Ezzedine Ghazouani[3], Chakib Mazigh[1], Zied Aouni[1*]

[1]Biochemistry Department, Research Unit, Military Hospital of Tunis, Tunis, Tunisia
[2]Endocrinology Department, Research Unit, Military Hospital of Tunis, Tunis, Tunisia
[3]Immunology Department, Military Hospital of Tunis, Tunis, Tunisia
[4]Epidemiology Department, Research Unit, Military Hospital of Tunis, Tunis, Tunisia
Email: *aouni_zied@yahoo.fr

Abstract

Aims: This study aims to determine the inflammatory status and evaluate the correlation between dietary intake and inflammatory biomarkers in a Tunisian obese group. Material and Methods: This is an open cross-sectional study that includes 81 individuals divided into two groups: a group of 42 obese patients recruited from the endocrinology department and a control group of 39 non-obese healthy subjects. All participants received a food survey, anthropometric measurements and blood sampling. Pro-inflammatory cytokines (IL-6, IL-8, TNF-α), and hs-CRP were measured in patients and controls. Results: Dietary data revealed significant increases in food intake in obese patients compared to controls. The results of the laboratory parameters showed a statistically significant increase in IL-8, TNF-α and blood glucose in obese compared to controls. The analysis of correlations among the parameters studied showed that the plasma level of IL-6 was positively correlated with dietary fat intake ($r = 0.70$; $p < 10^{-3}$) and carbohydrate ($r = 0.54$; $p = 0.03$) and the dietary intake expressed in calories ($r = 0.64$; $p < 10^{-3}$). Conclusion: dietary imbalances in obese were observed and characterized by an excessive intake of calories, fat and carbohydrates. The excessive carbohydrate and fat intake is associated with increased IL-6 and TNF-α plasma levels.

Keywords

Obesity, Dietary Intake, Inflammatory Biomarkers

---

*Corresponding author.

1. Introduction

Obesity is the epidemic of the 21st century. In developing countries, the number of obese people is increasing, and obesity is occurring at younger ages [1]. The fundamental cause of obesity and overweight is an energy imbalance between calories consumed and calories expended. As more is understood about obesity, the complexity of this chronic disorder becomes more apparent, exhibiting a multi-factorial etiology. Lifestyle factors such as diet and exercise continue to be recognized to play an important role in the development and progression of obesity and its comorbidities. However, genetic variation is also known to contribute to the obese phenotype [2]. The World Health Organization (WHO) has reported that obesity has been growing at an alarming rate, accounting for approximately 35% of the population. Obesity and overweight increase the risk of several serious chronic diseases, such as type 2 diabetes, cardiovascular disease, hypertension and stroke, hypercholesterolemia, and hypertriglyceridemia [3].

A common denominator that links these diseases to obesity is inflammation. While signals that initiate the inflammatory process remain unclear, emerging evidence suggests that nutrients and the modifications they cause in adipose tissue during situations of nutritional overload can activate immune sensors [4].

Adipose tissue, the main feature of obesity, was considered as an inert tissue mainly devoted to fat storage: However, it is now recognized as an active tissue in the regulation of physiological and pathological process, including immunity and inflammation. Adipose tissue produces and releases a variety of adipokines and cytokines, including leptin, adiponectin, TNF-α, IL-6... [5]. Many studies have reviewed the role of diet and dietary factors on inflammation state and its relationship to obesity [6] [7].

In our study, we aimed to determine the inflammatory status and evaluate the correlation between dietary intake and inflammatory biomarkers in a Tunisian obese group.

2. Materials and Methods

This is a prospective open cross sectional study conducted at the Biochemistry department in collaboration with the Endocrinology Service in Military Hospital of Tunis.

2.1. Study Population

Our population consists of 80 subjects divided into two groups: a group of obese subjects consisted of 41 individuals admitted to the endocrinology department. Weight and height were measured on barefoot and lightly clothed subjects. Body mass index (BMI; kg/m^2) was calculated and obesity was defined as BMI $\geq$ 30 kg/m^2. And a control group containing 39 healthy individuals whose clinical and anthropometric measures have eliminated the diagnosis obesity. The study objectives and procedure were explained to all participants, before obtaining their consent to enroll into the study.

2.2. Data Collection

All patients and controls have received a complete physical examination with determination of anthropometric parameters (weight, height, waist circumference and hip circumference). The nutritional profile of obese subjects and controls was established through a food survey. They were asked to complete a week dietary record, and to report exhaustively the exact amount of foods and beverages ingested. The same dietitian calculated the total daily intake of calories, carbohydrates, lipids and proteins by BILNUT software using a food composition data base. The BILNUT method range from detailed individual weighed records collected over a variable period of time to food frequency questionnaires and dietary recalls.

2.3. Blood Analyses

The hs-CRP was performed by a particle enhanced immunonephelometry method using polystyrene particles coated with monoclonal antibodies specific to human CRP on the BN Pro Spec analyser (Siemens). The result is evaluated by comparison with a standard of known concentration. Proinflammatory cytokines (IL-6, IL-8 and TNF-α) were measured by immunometric method with detection by chemiluminescence on Immulite system (Siemens).

2.4. Statistical Analysis

Data were entered and analyzed by SPSS 19.0 software release. The results were expressed as the number of cases and percentages for categorical variables and mean and standard deviation for quantitative variables. The comparative study on independent series was performed using the t test for quantitative variables and Chi-square test for categorical variables. The value of p = 0.05 is set as a threshold value below which a difference is taken as statistically significant.

3. Results

This study analyses a total of 81 subjects (42 obese patients and 39 non-obese healthy subjects).

Anthropometric and biochemical parameters for obese patients and controls are shown in **Table 1**.

The two study groups were matched for age and sex. It was noted that 92.7% of obese subjects had a family history of cardiovascular disease. Smoking was less common in obese compared to controls (17.1% vs. 31.6%), but without statistically significant difference.

Among the modifiable cardiovascular risk factors, hypertension was found in 36.6% of obese vs 5.4% of controls (p = 10^{-3}). Dyslipidemia was observed in 14.6% of obese and 4.3% of controls. Similarly, 22% were diabetic obese compared with 4.9% of controls (p = 0.04).

The plasma levels of hs-CRP were significantly higher in obese (p < 10^{-3}). We observed that the mean levels of TNF-α were significantly higher in obese compared to controls (p = 0.028). Similarly, a significant increase of the mean values of IL-8 was observed in the obese group (p = 0.013). The plasma levels of IL-6 were higher in obese but this increase was not significant (p = 0.3).

The daily intake of various nutrients is given in the **Table 2**.

Table 1. Anthropometric and biochemical parameters for obese patients and controls.

	Obese (n = 41)	Controls (n = 39)	p
Age	43.44 ± 10.34	41.35 ± 11.42	0.21
Gender M/W (%)	16.7/83.3	17.9/82.1	NS
BMI	39.17 ± 7.35	24.38 ± 3.78	<10^{-3}
Tobacco (%)	17.1	31.6	0.015
Hypertension (%)	36.6	5.4	0.001
Dyslipidemia (%)	14.6	4.3	0.018
Diabetes (%)	22	4.9	0.03
hs-CRP (mg/l)	5.46 ± 4.8	1.63 ± 1.75	<10^{-3}
TNF α (pg/ml)	6.99 ± 2.13	6.00 ± 1.60	0.028
IL-6 (pg/ml)	2.78 ± 1.85	2.50 ± 0.84	0.3
IL-8 (pg/ml)	9.38 ± 4.90	6.73 ± 2.37	0.013

M/W: male/woman.

Table 2. The daily intake of various nutrients in obese and control subjects.

	Obese (n = 41)	Controls (n = 39)	p
Protides (g/24h)	87.19 ± 36.18	55.9 ± 14.9	<10^{-3}
Carbohydrates (g/24h)	298.5 ± 184.99	202.3 ± 61.4	0.1
Lipids (g/24h)	114.68 ± 82.68	70.5 ± 19.6	0.007
Calories (Kcal/24h)	2580 ± 1494.15	1704.4 ± 374.9	0.003

The analysis of the association between dietary intake and pro-inflammatory cytokines in obese showed that the plasma levels of IL-6 was positively correlated with dietary fat intake (r = 0.70; p < 10^{-3}) (**Figure 1**) and carbohydrate (r = 0.54; p = 0.03) (**Figure 2**) and the total dietary intake expressed in calories (r = 0.64; p < 10^{-3}).

4. Discussion

Obesity is associated with a chronic increase of a set of inflammatory and lipid markers. Obese individuals in our series have high values of circulating TNF α and IL-8 compared to the control population. The mean values of IL-6 found in obese are higher than in the control population. However, this increase was not statistically significant. Our results are in agreement with most studies [8] [9].

During aggravation of obesity, there is an hypertrophy of the adipocytes. Indeed, adipose tissue of obese patients is the seat of macrophage accumulation [10]. These macrophages are a source of production of adipokines such as resistin and visfatin [11] and pro-inflammatory cytokines. In response to reservations of excess lipids, adipocytes secrete increasing amounts of inflammatory cytokines such as IL-6 and TNF-α and chemokines. These promote migration of macrophages in adipose tissue which increases the release of cytokines [12].

In our study, obese patients have significantly higher CRP concentrations compared to controls. Maria João Neuparth *et al*. [13] reported significantly higher CRP values in obese subjects compared to control groups. These authors have shown that CRP values tend to increase in overweight subjects. hs-CRP is produced by hepatocytes in response to proinflammatory cytokines, in particular IL-6, [14]. It should be noted that the liver and lymphoid organs are the main producers of these inflammatory mediators sites, but in obese individuals, fat

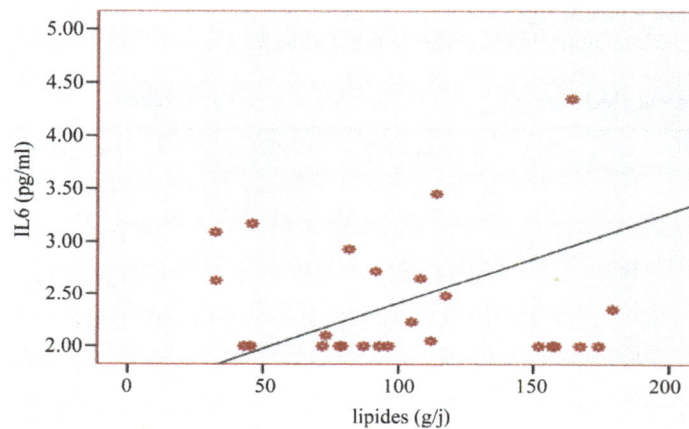

Figure 1. Correlation between lipids (g/j) and IL6 (pg/ml).

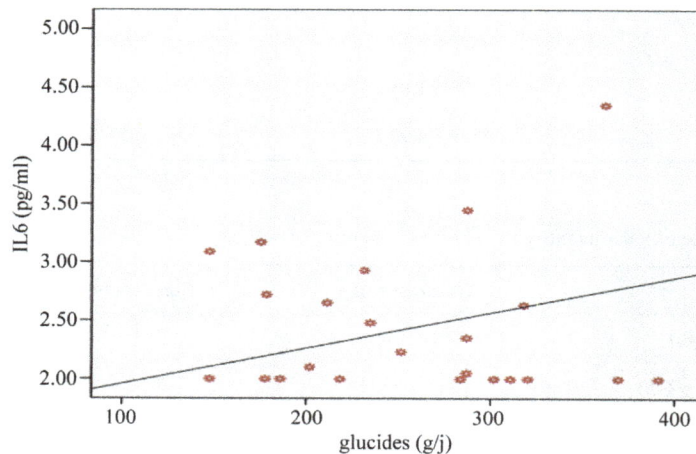

Figure 2. Correlation between glucides (g/j) and IL6 (pg/ml).

tissue becomes a major producer of these markers [15]. The nutritional profile of obese established through food survey was characterized by excessive calorie intake means. Furthermore, the distribution of energy nutrients in daily calorie intake is unbalanced in favor of an excess of lipid and carbohydrate consumption. These results are comparable to those of Fennira *et al.* [16] in a study of 108 nearby Tunisian obese adolescents.

In our study, we found a statistically significant correlation between IL-6 and dietary carbohydrate intake on the one hand and the contributions by the other lipids.

Several studies have examined the effect of different dietary fatty acids on the production of IL-6 and expression of the gene of IL-6 into the cell. In vitro studies have reported that incubation of the adipocytes with palmitic acid increases expression of the gene and production of IL-6. Furthermore, in mice fed a diet rich in fatty acids the expression of IL-6 gene is three times higher than in mice fed a diet low in fatty acids [2].

Food is an important factor in regulating the immune response. Overeating leads to immuno-activation due to a susceptibility to an inflammatory disease. Therefore, optimal nutrition is necessary for a healthy immune balance. But, a nutrient overload causes obesity which is a chronic inflammatory condition [17].

Increasing dietary intake of fatty acids, especially in people who have an overweight or obese is associated with increased concentrations of inflammatory markers, inducing inflammatory changes in adipocytes and macrophages and increasing the gene expression and adipocytokine production. It has been shown that when adipocytes are exposed to dietary fatty acids such as palmitic acid, the production of IL-6 and expression of mRNA increases. Similarly monocytes were activated directly when exposed to dietary fatty acids [2].

The same modest reduction in weight improves the complications related to obesity. Many studies show that reducing food intake and increasing physical activity are factors that reduce inflammation. When loosing weight, a reduction of many molecules of inflammation is observed, it is established for CRP, IL-6, IL-8 and TNF-α [18].

5. Conclusions

We have highlighted the existence of an inflammatory state in obesity marked by an increase in TNF α levels, IL-8 and hs-CRP.

Nutritionally, dietary imbalances in obese were observed characterized by an excessive intake of calories, fat and carbohydrates. A dietary impact of these errors on the metabolic profile was noted. According to the results of our work, excessive carbohydrate and fat intake is associated with increased IL-6 and TNF alpha. the reduction of inputs and the correction of dietary errors are unavoidable in the management of obesity. In this context, we recommend, to prevent obesity, to avoid foods that are high in "energy density" or that have a lot of calories in a small amount of food and focus on low-calorie, nutrient-dense foods, such as fruits, vegetables and whole grains.

However, our study has some limitations. The most important is the relatively small size of our study population.

Conflict of Interests

The author had no conflict of interests to report.

Acknowledgements

The authors thank all the technicians of the biochemistry lab in military hospital of Tunis, especially Mr. Zeddini Imed and Mrs. Baccour Ilhem, for their contributions to the realization of this work.

References

[1]   World Health Organization (2005) Fact Sheet: Obesity and Overweight. http://www.who.int/dietphysicalactivity/publications/facts/obesity/en/

[2]   Joffe, Y.T., Collins, M. and Goedecke, J.H. (2013) The Relationship between Dietary Fatty Acids and Inflammatory Genes on the Obese Phenotype and Serum Lipids. *Nutrients*, **5**, 1672-1705. http://dx.doi.org/10.3390/nu5051672

[3]   World Health Organization (2008) Obesity [Internet]. WHO, Geneva. http://www.who.int/topics/obesity/en/

[4]   Greenberg, A.S. and Obin, M.S. (2006) Obesity and the Role of Adipose Tissue in Inflammation and Metabolism. *American Journal of Clinical Nutrition*, **83**, 461S-465S.

[5]   Galic, S., Oakhill, J.S. and Steinberg, G.R. (2010) Adipose Tissue as an Endocrine Organ. *Molecular and Cellular Endocrinology*, **316**, 129-139. http://dx.doi.org/10.1016/j.mce.2009.08.018

[6]   Galland, L. (2010) Diet and Inflammation. *Nutrition in Clinical Practice*, **10**, 1164-1172. http://dx.doi.org/10.1177/0884533610385703

[7]   Calder, P.C., Ahluwalia, N., Brouns, F., Buetler, T., Clement, K., Cunningham, K., *et al* (2011) Dietary Factors and Low Grade Inflammation in Relation to Overweight and Obesity. *British Journal of Nutrition*, **106**, S5-S78. http://dx.doi.org/10.1017/s0007114511005460

[8]   Khosravi, R., Ka, K., Huang, T., Khalili, S., Hong Nguyen, B., Nicolau, B. and Simon, D. (2013) Tumor Necrosis Factor-α and Interleukin-6: Potential Interorgan Inflammatory Mediators Contributing to Destructive Periodontal Disease in Obesity or Metabolic Syndrome. *Mediators of Inflammation*, **2013**, 1-6. http://dx.doi.org/10.1155/2013/728987

[9]   Agarwal, N., Chitrika, A., Bhattacharjee, J. and Jain, S.K. (2011) Correlation of Tumour Necrosis Factor-α and Interleukin-6 with Anthropometric Indices of Obesity and Parameters of Insulin Resistance in Healthy North Indian Population. *JIACM*, **12**, 196-204.

[10] Pigeyre, M(2010). Évolution des concepts physiopathologiques de l'obésité. *La Presse Médicale*, **39**, 907-912. http://dx.doi.org/10.1016/j.lpm.2010.05.015

[11] Schlienger, J.-L.(2010) Conséquences pathologiques de l'obésité. *La Presse Médicale*, **39**, 913-920. http://dx.doi.org/10.1016/j.lpm.2010.04.018

[12] De Boer, M.D. (2013) Obesity, Systemic Inflammation, and Increased Risk for Cardiovascular Disease and Diabetes among Adolescents: A Need for Screening Tools to Target Interventions. *Nutrition*, **29**, 379-386. http://dx.doi.org/10.1016/j.nut.2012.07.003

[13] Neuparth, M.J., Proença, J.B., Santos-Silva, A. and Coimbra, S. (2013) Adipokines, Oxidized Low-Density Lipoprotein, and C-Reactive Protein Levels in Lean, Overweight, and Obese Portuguese Patients with Type 2 Diabetes. *ISRN obesity*, **2013**, Article ID: 142097. http://dx.doi.org/10.1155/2013/142097

[14] Kaur, J. (2014) A Comprehensive Review on Metabolic Syndrome. *Cardiology Research and Practice*, **2014**, 1-22. http://dx.doi.org/10.1155/2014/281483

[15] Caldar, P.C., Ahluwalia, N., Brouns, F., Buetler, T., Clement, K. and Cunningham, K. (2011) Dietary Factors and Low-Grade Inflammation in Relation to Overweight and Obesity. *BJN*, **106**, S1-S78. http://dx.doi.org/10.1017/s0007114511005460

[16] Fennira, E., Mahjoub, F., Abdesslem, H., Chaari, C., Gamoudi, A., Amrouche, C., *et al.* (2014) Alimentation de l'adolescent obèse tunisien: A propos de 108 cas. *Nutrition Clinique et Métabolisme*, **28**, S155-S156. http://dx.doi.org/10.1016/s0985-0562(14)70809-x

[17] Lee, H., In, S. and Choue, R. (2013) Obesity, Inflammation and Diet. *Pediatric Gastroenterology, Hepatology, and Nutrition*, **3**, 143-152. http://dx.doi.org/10.5223/pghn.2013.16.3.143

[18] Clément, K. and Vignes, S. (2009) Inflammation, adipokines et obésité. *La Revue de Médecine Interne*, **30**, 824-832. http://dx.doi.org/10.1016/j.revmed.2009.03.363

Abbreviations

IL-6: Interleukin-6;
IL-8: Interleukin-8;
TNF-α: Tumour Necrosis Factor Alpha;
hsCRP: High Sensitivity C Reactive Protein.

11

Influence of Antirisk Factors of Cardiovascular Diseases on Intracellular Metabolism of Neutrophils in Men with Obesity

Andrey Kratnov, Elena Timganova

Department of Therapy, Yaroslavl State Medical University, Yaroslavl, Russia
Email: kratnov@mail.ru

Abstract

Background: The factor promoting development of oxidative stress at obesity can be the neutrophils. Objective: To study the influence antirisk factors of cardiovascular diseases on intracellular metabolism of neutrophils in men with peripheral obesity. Methods: In 103 male patients aged 23 to 64 years without coronary heart disease, we studied the presence obesity, antirisk factors of cardiovascular diseases, and the metabolic activity of neutrophils. Results: It is identified that obesity in men associates with more rare use of crude vegetables or fruits every day, and also low physical activity. The daily uses of crude vegetables or fruits, and also the increase of physical activity in obese men promote increase intracellular activity of antioxidative protection at neutrophils. Conclusion: The antirisk factors of cardiovascular diseases increase activity antioxidative protection of neutrophils in men with peripheral obesity, reducing the probability of development of oxidative stress.

Keywords

Obesity, Neutrophils, Reactive Forms of Oxygen, Antioxidance

1. Introduction

The data are received that in the USA in 2013, 154.7 million adult people and 23.9 million children are having overweight or obesity [1]. It is believed that by 2015 year approximately 2.3 billion adult people will have overweight and more than 700 million will have obesity. It is shown that the risk of premature death in persons with 40% of overweight is 2 times higher in comparison with the people, who have average body weight [2].

Today it is proved, that oxidative stress, caused by non-controlled production of free radicals, plays the important role in the development of atherosclerotic vascular lesions, which is the main cause of development of cardiovascular diseases [3]. The source of active forms of oxygen at obesity belonging to the basic modifiable risk factors of cardiovascular diseases can be the neutrophils. In patients with III degree of obesity, the increase of formation of oxygen radicals of neutrophils is accompanied by the decrease in activity intracellular antioxidative protection that can promote development of oxidative stress [4]. The INTERHEART case—control study, which had the benefit of a very large sample size, in addition to the risk factors of cardiovascular diseases also revealed antirisk factors—sufficient use of vegetables and fruits, regular reception of small doses of alcohol, and regular physical activity [5].

The objective was to study the influence of antirisk factors of cardiovascular diseases on intracellular metabolism of neutrophils in men with peripheral obesity without coronary heart disease.

2. Participants and Methods

2.1. Participants

103 male aged 23 to 64 years (mean ± SD age: 47.1 ± 8.1 years) which were hospitalized in hospital for professional survey have been examined. In order to exclude coronary heart disease in all patients, the electrocardiography was performed, along with bicycle ergometry, Holter electrocardiography monitoring, and echocardiography. For the diagnosis of peripheral obesity, body mass index was calculated. The consumption the crude vegetables or fruits every day, intake of alcohol, physical loadings of medium intensity at work, and employment by sport or presence active leisure in participants by means of questionnaire was studied.

2.2. Methods

The material for this study was peripheral blood analysis which was performed at admission of patients to the hospital with the consent of the Ethical Committee. Neutrophils were isolated from heparinised blood in Ficoll-Verographin double density gradient 1.077 and 1.092 g/cm^3. The second interface cells contained 95% of neutrophils. The number of neutrophils in the cell suspension was counted in a cell with Goryaev vivo staining with methylene blue in 3% acetic acid (Turk dye) to determine viable cells. Viability of phagocytes, estimated by trypan test was more than 90%. In order to achieve a concentration of 5×10^6 neutrophils in 1 ml of cell suspension was diluted with medium 199.

The test of spontaneous and stimulated nitro blue tetrasolium reduction (**NBT-test**) was performed by means of quantitative spectrophotometric method using 0.2% nitro blue tetrazolium in phosphate buffer, fixing neutrophils with methanol and dissolving in mixture of reduced diformazan potassium hydroxide and dimethylsulfoxide 3:5 volume mixture [6]. Suspension of phytohemagglutinin (*Phaseolus vulgaris*, "PanEco", USA) was used as inducer of neutrophils redox metabolism.

Myeloperoxidase activity in neutrophils was studied using a 0.04% solution ortofenilendiamin in phosphate buffer pH 5.0, with the addition of 0.33% hydrogen peroxide solution at a ratio of 20:1 by volume. The reaction was stopped after 10 minutes of 10% sulphuric acid solution. Photometry was carried out at $\lambda = 492$ nM [7].

The determination of glutatione reductase activity in neutrophils was evaluated by method on degree of oxidation of NADH. In the control and skilled tests containing 0.5 ml of suspension neutrophils 1.5 ml of distilled water, 0.1 ml NADH and 0.3 ml buffer pH 8 was added. The reaction started by addition 0.2 ml of 0.033 mM solution oxidized glutathione. The tests were left at temperature 37°C for 30 minutes. To stop the reaction the test was placed in refrigerator for 10 minutes at temperature 4°C. Photometry was carried out at $\lambda = 340$ nM [8].

The determination of catalase activity in neutrophils was based on the ability of hydrogen peroxide to form salts with molybdenum stable colored complex. The reaction was run by adding 0.03% hydrogen peroxide solution and was stopped after 10 minutes, adding a 4% solution of ammonium molybdate. In control test instead of neutrophils distilled water was brought. The color intensity was measured at $\lambda = 410$ nM against a control sample of distilled water [9].

2.3. Statistical Analyses

Statistical data processing was performed using the package Statistica 8.0 (StatSoft, Inc., USA). The data for categorical variables are expressed as absolute values and percents, and the data for continuous variables are expressed as the median with the 25% - 75% inter quartile range. Differences between groups were considered statistically significant at $P < 0.05$.

3. Results

3.1. General Characteristics of the Study Participants

Obesity was encountered in 79 (76.7%) evaluable patients, of whom 49 (62%) revealed I degree of obesity (body mass index 30 - 34.9 kg/m^2), 23 (29.1%)—II degree of obesity (body mass index 35 - 39.9 kg/m^2), and 7 (8.9%) patients—III degree of obesity (body mass index $\geq$ 40 kg/m^2). The 31 (30%) men were used the crude vegetables or fruits every day. The alcohol was taken 97 (94.2%) patients, from which 12 (12.4%) men some times a week and 32 (32.9%) men some times a month was intake. The 92 (89.3%) participant had physical loadings of medium intensity at work, and 32 (31%) men were engaged sport or had active leisure.

The comparative characteristics of the study participants are presented in **Table 1**. The alcohol some times a month by men with obesity used authentically more often ($P < 0.05$). Obese men authentically less often had physical loadings of medium intensity at work ($P < 0.05$), they were engaged sports or had active leisure, and also used the crude vegetables or fruits every day less often.

3.2. Characteristics of the Obese Men Depending on the Use of Crude Vegetables or Fruits Every Day

The use of crude vegetables or fruits every day by men with obesity was accompanied authentically higher parameters of the spontaneous NBT-test (107.8 > 95.7 mM NBT reduced; $P = 0.04$) and catalase activity (344.3 > 333.7 mCat/l; $P = 0.03$) at neutrophils (**Table 2**). In men using crude vegetables or fruits every day also was observed authentically lower levels of glucose (4.8 < 5.2 mM/l; $P = 0.02$) and triglycerides (2 < 2.7 mM/l; $P = 0.01$) in blood.

3.3. Characteristics of the Obese Men Depending on the Employment by Sports or Presence Active Leisure

In obese men which were engaged sports or had active leisure has been revealed authentically higher glutathione reductase activity (314.9 > 298.8 nM·l^{-1}·sec^{-1}; $P = 0.01$) at neutrophils (**Table 3**), and also lower level of uric acid in blood (6.5 < 7 mg/dl; $P = 0.02$).

Presence of physical loadings of medium intensity at work and intake of alcohol did not cause authentically changes of intracellular metabolism of neutrophils.

Table 1. Comparative characteristics of the study participants.

Parameter	No Obesity (n = 24)	Obesity (n = 79)	P
The use of crude vegetables or fruits every day	8 (33.3)	23 (29.1)	>0.05
The intake of alcohol:	22 (91.6)	75 (94.9)	>0.05
- Some times a week	3 (13.7)	9 (12)	>0.05
- Some times a month	3 (13.7)	29 (38.7)	0.02
Physical loadings of medium intensity at work	24 (100)	68 (86)	0.02
Employment by sports or presence active leisure	9 (37.5)	23 (29.1)	>0.05

Table 2. Comparative characteristics of the obese men depending on the use of crude vegetables or fruits every day.

Parameter	The use of crude vegetables or fruits every day		P
	No (n = 49)	Yes (n = 20)	
Spontaneous NBT-test, mM	95.7 (77.8; 107.8)	107.8 (94.5; 112.8)	0.04
Stimulated NBT-test, mM	107.1 (88.2; 112.4)	108.5 (107.1; 113.5)	>0.05
Myeloperoxidase, SED	5.4 (4; 7.4)	5.5 (4.5; 7.7)	>0.05
Glutatione reductase, nM·l^{-1}·sec^{-1}	302.8 (281.4; 365.8)	304.4 (284.8; 366.5)	>0.05
Catalase, mCat/l	333.7 (241.7; 392.9)	344.3 (285.8; 400.9)	0.03

Table 3. Comparative characteristics of the obese men depending on the employment by sports or presence active leisure.

Parameter	Employment by sports or presence active leisure		P
	No (n = 46)	Yes (n = 23)	
Spontaneous NBT-test, mM	95.7 (78.8; 108.5)	106.7 (88.9; 109.2)	>0.05
Stimulated NBT-test, mM	107.8 (94.2; 112.4)	108.7 (93.9; 112.9)	>0.05
Myeloperoxidase, SED	5.4 (4; 7.2)	5.8 (4.3; 7.5)	>0.05
Glutatione reductase, $nM \cdot l^{-1} \cdot sec^{-1}$	298.8 (273.3; 337.7)	314.9 (296.1; 393.9)	0.01
Catalase, mCat/l	333.7 (199.8; 382.9)	348.3 (302.4; 404.7)	>0.05

4. Discussion

The main argument of an increased interest to obesity is its connection with an atherosclerosis and risk of development of cardiovascular diseases. In recent years growth of heart attacks is observed among youth and people of middle age. Believe that the reason this problem is increase among youth of persons with excessive weight which provokes heart complications. The obesity and hyperglycemia correlate with findings of atherosclerotic plaques in coronary arteries and abdomen part of the aorta in young people at the age of 15 - 34 years [10]. It is shown, that the increase in thickness of complex of intima-media which reflects progressing of atherosclerosis and associates with increase in risk of cardiovascular complications, depends on body weight [11]. Does not cause doubts that in pathophysiology of atherosclerosis play crucial role the subclinical chronic inflammation which present already at early stages. Low oxidative stress modulates in endothelia the expression of the gene inducing atherogenous factor that leads to formation of atherosclerotic plaque. Further existence endothelial oxidative stress conducts to continuous accumulation of lipids, strengthens inflammation, destruction of matrix and remodeling of vascular wall in the atherosclerotic plaque [12]. As adipose tissue produces proinflammatory cytokines, therefore, the obesity can be also considered how inflammation. It is proved, that adipose tissue represents the active metabolic and endocrine organ producing adipocytokines (peptide hormones) and adipokines, one of which—leptin is structurally similar to proinflammatory cytokines—interleukin-6 and interleukin-12. There are data, that leptin stimulates secretion of cytokines and strengthens the expression molecules of adhesion in phagocytes, promotes development of oxidative stress [13] [14].

The atherosclerosis is disease with multifactorial etiology, and development of coronary heart disease depends on degree of expressiveness of various factors, which can strengthen each other or act in role of antagonists. Probably that such protective factors as physical activity, antioxidants, and social support can counteract influence of classical risk factors of cardiovascular diseases. It is known, that in regulation of free radical processes in cell play the antioxidative mechanisms, dependent as from antioxidative enzymes, and natural low-molecular formations, which contents in organism of the person is caused by food stuffs. The meta-analysis of numerous researches testifies not only the reduction of antioxidative protection in patients with coronary heart disease, but also the change of its activity depending on smoking, physical activity, and diet [15]. In the present research it is revealed, that men with peripheral obesity less often used of crude vegetables or fruits every day, they had lower physical activity. The use of crude vegetables or fruits every day by obese men was accompanied lower levels of glucose and triglycerides in blood, and also higher antioxidative activity protection at neutrophils. Growth of activity of antioxidative enzymes at neutrophils also was promoted by increase in physical activity in obese men. Results of the research NHANES III, testifying to influence of physical activity on chronic subclinical inflammation, revealed that physical activity back correlates with the quantity of leucocytes and the contents of fibrinogen in blood [16].

5. Conclusion

In summary, the use of crude vegetables or fruits every day, and also employment by sports or presence active leisure in men with peripheral obesity promote increase in activity of antioxidative protection at neutrophils, which can reduce the risk of development of oxidative stress.

References

[1]   Go, A.S., Mozaffarian, D., Roger, V.L., *et al.* (2013) Heart Disease and Stroke Statistics—2013 Update: A Report

from the American Heart Association. *Circulation*, **127**, e6-e245. http://circ.ahajournals.org/lookup/doi/10.1161/CIR.0b013e31828124ad

[2] Malnick, S.D.H. and Knobler, H. (2006) The Medical Complications of Obesity. *QJM: An International Journal of Medicine*, **99**, 565-579. http://dx.doi.org/10.1093/qjmed/hcl085

[3] Heitzer, T., Schlinzig, T., Krohn, K., *et al.* (2001) Endothelial Dysfunction, Oxidative Stress, and Risk of Cardiovascular Events in Patients with Coronary Artery Disease. *Circulation*, **104**, 2673-2678. http://circ.ahajournals.org/content/104/22/2673.full

[4] Kratnov, A.E. (2014) Activity of Intracellular Metabolism at Neutrophils in Patients with Metabolic Syndrome. *Research in Endocrinology*, **2014**, Article ID: 963868. http://tinyurl.com/nv4vylt

[5] Yusuf, S., Hawken, S., Ôunpuu, S., *et al.* (2004) Effect of Potentially Modifiable Risk Factors Associated with Myocardial Infarction in 52 Countries (the INTERHEART Study): Case-Control Study. *Lancet*, **364**, 937-952. http://dx.doi.org/10.1016/S0140-6736(04)17018-9

[6] Gentle, T.A. and Thompson, R.A. (1990) Neutrophil Function Tests in Clinical Immunology. In: Gooi, H.G. and Chapel, H., Eds., *Clinical Immunology. A Practical Approach*, 2nd Edition, Oxford University Press, New York.

[7] Saidov, M.Z. and Pinegin, B.V. (1991) Spectrophotometric Analysis of Myeloperoxidase Activity in Phagocytes. *Laboratornoe delo*, **3**, 56-59.

[8] Kratnov, A.E., Potapov, P.P., Vlasova, A.V., *et al.* (2005) The Activity of Glutathione Reductase in Neutrophils of Patients with Mucoviscidosis. *Klinicheskaia laboratornaia diagnostika*, **2**, 33-36. http://scholar.qsensei.com/content/11s7vg

[9] Mamontova, N.S, Beloborodova, E.I. and Tucalova, L.I. (1994) Activity of Catalase at Chronic Dipsomania. *Klinicheskaia laboratornaia diagnostika*, **1**, 27-28.

[10] Strong, J.P., Malcom, G.T., McMahan, C.A., *et al.* (1999) Prevalence and Extent of Atherosclerosis in Adolescents and Young Adults: Implications for Prevention from the Pathobiological Determinants of Atherosclerosis in Youth Study. *JAMA*, **281**, 727-735. http://jamanetwork.com/ on 12/12/2014

[11] Bosevski, M., Georgievska-Ismail, L.J., Tosev, S. and Borozanov, V. (2009) Risk Factors for Development of Peripheral and Carotid Artery Disease among Type 2 Diabetes Patients. *Prilozi*, **30**, 81-90. http://manu.edu.mk/prilozi/5bm.pdf

[12] Spagnoli, L., Bonanno, E., Sangiorgi, G. and Mauriello, A. (2007) Role of Inflammation in Atherosclerosis. *Journal of Nuclear Medicine*, **48**, 1800-1815. http://10.2967/jnumed.107.038661

[13] Das, U.N. (2001) Is Obesity an Inflammatory Condition? *Nutrition*, **17**, 953-966. http://dx.doi.org/10.1016/S0899-9007(01)00672-4

[14] Cave, M.C., Hurt, R.T., Frazier, T.H., Matheson, P.J., Garrison, P.N., McClain, C.J., *et al.* (2008) Obesity, Inflammation, and the Potential Application of Pharmaconutrition. *Nutrition in Clinical Practice*, **23**, 16-34. http://10.1177/011542650802300116

[15] Flores-Mateo, G., Carrillo-Santisteve, P., Elosua, R., Guallar, E., Marrugat, J., Bleys, J., *et al.* (2009) Antioxidant Enzyme Activity and Coronary Heart Disease: Meta-Analyses of Observational Studies. *American Journal of Epidemiology*, **170**, 135-147. http://aje.oxfordjournals.org/content/170/2/135.full http://dx.doi.org/10.1093/aje/kwp112

[16] Ford, E.S., Ahluwalia, I.B. and Galuska, D.A. (2000) Social Relationships and Cardiovascular Disease Risk Factors: Findings from the Third National Health and Nutrition Examination Survey. *Preventive Medicine*, **30**, 83-92. http://dx.doi.org/10.1006/pmed.1999.0606

12

Nobiletin Prevents Body Weight Gain and Bone Loss in Ovariectomized C57BL/6J Mice

Young-Sil Lee[1], Midori Asai[1], Sun-Sil Choi[1], Takayuki Yonezawa[1], Toshiaki Teruya[2], Kazuo Nagai[1], Je-Tae Woo[3,4], Byung-Yoon Cha[1*]

[1]Research Institute for Biological Functions, Chubu University, Kasugai, Japan
[2]Faculty of Education, University of the Ryukyus, Nishihara, Japan
[3]Department of Biological Chemistry, Chubu University, Kasugai, Japan
[4]Department of Research and Development, Erina Co., Inc., Tokyo, Japan
Email: [*]bycha@isc.chubu.ac.jp

Abstract

Obesity and osteoporosis are associated with estrogen deficiency following menopause. Therefore, it is important to prevent and treat both disorders to maintain a healthy life in postmenopausal women. Nobiletin, a polymethoxylated flavone, exhibits various pharmacologic effects, including anti-tumor and anti-inflammatory activities. Therefore, in this study, we examined the effects of nobiletin on obesity, obesity-related metabolic disorders, and bone mass in ovariectomized (OVX) mice. Mice were divided into four groups and underwent sham operation or OVX. OVX mice were treated with 50 or 100 mg/kg nobiletin, or received vehicle alone (0.3% carboxyl methyl cellulose/0.5% dimethyl sulfoxide). Nobiletin decreased body weight gain and white adipose tissue weight in OVX mice. Nobiletin also decreased triglyceride levels, and tended to reduce plasma total cholesterol and glucose levels. Additionally, nobiletin prevented the reduction in bone mineral density of the trabecular region of the femur in OVX mice. Taken together, our results suggest that nobiletin improves adiposity, dyslipidemia, hyperglycemia, and prevents bone loss in OVX mice. Therefore, nobiletin is expected to have beneficial effects for the prevention and improvement of metabolic disorders and osteoporosis in postmenopausal women.

Keywords

Nobiletin, Ovariectomy, Obesity, Lipid and Glucose Metabolism, Bone Mineral Density

---

[*]Corresponding author.

1. Introduction

Estrogen is an important factor for protection against obesity in females. Estrogen deficiency leads to osteoporosis, as well as body weight gain [1] [2]. Recent studies have shown that postmenopausal women have greater body fat and visceral fat compared with premenopausal women [1]-[4]. Obesity is associated with several metabolic disorders including dyslipidemia, insulin resistance, and cardiovascular disease [1] [2]. Because osteoporosis and obesity are major health problems in postmenopausal women, it is important to identify strategies to prevent or treat these disorders and maintain a healthy life in postmenopausal women.

Natural phytoestrogens are increasingly being used to prevent or improve metabolic disorders, and are thought to reduce the risk of osteoporosis in postmenopausal women [5] [6]. Additionally, phytoestrogens seem to lack the undesirable side effects associated with estrogen. Therefore, there is growing interest in using natural compounds to prevent and improve metabolic disorders and osteoporosis in postmenopausal women.

Nobiletin is a polymethoxylated flavone present in some citrus fruits such as Citrus depressa (shiikuwasa) and Citrus sinensis (orangens) [7] [8]. Nobiletin was reported to exhibit biological effects via its anti-inflammatory, anti-tumor, and neuroprotective properties [9]-[11]. It was also recently reported that nobiletin can regulate bone metabolism by inhibiting osteoclast formation and bone resorption induced by interleukin (IL)-1 in osteoblasts, and preventing bone loss in OVX mice [12]. Recent reports have also revealed that nobiletin may be able to regulate lipid metabolism. Nobiletin enhances lipolysis and suppresses adipogenesis, although it is also reported that nobiletin induces adipocyte differentiation [13]-[15]. Our previous studies revealed that nobiletin reduces adiposity, plasma triglyceride (TG) levels, and insulin resistance in high-fat diet (HFD)-induced obese mice [16]. In the present study, we investigated the effects of nobiletin on obesity and bone mass in OVX mice.

2. Materials and Methods

2.1. Isolation of Nobiletin

Nobiletin was isolated and identified as described in our previous report [16].

2.2. Animals and Experimental Design

Female C57BL/6J mice were purchased from Japan SLC (Shizuoka, Japan) at 6 weeks of age. The mice were housed under temperature—($23°C \pm 3°C$) and humidity-controlled conditions with a 12-h light/dark cycle, and were given free access to food and water throughout the experiment. After acclimatization for 1 week with a standard rodent normal-fat diet (CRF-1; Charles River, Japan), the mice underwent either sham-operation (sham, $n = 8$) or ovariectomy (OVX, $n = 24$). After surgery, mice were allowed to recover under normal conditions. Two days later, the OVX mice were randomly divided into three groups ($n = 8$ mice/group) and treated with 50 (OVX + 50NOB) or 100 (OVX + 100NOB) mg/kg nobiletin, or vehicle (OVX control group). The vehicle was 0.3% carboxyl methyl cellulose/0.5% dimethyl sulfoxide. Nobiletin and vehicle were administered by oral gavage once daily for 12 weeks. Mice in the sham control group were administered with vehicle alone. Body weight and food intake for each mouse was measured two times per week during the study. The study was approved by The Animal Experimental Committee of Chubu University, and the mice were maintained in accordance with their guidelines.

2.3. Plasma, Tissue, and Bone Sampling

At the end of the 12-week study, the mice were anesthetized with a high dose of ether. Plasma samples were obtained by centrifuging blood samples at $5000 \times g$ for 15 min at 4°C. The resulting plasma samples were stored at −80°C until analysis. Liver, white adipose tissues (WAT; reproductive, perirenal, and mesenteric WAT), and the uterus were immediately excised, rinsed, and weighed. The femurs were also excised, soft tissue was carefully removed from the bone without damaging trabecular tissue, and the femoral bones were fixed in 70% ethanol.

2.4. Plasma Biochemistry

Plasma total cholesterol (T-CHO), TG, and glucose levels were determined using commercially available enzyme assay kits (Cholesterol E-Test, Triglyceride E-Test, and Glucose C II-Test, respectively; Wako Pure Chemical Industries, Osaka, Japan) according to the manufacturer's protocols.

2.5. Peripheral Quantitative Computed Tomography (pQCT) Analysis

Isolated bones were measured by pQCT (XCT Research, SA$^+$, Stratec Medizintechnik GmbH, Pforzheim, Germany) with a tube voltage of 50.5 kV and a tube current of 0.281 mA. The scan speed was 5 mm/s with a voxel resolution of 0.07 mm. The analytical parameters for cortical bone mineral density (BMD) were set as a threshold of 690 mg/cm^3 and a peel mode of 20. Trabecular BMD was <395 mg/cm^3 with a peel mode of 20. A femur slice located 0.6 mm from the distal end of the growth plate was used to measure trabecular and cortical BMD. Trabecular bone was defined by setting an internal area of 35% of the total cross-sectional area. Total BMD, trabecular BMD, and cortical BMD were calculated using pQCT software (Makejob; StratecMedizintechnik GmbH).

2.6. Statistical Analysis

Data are expressed as means ± standard error of the mean. Differences in mean values between each group were analyzed by one-way analysis of variance, followed by Dunnett's test. Values of $p < 0.05$ were considered to indicate statistical significance. All analyses were conducted using IBM-SPSS version 20 (IBM, New York, NY, USA).

3. Results

3.1. Effects of Nobiletin on Body Weight Gain and Food Intake

Body weight gain and food intake are shown in **Figure 1**. Body weight gain was significantly greater in the OVX group than in the sham group ($p < 0.005$). Body weight gain was significantly lower in the OVX + 100NOB group than in the OVX group ($p < 0.05$) but was not significantly differentbetween the OVX + 50NOB and OVX groups. Food intake was comparable among all four groups.

3.2. Effects of Nobiletin on Organ Weight

Organ weight is shown in **Figure 2**. Uterus weight was significantly lower in the OVX group than in the sham group ($p < 0.005$), indicating that the mice were estrogen deficient. Uterus weight tended to be higher in the OVX + 100NOB group than in the OVX group, although did not significantly. Liver weight did not differ among the four groups. WAT weight was significantly higher in the OVX group compared with the sham group ($p < 0.005$). The reproductive, perirenal, and total WAT weights were significantly lower in the OVX + 100NOB group than in the OVX group (all, $p < 0.05$). However, there was no difference in WAT weights between the OVX + 50NOB group and the OVX group.

3.3. Effects of Nobiletin on Plasma Biochemistry

Figure 3 shows the effects of nobiletin on plasma biochemistry. Plasma T-CHO levels were significantly higher in the OVX group than in the shamgroup ($p < 0.05$). Plasma T-CHO levels were decreased in the OVX + 100NOB group compared with the OVX group, although not significantly. Plasma TG levels were significantly

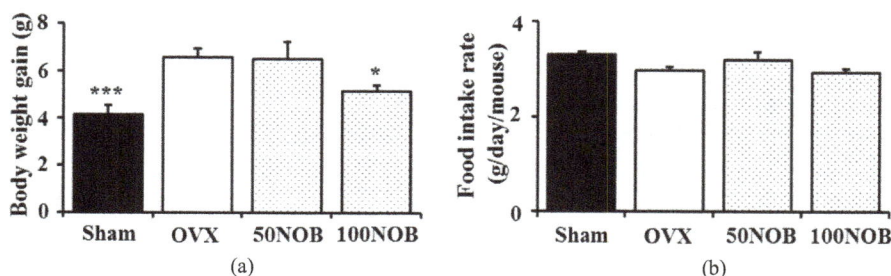

Figure 1. Effects of nobiletin on body weight gain (a) and food intake (b). Sham: sham-operated mice; OVX: ovariectomized mice; 50NOB: OVX + 50 mg/kg nobiletin; 100NOB: OVX + 100 mg/kg nobiletin. Values are means ± standard error of the mean ($n = 8$ mice/group). $^*p < 0.05$ and $^{***}p < 0.005$ vs the OVX group.

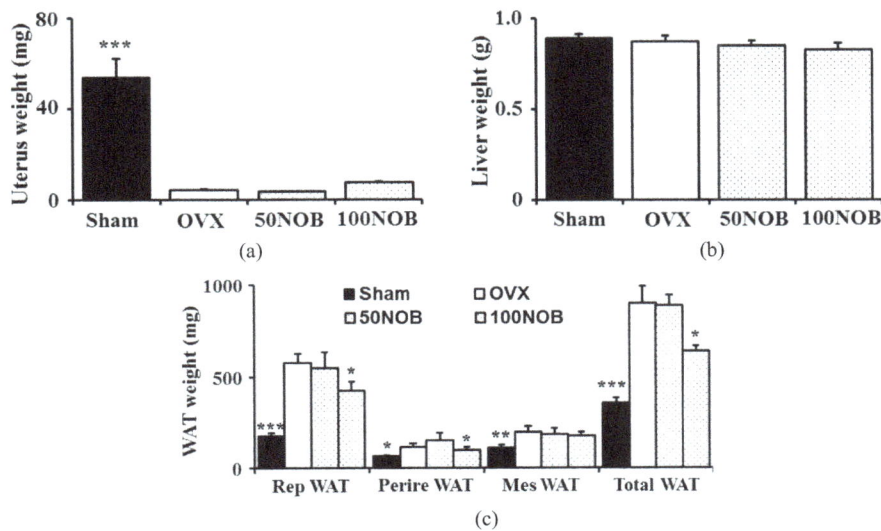

Figure 2. Effects of nobiletin on uterus weight (a), liver weight (b) and white adipose tissue (WAT) weight (c). RepW: reproductive WAT; PeriW: perirenal WAT; MesW: mesenteric WAT; TotalW: total WAT weight; Sham: sham-operated mice; OVX: ovariectomized mice; 50NOB: OVX + 50 mg/kg nobiletin; 100NOB: OVX + 100 mg/kg nobiletin. Values are means ± standard error of the mean ($n = 8$ mice/group). $^*p < 0.05$, $^{**}p < 0.01$, and $^{***}p < 0.005$ vs the OVX group.

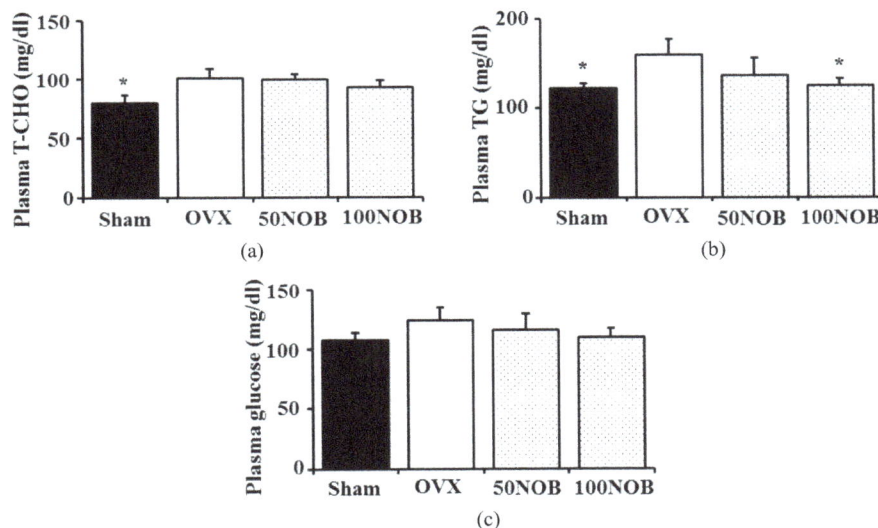

Figure 3. Effects of nobiletin on plasma total cholesterol (T-CHO; (a)), triglyceride (TG; (b)), and glucose (c) levels. Sham: sham-operated mice; OVX: ovariectomized mice; 50NOB: OVX+50 mg/kg nobiletin; 100NOB: OVX + 100 mg/kg nobiletin. Values are means ± standard error of the mean ($n = 8$ mice/group). $^*p < 0.05$ vs the OVX group.

higher in the OVX group than in the sham group ($p < 0.05$). Plasma TG levels were lower in the OVX + 100NOB group, but not in the OVX + 50NOB group, compared with the OVX group. Plasma glucose levels did not differ between the sham and OVX groups, although they tended to be lower in the OVX + 100NOB group than in the OVX group.

3.4. Effects of Nobiletin on BMD

Figure 4 shows the effects of nobiletin on BMD in OVX rats. Total femoral BMD and trabecular BMD were

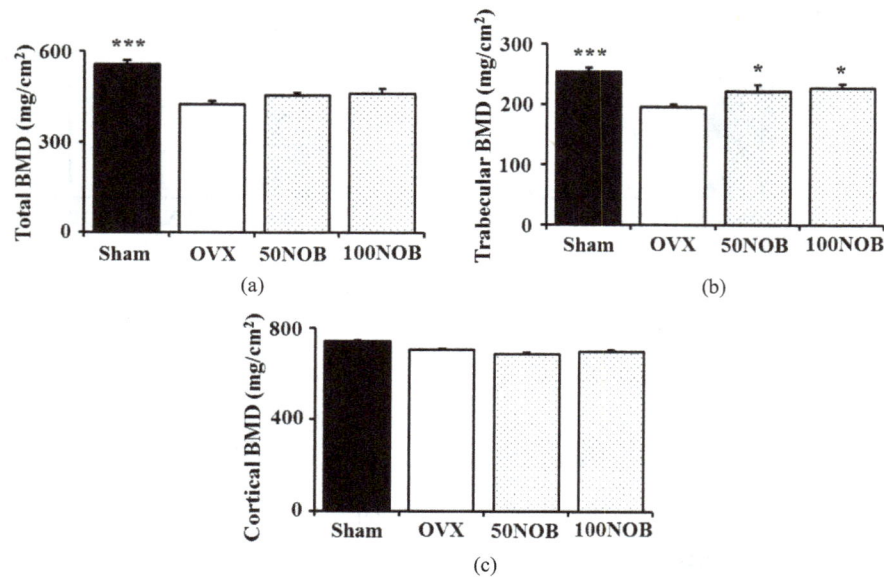

Figure 4. Effects of nobiletin on total femoral bone mineral density (BMD; (a)), trabecular BMD (b), and cortical BMD (c). Sham: sham-operated mice; OVX: ovariectomized mice; 50NOB: OVX + 50 mg/kg nobiletin; 100NOB: OVX + 100 mg/kg nobiletin. NFD: normal-fat diet; HFD: high-fat diet. Values are means ± standard error of the mean (n = 8). $^{*}p$ < 0.05 and $^{***}p$ < 0.005 vs the OVX group.

significantly lower in the OVX group than in the sham group (both, p < 0.005). The decrease in total femoral BMD caused by OVX was attenuated by both doses of nobiletin, although this not significantly. Trabecular BMD was significantly greater in both OVX + NOB groups than in the OVX group (both, p < 0.05). Cortical BMD did not differ among the four groups.

4. Discussion

In the present study, we examined whether nobiletin could reduce obesity, obesity-related metabolic disorders, and osteoporosis in OVX mice. To our knowledge, the present study is the first to show that nobiletin prevents the increases in body weight, WAT weight, and plasma TG, as well as bone loss, in OVX mice.

In the present study, nobiletin reduced increases in body weight gain and WAT weight in OVX mice. It has been reported that estrogen is capable of preventing obesity in females. OVX mice are characterized by increased food intake and decreased energy expenditure, which lead to obesity [17]. It was reported that treating OVX mice with estradiol prevented the development of obesity [18].

In the present study, food intake was similar in the sham and OVX groups, and was not affected by nobiletin. Therefore, the reduction in body weight gain and WAT weight in this study were not caused by changes in food intake. Recent studies and our own *in vivo* data indicate that nobiletin regulates adipogenesis and lipolysis. For example, nobiletin enhances lipolysis in differentiated adipocytes by activating the cAMP-cAMP response element-binding pathway and suppresses lipid accumulation by downregulating peroxisome proliferator-activated receptor (PPAR)γ, and activating AMP-activated protein kinase. However, it was reported that nobiletincan induce adipocyte differentiation [13]-[15]. Furthermore, we previous reported that nobiletin increased the expression of energy expenditure-related genes, such as PPARα and carnitine palmitoyltransferase I, in HFD-induced obese mice [16]. Based on these earlier findings, it is likely that increased lipolysis and energy expenditure may be involved in the reduced body weight gain and WAT weight in nobiletin-treated mice. Further studies are needed to examine the effects of nobiletin on the expression of lipid metabolism-related genes.

Obesity-related metabolic disorders, such as hyperlipidemia, hyperglycemia, and glucose intolerance, are significant problems in postmenopausal women. In the present study, nobiletinreduced plasma TG levels and tended to reduce plasma T-CHO and glucose levels in OVX mice. In our previous study, we showed that nobiletin improved hypertriglyceridemia [16]. These results suggest that nobiletin may improve obesity-related metabolic disorders, such as hyperlipidemia, in postmenopausal women.

Osteoporosis is a skeletal disease characterized by a reduction in bone strength, increasing the risk of fracture. Osteoporosis in postmenopausal women is caused by a decrease in estrogen levels and an increase in bone resorption [19]. In our present study, we showed that nobiletin inhibited the decrease in trabecular BMD of OVX mice and showed tendency to increase total femoral BMD in OVX mice. Previous studies have shown that nobiletin suppresses osteoclast formation and bone resorption by inhibiting nuclear factor-κB-dependent transcription and prostaglandin E production in osteoblasts via the activity of IL-1. This report also showed that nobiletin prevents bone loss in OVX mice [12] (Harada *et al.* 2011). Based on our results and this earlier report, nobiletin is expected to prevent osteoporosis in postmenopausal women.

5. Conclusion

In conclusion, treatment with nobiletin decreased body weight gain, WAT weight, and plasma TG levels in OVX mice. Nobiletin tended to decrease plasma T-CHO levels and glucose levels in OVX mice, and prevented the decrease in BMD following OVX. These results suggest that nobiletin may improve adiposity, hypertriglyceridemia, and bone metabolism in OVX mice, as a model of the postmenopausal state. Therefore, nobiletin may have beneficial effects for the prevention and treatment of metabolic disorders and osteoporosis in postmenopausal women.

References

[1]   You, T., Ryan, A.S. and Nicklas, B.J. (2004) The Metabolic Syndrome in Obese Postmenopausal Women: Relationship to Body Composition, Visceral Fat, and Inflammation. *The Journal of Clinical Endocrinology Metabolism*, **89**, 5517-5522.
        http://press.endocrine.org/doi/abs/10.1210/jc.2004-0480?url_ver=Z39.88-2003&rfr_id=ori:rid:crossref.org&rfr_dat=cr_pub=pubmed&
        http://dx.doi.org/10.1210/jc.2004-0480

[2]   Kaaja, R.J. (2008) Metabolic Syndrome and the Menopause. *Menopause International*, **14**, 21-25.
        http://min.sagepub.com/content/14/1/21.abstract
        http://dx.doi.org/10.1258/mi.2007.007032

[3]   Cooke, P.S. and Naaz, A. (2004) Role of Estrogens in Adipocyte Development and Function. *Experimental Biology and Medicine* (Maywood), **229**, 1127-1235. http://ebm.sagepub.com/content/229/11/1127.abstract

[4]   Lobe, R.A. (2008) Metabolic Syndrome after Menopause and the Role of Hormones. *Maturitas*, **60**, 10-18.
        http://www.maturitas.org/article/S0378-5122(08)00039-X/abstract
        http://dx.doi.org/10.1016/j.maturitas.2008.02.008

[5]   Anderson, J.W., Johnstone, B.M. and Cook-Newell, M.E. (1995) Meta-Analysis of the Effects of Soy Protein Intake on Serum Lipids. *The New England Journal of Medicine*, **333**, 276-282.
        http://www.nejm.org/doi/full/10.1056/NEJM199508033330502
        http://dx.doi.org/10.1056/NEJM199508033330502

[6]   Messina, M.J. (2002) Soy Foods and Soybean Isoflavones and Menopausal Health. *Nutrition in Clinical Care*, **5**, 272-282. http://onlinelibrary.wiley.com/doi/10.1046/j.1523-5408.2002.05602.x/abstract
        http://dx.doi.org/10.1046/j.1523-5408.2002.05602.x

[7]   Mercader, J., Wanecq, E., Chen, J. and Carpéné, C. (2011) Isopropylnorsynephrine Is a Stronger Lipolytic Agent in Human Adipocytes than Synephrine and Other Amines Present in Citrus Aurantium. *Journal of Physiology and Biochemistry*, **67**, 443-452. http://link.springer.com/article/10.1007%2Fs13105-011-0078-2

[8]   Nagata, U., Sakamoto, K., Shiratsuchi, H., Ishi, T., Yano, M. and Ohta, H. (2006) Flavonoid Composition of Fruit Tissues of Citrus Species. *Bioscience, Biotechnology, and Biochemistry*, **70**, 178-192.
        https://www.jstage.jst.go.jp/article/bbb/70/1/70_1_178/_article

[9]   Murakami, A., Nakamura, Y., Torikai, K., *et al.* (2000) Inhibitory Effect of Citrus Nobiletin on Phorbol Ester-Induced Skin Inflammation Oxidative Stress, and Tumor Promotion in Mice. *Cancer Research*, **60**, 5059-5066.
        http://cancerres.aacrjournals.org/content/60/18/5059.long

[10]   Silalahi, J. (2002) Anticancer and Health Protective Properties of Citrus Fruit Components. *Asia Pacific Journal of Clinical Nutrition*, **11**, 79-84. http://onlinelibrary.wiley.com/doi/10.1046/j.1440-6047.2002.00271.x/abstract
        http://dx.doi.org/10.1046/j.1440-6047.2002.00271.x

[11]   Nakajima, A., Yamakuni, T., Haraguchi, M., Omae, N., Song, S.Y., Kato, C., *et al.* (2007) Nobilein, a Citrus Flavonoid

that Improves Memory Impairment, Rescues Bulbectomy-Induced Cholinergic Neurodegeneration in Mice. *Journal of Pharmacological Sciences*, **105**, 122-126. https://www.jstage.jst.go.jp/article/jphs/105/1/105_1_122/_article

[12] Harada, S., Tominari, T., Matsumoto, C., Hirata, M., Takita, M., Inada, M. and Miyaura, C. (2011) Nobiletin, a Polymethoxy Flavonoid, Suppresses Bone Resorption by Inhibiting NFκB-Dependent Prostaglandin E Synthesis in Osteoblasts and Prevents Bone Loss Due to Estrogen Deficiency. *Journal of Pharmacological Sciences*, **115**, 89-93. https://www.jstage.jst.go.jp/article/jphs/115/1/115_10193SC/_article http://dx.doi.org/10.1254/jphs.10193SC

[13] Saito, T., Abe, D. and Sekiya, K. (2007) Nobiletin Enhances Differentiation and Lipolysis of 3T3-L1 Adipocytes. *Biochemical and Biophysical Research Communications*, **357**, 371-376. http://www.sciencedirect.com/science/article/pii/S0006291X07006109

[14] Kanda, K., Nishi, K., Kadota, A., Nishimoto, S., Liu, M.C. and Sugahara, T. (2011) Nobiletin Suppresses Adipocyte Differentiation of 3T3-L1 Cells by an Insulin and IBMX Mixture Induction. *Biochimica et Biophysica Acta*, **1820**, 461-468. http://www.sciencedirect.com/science/article/pii/S0304416511002923

[15] Choi, Y., Kim, Y., Ham, H., Park, Y., Jeong, H.S. and Lee, J. (2011) Nobiletin Suppresses Adipogenesis by Regulating the Expression of Adipogenic Transcription Factors and the Activation of AMP-Activated Protein Kinase (AMPK). *Journal of Agricultural and Food Chemistry*, **59**, 12843-12849. http://pubs.acs.org/doi/abs/10.1021/jf2033208 http://dx.doi.org/10.1021/jf2033208

[16] Lee, Y.S., Cha, B.Y., Saito, K., Yamakawa, H., Choi, S.S., Yamaguchi, K., *et al.* (2010) Nobiletin Improves Hyperglycemia and Insulin Resistance in Obese Diabetic *ob/ob* Mice. *Biochemical Pharmacology*, **79**, 1674-1683. http://www.sciencedirect.com/science/article/pii/S0006295210000936 http://dx.doi.org/10.1016/j.bcp.2010.01.034

[17] Roger, N.H., Perfield II, J.W., Strissel, K.J., Obin, M.S. and Greenberg, A.S. (2009) Reduced Energy Expenditure and Increased Inflammation Are Early Events in the Development of Ovariectomy-Induced Obesity. *Endocrinology*, **150**, 2161-2168. http://press.endocrine.org/doi/abs/10.1210/en.2008-1405?url_ver=Z39.88-2003&rfr_id=ori:rid:crossref.org&rfr_dat=cr_pub=pubmed http://dx.doi.org/10.1210/en.2008-1405

[18] Kolta, S., De Vernejoul, M.C., Meneton, P., Fechtenbaum, J. and Roux, C. (2003) Bone Mineral Measurements in Mice: Comparison of Two Devices. *Journal of Clinical Densitometry*, **6**, 251-258. http://www.sciencedirect.com/science/article/pii/S109469500660276X http://dx.doi.org/10.1385/JCD:6:3:251

[19] Riggs, B.L. (1992) Osteoporosis. In: Wyngaarden, J.B., Ed., *Textbook of Medicine*, 19th Edition, Saunders, Philadelphia, 1426-1430.

13

Changes in Adenosine Metabolism in Asthma. A Study on Adenosine, 5'-NT, Adenosine Deaminase and Its Isoenzyme Levels in Serum, Lymphocytes and Erythrocytes

Jitender Sharma[1], Bala K. Menon[2], Vannan K. Vijayan[3,4], Surendra K. Bansal[1*]

[1]Department of Biochemistry, Vallabhbhai Patel Chest Institute, University of Delhi, Delhi, India
[2]Department of Respiratory Allergy and Applied Immunology, Vallabhbhai Patel Chest Institute, University of Delhi, Delhi, India
[3]Department of Pulmonary Medicine, Vallabhbhai Patel Chest Institute, University of Delhi, Delhi, India
[4](Present Address) Bhopal Memorial Hospital and Research Centre, Bhopal, India
Email: [*]bansalsurendrak@yahoo.com

Abstract

Background: Adenosine deaminase (ADA) and 5'-nucleotidase (5'-NT) play a crucial role in adenosine metabolism in healthy individuals. Adenosine is an inflammatory mediator of asthma. Changes in adenosine metabolism and role of ADA and 5'-NT in regulating adenosine level in asthmatics and correlation of these changes with severity of asthma are not clearly understood. Methods: In this study, we screened 5217 patients, of which 2416 were diagnosed with asthma. Further, of 2416 asthmatics, only 45 patients who strictly fulfilled the selection criteria were enrolled in the study. The patients were classified into mild, moderate and severe persistent groups; each group consisted of fifteen patients. Fifteen healthy subjects served as controls. Adenosine levels and activities of 5'-NT, total ADA, ADA1 and ADA2 in serum, lymphocytes and erythrocytes were determined. The data were analysed statistically and $p < 0.05$ was considered significant. Results: In asthma, adenosine levels in serum, lymphocytes and erythrocytes were found to be raised significantly. A significant reciprocal correlation existed between adenosine levels in serum, lymphocytes and erythrocytes of asthmatics and FEV1%. The 5'-nucleotidase activity in serum and lymphocytes was raised in moderate and severe persistent groups and an inverse correlation existed between 5'-nucleotidase activity and FEV1% whereas in erythrocytes it was raised only in severe persistent group and FEV1% had no correlation with the 5'-nucleotidase activity. The activities of total ADA, ADA1 and ADA2 were decreased in serum and lymphocytes of moderate and severe persistent asthmatics and a positive correlation existed between total ADA and FEV1%. In eryth-

---

rocytes, total ADA activity increased in mild persistent group but remained unchanged in moderate and severe persistent groups. Conclusion: The present study suggests that adenosine levels tend to increase in serum, lymphocytes and erythrocytes with the severity of bronchial asthma. The balance between ADA and 5'-NT determines the levels of adenosine in serum and lymphocytes which may result in pathogenesis of asthma, or *vice versa*.

Keywords

Asthma, Adenosine, Metabolism, Adenosine Deaminase, 5'-Nucleotidase

1. Introduction

Bronchial asthma is one of the most common chronic diseases globally and currently affects nearly 300 million people [1]. Prevalence of asthma in Indian population is 2.38% as per a study conducted by Jindal in 2007 [2]. Airway inflammation plays a cardinal role in pathogenesis of bronchial asthma and airway hyperresponsiveness is the characteristic physiologic abnormality that determines excessive bronchoconstrictor response to multiple inhaled triggers [3]. There is good evidence that the specific pattern of airway inflammation in asthma is associated with airway hyperresposiveness that is further correlated with variable airflow obstruction [4]. Several cell types such as lymphocytes, mast cells, macrophages, eosinophils, neutrophils and epithelial cells produce inflammatory changes by release of various mediators like adenosine, histamine, kinin, leukotrienes, prostaglandins, PAF, chemokines and cytokines which interact in a complex way to produce airway inflammation [4]. Severity of asthma is based on the frequency and intensity of symptoms. The mildest grade is characterized by acute attacks upon allergen exposure, and with symptoms reversed by β-adrenergic agonists [5]; lung function is normal between acute attacks. More severe grades of asthma are characterized by sustained increase in airway resistance (the late-phase response), impaired basal lung function and heightened airways responsiveness to non-specific irritants and cellular inflammation comprising of increased number of mast cells and eosinophils in the bronchial mucosa [6].

Adenosine is a ubiquitous purine nucleoside, playing a fundamental role in many biological processes such as energy generation and protein metabolism, but in the last two decades, it has become clear that adenosine is a mediator involved in the pathogenesis of many inflammatory disorders including bronchial asthma. It has been known for a long time that inflammatory tissue damage is accompanied by accumulation of extracellular adenosine in inflamed areas due to its release from non-immune and immune cells; local tissue hypoxia in inflamed areas represents one of the most important conditions leading to adenosine release and accumulation [7] [8]. Also, contributing to the accumulation of adenosine is the release of rapidly metabolized ADP and ATP from various cells including platelets, mast cells, and endothelial cells [9]. Adenosine, thus accumulated then interacts with specific G-protein coupled adenosine receptors (ARs) viz. A_1R, $A_{2A}R$, $A_{2B}R$, A_3R on inflammatory and immune cells to regulate their functions [10].

Evidence for role of adenosine in bronchial asthma was first demonstrated more than twenty years ago when a group of asthma patients exhibited bronchoconstriction in response to aerosolized adenosine while normal individuals didn't display response [11]. Adenosine acts through its A_{2B} and A_3 receptors to cause degranulation of mast cells and the release of vasoactive, pro-inflammatory and nociceptive mediators that include histamine, cytokines and proteolytic enzymes [12]-[15]. These mediators can cause bronchoconstriction in asthmatics. In addition to increase in mast cells activation, adenosine promotes release of inflammatory cytokines from smooth muscles, leukocytes chemotaxis via adenosine A2B receptors and eosinophils recruitment and activation via adenosine A3 receptors [16]. Adenosine seems to play an important role in modulation of T lymphocyte functions. Both peripheral cytotoxicT lymphocytes (CTLs) and T helper (Th) cells express A2A, A2B and A3 receptors, but A2A receptors are proposed to be the predominantly expressed in peripheral T lymphocytes [17], probably, extracellular adenosine effect on these cells is mediated through A2A receptors [18]. Moreover, cytokine production by activated Th cells is modulated by extracellular adenosine through A2A receptors [17]. Patients with bronchial asthma also reveal appreciable alterations of erythrocyte morphology and decreased membrane microviscosity which is related with severity of bronchial asthma [19] [20]. Adenosine levels are increased in the bronchoalveolar lavage (BAL) fluid of asthmatics compared to normal subjects, suggesting that there is an imbalance in the homeostatic mechanisms involved in purine metabolism [21]. Furthermore, adenosine levels are increased in the lung lavage fluid after specific allergen challenge in sensitised rabbits [22]. Inhalation of allergen in atopic asthmatics increases adenosine plasma levels up to 3-fold [23]. Elevated concentrations of adenosine in the lungs of adenosine deaminase deficient mouse models have produced a lung phenotype with features of asthma [24]. The specific cellular source of adenosine in bronchoalveolar lavage fluid is unknown, but is likely to include mast cells along with epithelial cells, neutrophils, lymphocytes and platelets [25].

Adenosine bioavailability is a key determinant of its action. The processes related to its production, release, cellular uptake and metabolism determine the bioavailability of adenosine at receptor sites [26]. Adenosine occupies an interesting central position in purine metabolism. It may be subjected to three metabolic fates: phosphorylation to the nucleotide level, deamination to inosine, or conversion to the base level by adenosine phosphorylase. But adenosine phosphorylase has been found only in bacterial systems [27] [28]. Phosphorylation is favoured at low concentrations while deamination predominates at higher adenosine concentrations [29]. Under normal conditions adenosine is derived from intracellular adenosine monophosphate (AMP) that is present at low levels in the cell, mostly derived from the catabolism of high energy adenosine phosphates (ATP, ADP) [30]. Intracellular (AMP) is formed and shortly reconverted to ADP and ATP as part of the energy cycle. However, under conditions of high-energy demand, AMP cannot be reconverted and it is metabolised to adenosine by 5′-nucleotidase (plasma membrane bound mainly as well as cytoplasmic) [31]. Intracellular levels of adenosine are kept low by its conversion to AMP by the enzyme adenosine kinase and to inosine by adenosine deaminase, but when energy demands are greater as in inflammation, deamination predominates [32]. Extracellular adenosine diffuses back into the cell through the operation of an energy-independent nucleoside transporter [33]. 5′-nucleotidase (5′-NT, E.C. 3.1.3.5) catalyzes the hydrolysis of the phosphoric ester bond of 5′-ribonucleotides to the corresponding ribonucleoside and phosphate. The main function of 5′-NT is the hydrolysis of AMP to adenosine. Adenosine deaminase (ADA, EC 3.5.4.4), a key enzyme in the purine salvage pathway, catalyzes the irreversible hydrolytic deamination of adenosine and 2′-deoxyadenosine to inosine and 2′-deoxyinosine, respectively. Two different isoenzymes of ADA designated as ADA1 and ADA2 were found in mammals and lower vertebrates [34].

The production, release and metabolism of adenosine depend ultimately on the relevant enzyme activities influencing its metabolism. Adenosine deaminase and 5′-nucleotidase are the two key enzymes regulating adenosine level inside the cell as well as in plasma. We hypothesized that the decreased activity of adenosine deaminase or increased activity of 5′-nucleotidase or both may result in elevated level of adenosine. Since studies measuring activities of these enzymes and correlating it with adenosine levels in bronchial asthma patients are lacking, we proposed the present study to examine the activities of adenosine deaminase, its isoenzymes, 5′-nucleotidase and adenosine levels in serum, erythrocytes and lymphocytes to understand the metabolism of adenosine in bronchial asthma.

2. Materials and Methods

2.1. Plan of Study

The study included a total number of 60 subjects of bronchial asthma and healthy controls. The asthmatic patients were classified into three groups consisting of 15 patients each viz. mild persistent, moderate persistent and severe persistent as per the EPR 3 guidelines [35]. The control group consisted of 15 healthy subjects. Blood (10 ml) was collected, serum, lymphocytes and erythrocytes separated, and adenosine levels, assay of activities of 5′-NT, ADA, ADA1 and ADA2 were performed and correlated with FEV1 (% of predicted). The study was approved by the Ethics Committee of Vallabhbhai Patel Chest Institute, University of Delhi, Delhi, India. Informed and written consent was taken from each subject.

2.2. Study Population

The patients were selected from those attending the outpatient department of Vallabhbhai Patel Chest Institute. During the period of this study, 5217 patients attended outpatient department, out of which 2416 were diagnosed as patients of bronchial asthma. We selected 45 patients from 2416 asthmatics according to our inclusion and exclusion criteria. Inclusion criteria for asthmatics: Patients with reversible airflow obstruction and pulmonary function test as per the EPR 3 guidelines [35], with age between 18 and 60 years of either sex. Exclusion criteria: smokers, patients having other respiratory and systemic disease, on oral corticosteroids, and pregnant or lactating females. Fifteen age and sex matched healthy subjects were included in the study.

2.3. Chemicals and Reagents

Adenosine deaminase, EHNA [Erythro-9(2-hydroxy-3-nonyl) adenine], histopaque (specific gravity −1.077), and 4-methylaminophenol sulphate were purchased from Sigma Chemical Co. St Louis, USA. Adenosine, adenosine monophosphate, nickel chloride, potassium bisulphate, and sodium nitroprusside were procured from Sisco Research Laboratories PVT. LTD. (Mumbai, India). Ammonium molybdate, ammonium sulphate, disodium hydrogen phosphate, EDTA (Ethylenediaminetetraacetic acid) disodium, manganese sulphate, perchloric acid 70%, phenol, potassium carbonate, sodium acetate, sodium dihydrogen phosphate, sodium hydroxide, sodium hypochlorite, sodium veronal, sulphuric acid 96%, trichloroacetic acid and triethanolamine hydrochloride were purchased from Qualigens Fine Chemicals (Mumbai, India). All other chemicals used were of analytical grade.

2.4. Preparation of Serum and Lysate of Lymphocytes and Erythrocytes

Venous blood (10 ml) was collected under aseptic conditions in two tubes, 7 ml of it was collected in tube containing EDTA (1 mg/ml) as anticoagulant and remaining 3 ml was taken in other tube without anticoagulant to isolate the serum. Lymphocytes were isolated by the method of Boyum [36] with some modifications. Venous blood (7 ml) was diluted in the ratio of 1:1 with physiological saline (0.15 M NaCl), carefully layered over 7 ml histopaque (specific gravity 1.077) and centrifuged at 2000 rpm (670 × g) in a refrigerated centrifuge (Plasto Craft, 4 R-V/FM, India) at 4°C using swing out rotor (no. 15) for 15 minutes. The opaque ring at the interface containing lymphocytes was collected with a sterile Pasteur pipette, diluted with physiological saline and centrifuged at 1500 rpm (500 × g) in a refrigerated centrifuge (Plasto Craft, 4 R-V/FM, India) at 4°C for 10 min. The pellet containing lymphocytes was washed twice with physiological saline. Contaminating erythrocytes were removed by giving osmotic shock to the pellet by the method of Bansal et al. [37]. The cell suspension was centrifuged again, the pellet washed twice with physiological saline and resuspended in physiological saline. The lymphocytes were counted using automated cell counter (Sysmex PoCH-100i). After removal of opaque ring at the interface containing lymphocytes and discarding the supernatant, packed erythrocytes were washed with 5 volumes of physiological saline (0.15 M NaCl) and centrifuged at 3000 rpm (650 × g) in a refrigerated centrifuge (Plasto Craft, 4 R-V/FM, India) using angular rotor (no. 9) at 4°C for 10 minutes. Pellet was washed three times similarly. Supernatant was discarded each time. The packed cells were resuspended in 0.15 M saline. The erythrocytes were counted using automated cell counter (Sysmex PoCH-100i). To assess the overall viability of lymphocytes, the cell suspension was washed two times with PBS (137 mM NaCl, 2.7 mM KCl, 10 mM Na_2HPO_4, 2 mM KH_2PO_4, pH 7.4) and treated with a 0.4% solution of trypan blue for 2 to 3 min. Lymphocytes and erythrocytes were suspended in phosphate buffer (50 mM NaH_2PO_4 and $Na_2HPO_4 \cdot 12H_2O$, pH 6.5) for adenosine deaminase and its isoenzymes assay, in veronal buffer (40 mM $C_8H_{11}O_3N_2Na$, pH 7.5) for 5'-nucleotidase assay and in triethanolamine buffer (0.1 M $C_6H_{15}NO_3$, pH 7.4) for adenosine estimation. Lymphocytes suspended in respective buffer to obtain a suspension of 20×10^6 cells/ml were sonicated by an ultrasonicator using a microtip by giving five bursts of 30 seconds each at an interval of one minute at 0°C in an ice bath. The cell lysis was confirmed by light microscopy. Venous blood (3 ml) collected in tube without anticoagulant was allowed to clot and then centrifuged at 2700 rpm (900 × g) in a refrigerated centrifuge (Plasto Craft, 4 R-V/FM, India) using swing out rotor (no. 15) at 4°C for 10 minutes to obtain serum.

2.5. Adenosine Estimation

Adenosine estimation was done according to the method described by Mollering and Bergmeyer [38]. Samples were deproteinized with 70% PCA. In a 3 ml eppendorf tube 600 μl of sample and 600 μl of ice cold 70% PCA (1 M) was mixed thoroughly and centrifuged at 3080 rpm (1000 × g) in a refrigerated centrifuge (Hermle Labortechnik GmbH Germany Type Z 36 HK) using angular rotor (no. 8) for 15 minutes at 10°C. Then to 400 μl of supernatant, 20 μl K_2CO_3 solution (5 M) was added to neutralize the sample. The reaction was allowed to stand for 15 minutes in an ice bath, centrifuged at 3080 rpm (1000 × g) at 10°C for 15 minutes and supernatant saved for adenosine estimation. Triethanolamine buffer solution (0.1 M $C_6H_{15}NO_3$, pH 7.4) (1000 μl) and sample (200 μl) was pipetted into cuvette, mixed thoroughly, and extinction E_I was read at 265 nm wavelength, using UV-Vis spectrophotometer (Cary Bio 100 Varian). Then, 8 μl of adenosine deaminase (0.1 mg protein/ml) was added and it was kept at 37°C for 5 minutes in a water bath. Final extinction E_{II} was read after 5 minutes. The difference in extinction coefficient ($\Delta E = E_I - E_{II}$) was calculated. The extinction increase due to addition of adenosine deaminase suspension alone was determined by the addition of further 8 µl of adenosine deaminase suspension II at the end of the reaction. Then this extinction increase was added to the extinction difference (ΔE). The results were expressed in nmol adenosine/ml serum, nmol adenosine/million lymphocytes and nmol adenosine/billion erythrocytes.

2.6. 5´-Nucleotidase (5´-NT) Assay

5´-nucleotidase activity was determined by the method described by Gerlach and Hiby [39]. Five tubes were taken and labelled, I as blank, II as standard, III without Ni^{2+}, IV with Ni^{2+} and V as control, followed by pipetting in eppendorf tubes (3 ml): distilled water (800 µl) in I and II, veronal buffer (40 mM $C_8H_{11}O_3N_2Na$, pH 7.5) (520 µl in serum and 640 µl in lysates of lymphocytes and erythrocytes labelled tubes) in III and V tubes and veronal buffer (40 mM $C_8H_{11}O_3N_2Na$, pH 7.5) (440 µl in serum and 560 µl in lysates of lymphocytes and erythrocytes labelled tubes) in IV tube, manganese sulphate solution (20 mM) (40 µl) in III, IV and V tubes, nickel chloride solution (0.1 M) (80 µl) in IV tube, distilled water (80 µl) in V tube, serum (160 µl) and lysates of lymphocytes and erythrocytes (40 µl) in III, IV and V tubes, AMP solution (10 mM) (80 µl) in III and IV tubes followed by mixing and incubation for 30 minutes at 37°C in water bath. Then 11% TCA (0.68 M) (800 µl) was added followed by centrifugation at 5340 rpm (3000 × g) in refrigerated centrifuge (HermleLabortechnik GmbH Germany Type Z 36 HK) using angular rotor (no. 8) at 10°C for 5 minutes and supernatant (1000 µl) transferred in properly labelled respective test tubes. Then KH_2PO_4 standard (50 µg/ml) (60 µl *i.e.* 3 µg) was pulsed in II, III and IV test tube followed by pipetting of 3000 µl distilled water into I and V and 2940 µl into II, III and IV tubes, molybdate solution (40 mM) (800 µl), reducing agent (400 µl) added successively into each test tube and mixed and allowed to stand for 10 minutes followed by addition of acetate solution (2.5 M) (1600 µl) and distilled water (1200 µl) into each tube. The reaction was allowed to stand for 5 minutes followed by measurement of O.D. at 578 nm, using UV-Vis spectrophotometer (Cary Bio 100 Varian). The enzyme activity was expressed in U/l in case of serum, mU/million lymphocytes, and mU/billion RBC.

2.7. Adenosine Deaminase (ADA) and Its Isoenzymes Assay

Total adenosine deaminase (ADA) activity was determined by the method of Giusti [40] and its isoenzymes (ADA1, ADA2) activities were determined as described by Goodarzi *et al.* [41].

2.7.1. Adenosine Deaminase (ADA) Assay

Four test tubes were prepared and labelled as reagent blank, standard, control and sample and followed by pipetting in test tubes: phosphate buffer (50 mM NaH_2PO_4 and $Na_2HPO_4 \cdot 12H_2O$, pH 6.5) (420 µl) in reagent blank tube, ammonium sulphate standard solution (75 µM) (400 µl) and distilled water (20 µl) in standard tubes, buffered adenosine solution (21 mM adenosine, 50 mM phosphate, pH 6.5) (380 µl in serum and erythrocytes labelled tubes and 410 µl in lymphocytes labelled tube) in sample and control tubes, sample (40 µl serum, 40 µl erythrocyte lysate and 10 µl of lymphocyte lysate) in sample tube followed by thorough mixing and incubation for 60 minutes at 37°C in water bath. Phenol-nitroprusside solution (106 mM phenol, 0.17 mM sodium nitroprusside) (1200 µl) and alkaline hypochlorite solution (11 mM NaOCl, 125 mM NaOH) (1200 µl) in all the four test tubes and sample (40 µl serum, 40 µl erythrocyte lysate and 10 µl lymphocyte lysate) were added in control tube successively. The contents of the tube were mixed before pipetting into the next test tube followed by incubation for 30 minutes at 37°C in water bath. The O.D. was measured against distilled water at 630 nm, using UV Visible spectrophotometer (Cary Bio 100 Varian). Enzyme activity was expressed in U/l in case of serum, mU/million lymphocytes, and mU/billion RBC.

2.7.2. Adenosine Deaminase Isoenzymes (ADA1, ADA2) Assay

ADA isoenzymes were distinguished by their differential inhibition by EHNA[Erythro-9(2-hydroxy-3-nonyl) adenine], which is known to inhibit ADA1. Four test tubes were prepared and labelled as reagent blank, standard, control and sample and followed by pipetting in test tubes: phosphate buffer (50 mM NaH_2PO_4 and $Na_2HPO_4 \cdot 12H_2O$, pH 6.5) (420 µl) in reagent blank tube, ammonium sulphate standard solution (75 µM) (400 µl) and distilled water (20 µl) in standard tubes, buffered adenosine solution (42 mM adenosine, 50 mM phosphate, pH 6.5) (200 µl in serum, lymphocytes and erythrocytes labelled tubes) in sample and control tubes, EHNA solution (1 mM) (84 µl), sample (40 µl serum, 40 µl erythrocyte lysate and 10 µl of lymphocyte lysate) in sample tube and phosphate buffer (50 mM NaH$_2$PO$_4$ and Na$_2$HPO$_4$·12H$_2$O, pH 6.5) (96 μl in serum and erythrocyte labelled and 126 μl in lymphocyte labelled tubes) to make up the total volume equal (420 μl) followed by thorough mixing and incubation for 60 minutes at 37˚C in water bath. Phenol-nitroprusside solution (106 mM phenol, 0.17 mM sodium nitroprusside) (1200 μl) and alkaline hypochlorite solution (11 mM NaOCl, 125 mM NaOH) (1200 μl) in all the four test tubes and sample (40 μl serum, 40 μl erythrocyte lysate and 10 μl lymphocyte lysate) were added in control tube successively. The contents of the tube were mixed before pipetting into the next test tube followed by incubation for 30 minutes at 37˚C in water bath. The O.D. was measured against distilled water at wavelength 630 nm, using UV-V is spectrophotometer (Cary Bio 100 Varian). The ADA2 enzyme activity was expressed in U/l in case of serum, mU/million lymphocytes, and mU/billion RBC. ADA$_1$ activity was calculated by subtracting ADA$_2$ from total ADA activity.

2.8. Statistical Analysis

One way analysis of variance (ANOVA) and Tukey HSD test was applied for statistical analysis. The Pearson's test was used to determine correlation. Normally distributed data is displayed as mean and 95% confidence interval (CI). The p value of <0.05 was considered significant.

3. Results

3.1. Characteristics of Study Population

The characteristics of the study population are shown in **Table 1**.

Table 1. The clinicophysiological details of subjects.

Subject information parameters	Healthy controls	Bronchial asthma groups		
		Mild persistent (Group I)	Moderate persistent (Group II)	Severe persistent (Group III)
Age (years)	31.13 ± 9.79	31.93 ± 8.97	35.93 ± 10.46	34.53 ± 11.38
(Range)	(19 - 52)	(18 - 48)	(20 - 54)	(19 - 53)
Sex				
Male	6	4	8	8
Female	9	11	7	7
Duration of illness	-	1.60 ± 1.52	3.52 ± 3.30	5.33 ± 3.27
(Range)	-	(2 months - 6 years)	(6 months - 10 years)	(1 - 11 years)
Family history of asthma				
Positive	None	2	2	1
Absent		13	13	14
Diet				
Vegetarian	7	8	8	6
Non-vegetarian	8	7	7	9
FEV1% predicted	-	84.20 ± 3.28	71.40 ± 6.16	51.0 ± 5.75
(Range)		(80 - 89)	(61 - 78)	(36 - 57)
FEV1/FVC% predicted	-	88.60 ± 7.87	84.66 ± 10.8	69.26 ± 10.79
(Range)		(80.73 - 96.47)	(73.86 - 95.46)	(58.47 - 80.05)

Parameter values are mean ± S.D for n = 15 subjects. FEV1: forced expiratory volume in 1 sec.

3.2. Characteristics of Isolated Lymphocytes and Erythrocytes

Total number of lymphocytes obtained from peripheral blood of controls was 1.46 ± 0.03 (mean $\pm$ SEM) million/ml and of asthmatic patients was 1.79 ± 0.04 (mean $\pm$ SEM) million cells/ml. The differential cell counts of the isolated lymphocytes from blood revealed that $96.0\% \pm 0.45\%$ (mean $\pm$ SEM) of the cells were lymphocytes in the cell suspension. The viability of the cells was $96.00\% \pm 0.097\%$ (mean $\pm$ SEM). Total number of erythrocytes obtained from peripheral blood was 6.00 ± 0.12 (mean $\pm$ SEM) billion cells/ml in normal subjects and 5.51 ± 0.09 (mean $\pm$ SEM) billion/ml in asthma.

3.3. Adenosine Levels in Healthy Controls and Asthmatics

In asthma, adenosine levels in serum, lymphocytes and erythrocytes were found to be raised significantly as compared to healthy controls ($p < 0.0001$). The difference was statistically significant between control and mild persistent [($p < 0.001$) in serum and ($p < 0.0001$) in lymphocytes and erythrocytes], control and moderate persistent ($p < 0.0001$) and control and severe persistent asthmatics ($p < 0.0001$) in serum, lymphocytes and erythrocytes separately. Within the three groups of asthmatics, difference in adenosine levels were significant between mild persistent and severe persistent asthmatics in serum, lymphocytes and erythrocytes ($p < 0.05$). The difference between mild and moderate persistent and between moderate and severe persistent was found to be significant in lymphocytes ($p < 0.05$) and not significant in serum and erythrocytes (**Table 2**). The FEV1% was observed to have a negative correlation with the serum adenosine levels ($r = -0.4879$, $p < 0.001$) (**Figure 1(a)**), adenosine levels of lymphocytes ($r = -0.7097$, $p < 0.0001$) (**Figure 1(b)**), and with the erythrocytes' adenosine levels ($r = -0.5581$, $p < 0.0001$) (**Figure 1(c)**).

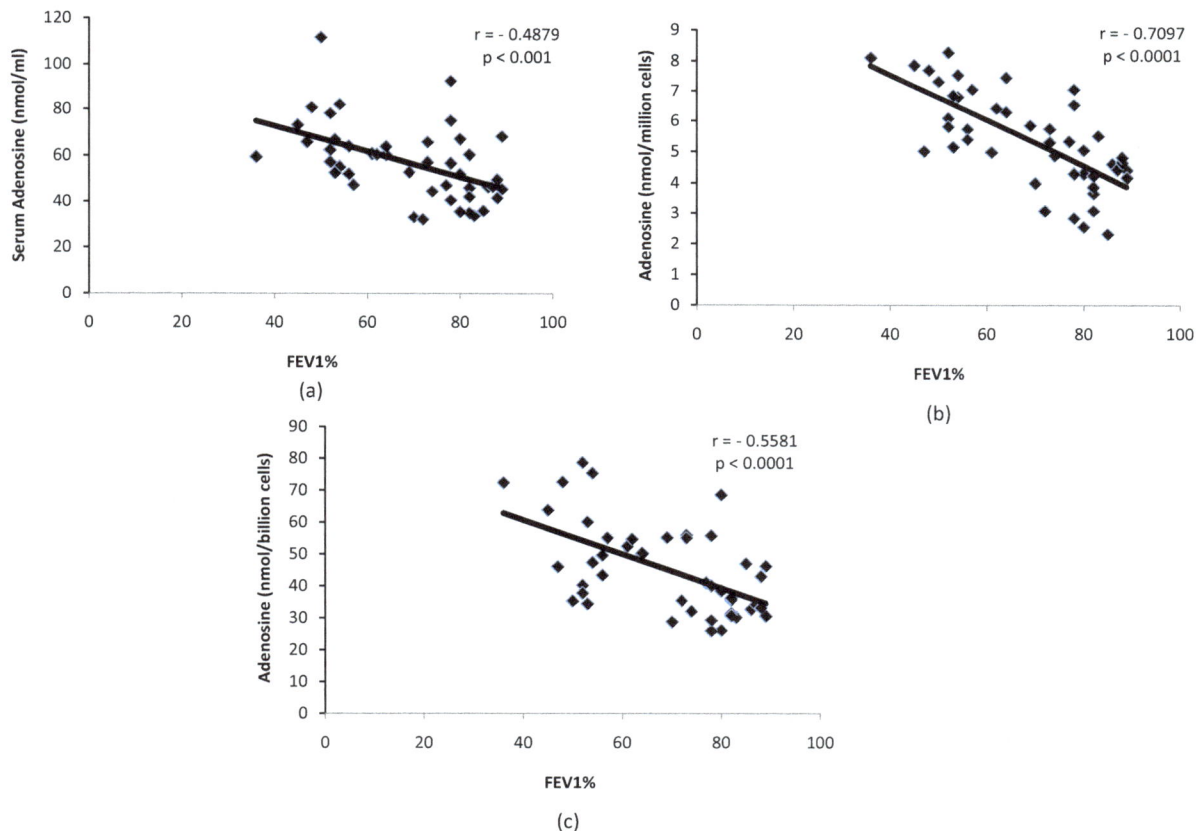

Figure 1. Relationship between FEV1% predicted and adenosine levels in (a) serum expressed as nanomoles/ml (b) lymphocytes expressed as nanomoles/million cells and (c) erythrocytes expressed as nanomoles/billion cells of asthmatic patients. FEV1: forced expiratory volume in one second.

Table 2. Adenosine levels in serum, lymphocytes and erythrocytes.

	Healthy controls	Bronchial asthma groups		
		Mild persistent (Group I)	Moderate persistent (Group II)	Severe persistent (Group III)
Serum[a]	27.82 ± 1.90	47.01 ± 2.83**	56.14 ± 4.06***	67.17 ± 4.20****†
(Range)	(16.61 - 41.83)	(33.62 - 67.98)	(32.11 - 92.63)	(47.36 - 111.60)
Lymphocytes[b]	2.54 ± 0.14	4.13 ± 0.23***	5.34 ± 0.35****†	6.71 ± 0.28****†‡
(Range)	(1.14 - 3.25)	(2.31 - 5.50)	(2.84 - 7.46)	(5.00 - 8.27)
Erythrocytes[c]	20.31 ± 1.40	37.57 ± 2.70***	44.11 ± 2.93***	54.11 ± 3.97****†
(Range)	(9.96 - 29.58)	(26.07 - 68.51)	(25.92 - 55.95)	(34.36 - 78.65)

[a]Expressed as nanomoles/ml (mean ± SEM). [b]Expressed as nanomoles/million lymphocytes (mean ± SEM). [c]Expressed as nanomoles/billion erythrocytes (mean ± SEM). **$p < 0.001$, ***$p < 0.0001$ in comparison with healthy controls. †$p < 0.05$ in comparison with Group I, ‡$p < 0.05$ in comparison with Group II. N = 15 in each group.

3.4. 5′-Nucleotidase Activity in Healthy Controls and Asthma Patients

In asthma, the 5′-NT activity was raised significantly in moderate persistent [($p < 0.0001$) in serum and ($p < 0.05$) in lymphocytes], and severe persistent [($p < 0.0001$) in serum and lymphocytes and ($p < 0.05$) in erythrocytes] asthmatics in comparison with the healthy controls but the difference was not significant statistically between mild persistent and healthy controls in serum, lymphocytes and erythrocytes. The difference was significant between mild and severe persistent asthmatics in serum and lymphocytes ($p < 0.05$) and between mild and moderate ($p < 0.05$) and between moderate and severe persistent ($p < 0.05$) asthmatics in lymphocytes (**Table 3**). Comparison among various groups of bronchial asthma revealed no statistically significant difference in erythrocytes. The FEV1% showed a negative correlation with the serum 5′-NT activity ($r = -0.4018$, $p < 0.05$) (**Figure 2(a)**) and with the 5′-NT activity in lymphocytes ($r = -0.8362$, $p < 0.0001$) (**Figure 2(b)**). No correlation between FEV1% and 5′-NT activity in erythrocytes ($r = -0.1399$) existed (**Figure 2(c)**).

3.5. Adenosine Deaminase and Its Isoenzymes Activity in Healthy Controls and Asthmatics

Total ADA and its isoenzymes (ADA1, ADA2) activities were assayed in serum, lymphocytes and erythrocytes (**Table 4**). In asthma, the total activity of ADA, ADA1 and ADA2 in serum decreased as compared to healthy controls. The difference was significant between control and moderate persistent asthmatics [($p < 0.0001$) for total ADA and ADA1, ($p < 0.001$) for ADA2], control and severe persistent asthmatics [($p < 0.0001$) for total ADA, ADA1 and ADA2]. However, the difference was not significant between mild persistent and healthy controls. Further, the decrease in total ADA, ADA1 and ADA2 was significant between mild and moderate persistent asthmatics and between mild and severe persistent asthmatics ($p < 0.05$). The FEV1% had a positive correlation with the serum total ADA ($r = 0.6127$, $p < 0.0001$), ADA1 ($r = 0.4630$, $p < 0.001$) and ADA2 ($r = 0.5804$, $p < 0.0001$) activity (**Figure 3**).

In lymphocytes, the total ADA and ADA1 activity decreased significantly in moderate persistent and severe persistent asthmatics in comparison with healthy controls ($p < 0.0001$). The difference was not significant between mild persistent asthmatics and healthy controls. Also, no significant difference in ADA2 activity was found between asthmatics and healthy controls. Comparison among bronchial asthma groups revealed significant decrease in total ADA and ADA1 in moderate persistent than in mild persistent and significant decrease in severe persistent than in moderate persistent and mild persistent ($p < 0.05$) (**Table 4**). There was a positive correlation ($r = 0.7015$, $p < 0.0001$) between FEV1 (% predicted) and total ADA activity (**Figure 4(a)**).

In erythrocytes, the total ADA, ADA1 and ADA2 activity in erythrocytes of bronchial asthma patients increased significantly in mild persistent asthmatics as compared to healthy controls ($p < 0.0001$), but became normal in moderate and severe persistent (**Table 4**). The difference was significant between mild and moderate persistent and between mild and severe persistent ($p < 0.0001$) but not between moderate and severe persistent asthmatics. A positive correlation ($r = 0.5473$, $p < 0.0001$) was observed between FEV1 (% predicted) and total ADA activity (**Figure 4(b)**).

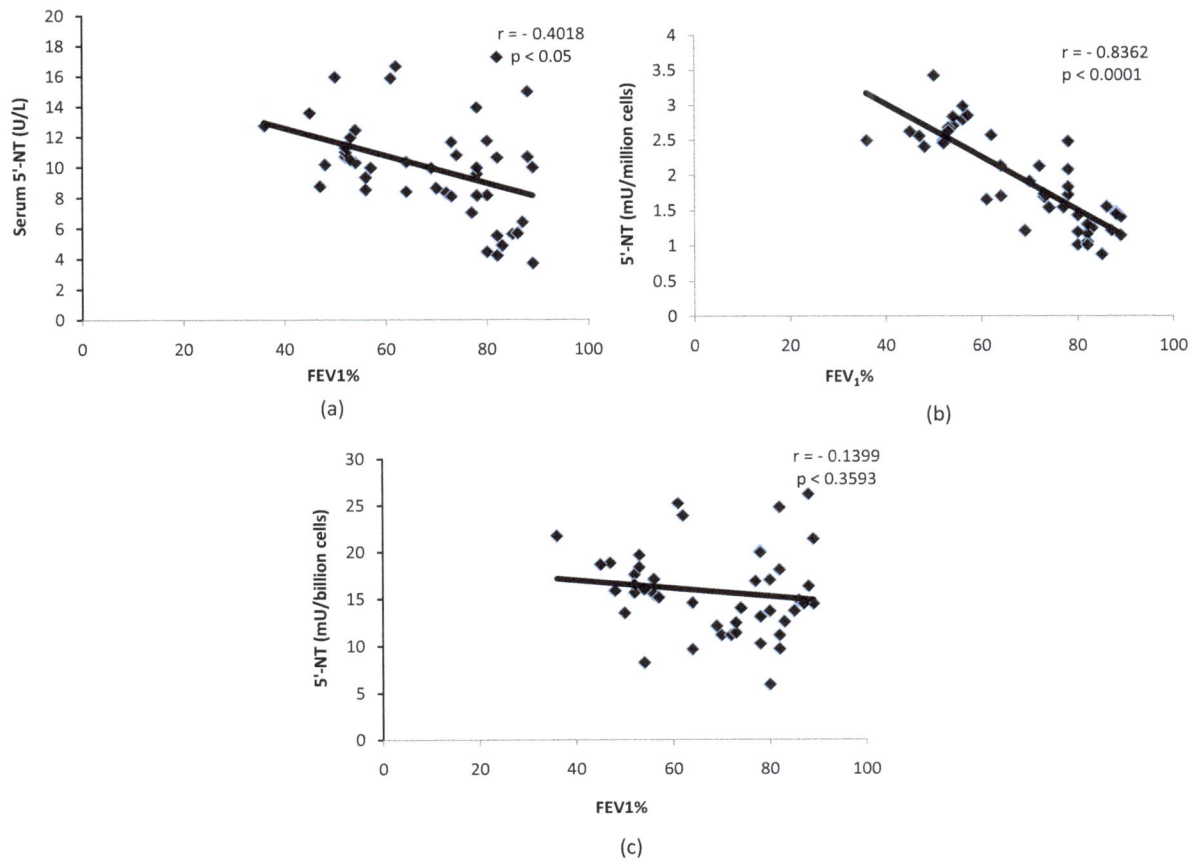

(a)

(b)

(c)

Figure 2. Correlation between FEV1% predicted and 5′-NT activity in (a) serum expressed as Units/l (b) lymphocytes expressed as milliunits/million cells and (c) erythrocytes expressed as milliunits/billion cells of asthmatic patients. FEV1: forced expiratory volume in one second. 5′-NT: 5′-nucleotidase.

Table 3. 5′-nucleotidase (5′-NT) activity in serum, lymphocytes and erythrocytes.

	Healthy controls	**Bronchial asthma groups**		
		Mild persistent (Group I)	**Moderate persistent (Group II)**	**Severe persistent (Group III)**
Serum[a]	6.26 ± 0.26	8.26 ± 1.07	$10.49 \pm 0.75^{***}$	$11.14 \pm 0.50^{***\dagger}$
(Range)	(4.28 - 7.63)	(3.70 - 17.27)	(7.02 - 16.66)	(8.53 - 15.94)
Lymphocytes[b]	1.53 ± 0.08	1.23 ± 0.05	$1.86 \pm 0.09^{*\dagger}$	$2.69 \pm 0.07^{***\dagger\ddagger}$
(Range)	(0.98 - 1.97)	(0.88 - 1.55)	(1.21 - 2.57)	(2.40 - 3.42)
Erythrocytes[c]	11.75 ± 0.68	15.60 ± 1.39	15.03 ± 1.29	$16.54 \pm 0.80^{*}$
(Range)	(7.49 - 15.48)	(5.86 - 26.17)	(9.61 - 25.18)	(8.20 - 21.74)

[a]Expressed as U/L (mean $\pm$ SEM). [b]Expressed as mU/million lymphocytes (mean $\pm$ SEM). [c]Expressed as mU/billion erythrocytes (mean $\pm$ SEM). $^{*}p < 0.05$, $^{***}p < 0.0001$ in comparison with healthy controls, $^{\dagger}p < 0.05$ in comparison with Group I, $^{\ddagger}p < 0.05$ in comparison with Group II. n= 15 in each group.

4. Discussion

Adenosine is a signalling molecule produced as a result of cell stress or damage [26]. Several studies demonstrate elevated adenosine levels in patients with chronic lung disease [42]. Adenosine levels are elevated in

Table 4. ADA and its isoenzymes activities.

	Healthy controls	Bronchial asthma groups		
		Mild persistent (Group I)	Moderate persistent (Group II)	Severe persistent (Group III)
Serum				
ADA[a]	11.16 ± 0.39	10.69 ± 0.32	$8.29 \pm 0.31^{****\dagger}$	$7.71 \pm 0.33^{****\dagger}$
(Range)	(8.82 - 14.37)	(7.91 - 20.4)	(6.46 - 10.57)	(8.53 - 15.94)
ADA1[a]	3.77 ± 0.20	3.53 ± 0.23	$2.24 \pm 0.16^{****\dagger}$	$2.43 \pm 0.18^{****\dagger}$
(Range)	(2.91 - 5.85)	(1.77 - 4.76)	(1.31 - 3.61)	(1.16 - 3.46)
ADA2[a]	7.39 ± 0.29	7.16 ± 0.19	$6.06 \pm 0.24^{**\dagger}$	$5.28 \pm 0.23^{****\dagger}$
(Range)	(5.58 - 9.48)	(6.14 - 8.56)	(5.07 - 8.42)	(3.36 - 6.38)
Lymphocytes				
ADA[b]	6.91 ± 0.19	7.39 ± 0.19	$5.57 \pm 0.29^{****\dagger}$	$4.53 \pm 0.21^{****\dagger\ddagger}$
(Range)	(5.58 - 7.95)	(5.79 - 8.24)	(4.07 - 7.46)	(2.88 - 5.79)
ADA1[b]	6.45 ± 0.17	6.84 ± 0.19	$5.10 \pm 0.25^{****\dagger}$	$4.21 \pm 0.19^{****\dagger\ddagger}$
(Range)	(5.30 - 7.32)	(5.26 - 7.89)	(3.74 - 6.70)	(2.65 - 5.47)
ADA2[b]	0.46 ± 0.05	0.55 ± 0.05	0.47 ± 0.05	$0.32 \pm 0.03^{\dagger}$
(Range)	(0.20 - 0.86)	(0.35 - 0.79)	(0.19 - 0.76)	(0.12 - 0.49)
Erythrocytes				
ADA[c]	3.77 ± 0.23	$6.55 \pm 0.27^{***}$	$3.74 \pm 0.27^{\dagger\dagger\dagger}$	$3.71 \pm 0.34^{\dagger\dagger\dagger}$
(Range)	(2.02 - 5.09)	(4.52 - 8.28)	(1.44 - 5.22)	(2.88 - 5.79)
ADA1[c]	3.60 ± 0.23	$6.24 \pm 0.26^{***}$	$3.57 \pm 0.26^{\dagger\dagger\dagger}$	$3.65 \pm 0.33^{\dagger\dagger\dagger}$
(Range)	(1.87 - 4.98)	(4.34 - 8.01)	(1.37 - 5.00)	(0.98 - 5.76)
ADA2[c]	0.17 ± 0.01	$0.31 \pm 0.03^{***}$	$0.17 \pm 0.01^{\dagger\dagger\dagger}$	$0.14 \pm 0.01^{\dagger\dagger\dagger}$
(Range)	(0.11 - 0.27)	(0.14 - 0.60)	(0.07 - 0.27)	(0.12 - 0.49)

[a]Expressed as U/L (mean ± SEM). [b]Expressed as mU/million lymphocytes (mean ± SEM). [c]Expressed as mU/billion erythrocytes (mean ± SEM). $^{**}p < 0.001$, $^{***}p < 0.0001$ in comparison with healthy controls, $^{\dagger}p < 0.05$, $^{\dagger\dagger\dagger}p < 0.0001$ in comparison with Group I, $^{\ddagger}p < 0.05$ in comparison with Group II. n = 15 in each group.

lavage fluid collected from asthmatics [21], in the exhaled breath condensate of patients with allergic asthma [43], in plasma of asthmatic subjects following bronchial provocation with allergen [44] and in patients with exercise-induced asthma [45]. Adenosine levels are controlled by the rates of adenosine biosynthesis and its catabolism. Adenosine is generated intracellularly and released through constitutively expressed nucleoside transporters. Extracellular adenosine is formed from the dephosphorylation of adenine nucleotides, a reaction catalysed by 5′-nucleotidase. Once produced, adenosine can engage cell surface adenosine receptors or be removed by metabolism to inosine by adenosine deaminase (ADA).

The 5′-nucleotidase (CD73) is the major enzyme for extracellular adenosine production [42]. 5′-nucleotidase levels are up-regulated in the lungs of mouse models with chronic lung disease including ADA-deficient mice and mice exposed to bleomycin [46]. In addition, bronchial epithelial cells from patients with cystic fibrosis exhibit increased CD73 activity [47]. These findings suggest that the up-regulation of 5′-nucleotidase is an important purinergic remodelling response in environments where adenosine has been shown to regulate the disease. In the current study, we observed that the enzymatic activity of 5′-nucleotidase was significantly increased in

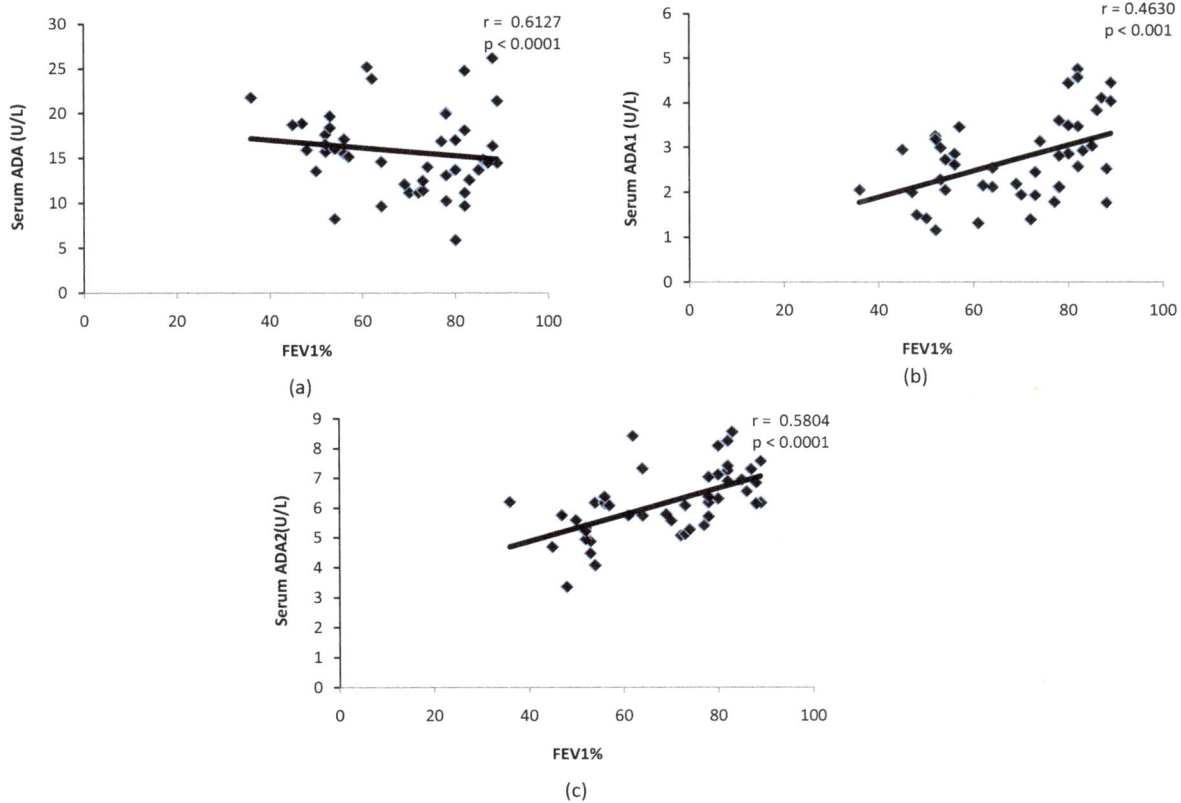

Figure 3. Relationship between FEV1% predicted and serum (a) total ADA activity (b) ADA1 and (c) ADA2 activity expressed as Units/l in asthma. FEV1: forced expiratory volume in one second. ADA: Adenosine deaminase.

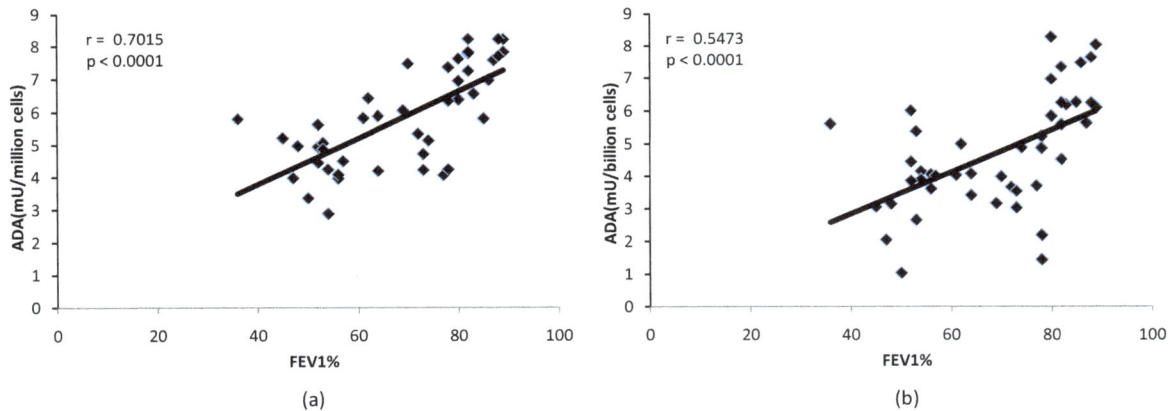

Figure 4. Correlation between FEV1% predicted and ADA activity in (a) lymphocytes expressed as milliunits/million cells and (b) erythrocytes expressed as milliunits/billion cells of asthmatic patients. FEV1: forced expiratory volume in one second. ADA: Adenosine deaminase.

serum as well as lymphocytes of both moderate persistent (Group II) and severe persistent asthma (Group III) groups (p < 0.0001). Consistent with this, adenosine levels in serum and lymphocytes in asthma patients were found to be raised significantly compared with subjects with preserved lung function. Further, in this study, the changes in 5′-nucleotidase activity in serum and lymphocytes showed a significant reciprocal correlation with FEV1 of asthma patients suggesting that as the severity of airway obstruction increases (shown by decrease in

FEV1), the level of 5'-nucleotidase activity was found to be increased. Similarly, raised adenosine levels in serum and lymphocytes showed a significant inverse correlation with FEV1 of asthma patients which suggest that with the increase in the severity of airway obstruction, levels of adenosine were found to be elevated. These findings suggest that 5'-nucleotidase enzyme might play a major role not only in the production of adenosine but also in the modulation of adenosine levels in serum and lymphocytes and the up-regulation of 5'-nucleotidase might be considered as an important purinergic response in bronchial asthma. In case of erythrocytes, adenosine levels were found to be increased in asthma patients but 5'-nucleotidase activity was raised only in severe persistent group and as no correlation was found between severity of asthma and 5'-nucleotidase activity, therefore it could be assumed that 5'-nucleotidase contributes little in regulating levels of adenosine in erythrocytes. These findings suggest that there is an increased production of adenosine in asthma and the increase in 5'-nucleotidase in serum and lymphocytes provides a novel and important means of determining the capacity of adenosine generation.

Adenosine deaminase (ADA) is the major enzyme of adenosine metabolism [48]. It deaminates adenosine to inosine. Elevated levels of adenosine have been shown to be associated with features of inflammation, alveolar remodelling, pulmonary fibrosis, and mucus secretion in lungs of a mice model over-expressing the Th2 cytokines viz. IL-4 or IL-13 [49] [50]. Interestingly, ADA transcripts and enzymatic activity are selectively down-regulated in the lungs of these mice suggesting a purinergic remodelling response directed at promoting adenosine accumulation. In our study, we observed that the total activity of adenosine deaminase was significantly decreased in serum of asthma patients. Total ADA activity decreased in all the three groups of asthmatics, which was however decreased significantly in moderate (Group II) and severe persistent (Group III) groups. The decrease in total ADA activity in serum of asthma patients was apparently primarily due to low ADA2 activity, although ADA1 activity also decreased in moderate and severe persistent groups. Further, a significant positive correlation between FEV1 of asthma patients and reduction in the total activity of ADA and its isoenzymes in serum indicates that with the increase in the severity of airway obstruction, activities of ADA and its isoenzymes (ADA1 and ADA2) decreased significantly or *vice versa*. In lymphocytes of asthma patients, total ADA activity was found to be decreased as compared to subjects with preserved pulmonary function in our study. The decrease in activity was found to be significant in moderate persistent (Group II) and severe persistent (Group III) asthma patients and no significant alteration in its activity was found in mild persistent (Group I) group. The decreased total ADA activity in bronchial asthma was largely due to reduced activity of the ADA isoenzyme ADA1 and the contribution of ADA2 was only minor. Further, fall in the activity of ADA and its isoenzymes in lymphocytes showed a significant positive correlation with FEV1 of asthma patients suggesting that with the increase in the severity of airway obstruction, activities of ADA and its isoenzyme (ADA1) were decreased significantly. Thus, fall in total activity of ADA along with raised adenosine levels in serum and lymphocytes and positive correlation of both with the severity of airway obstruction indicates that ADA enzyme might also act as a major regulator of adenosine levels in serum and lymphocytes of asthma patients. In case of erythrocytes, total ADA activity was found to be raised significantly only in mild persistent (Group I) group of asthma but the difference was not significant in moderate(Group II) and severe persistent (Group III) group when compared to healthy control. This increased activity of ADA was predominantly due to increased activity of the ADA isoenzyme, ADA1. ADA and its isoenzymes activities in erythrocytes showed a significant positive correlation with FEV1 of asthma patients. These findings suggest that determination of ADA, ADA1 and ADA2 in serum, and ADA or more specifically ADA1 in lymphocytes, might serve as a way of determining the capacity of adenosine generation.

Increased activity of 5'-nucleotidase and concomitant low activity of ADA along with raised levels of adenosine in asthma patients suggest that these two enzymes might play a crucial role in controlling levels of adenosine in serum. Elevation in serum adenosine level that was found in this study may lead to increased circulation of adenosine in lungs which may also reflect its increased level in lung of asthma patients (**Figure 5**). It is also known that the leakage of metabolites and enzymes from a tissue may cause an increase in the blood and may thus reflect the changes in a particular tissue in a particular condition. In the setting of tissue injury, the predominant source of extracellular adenosine arises from the breakdown of adenine nucleotides [51] [52]. Elevations in extracellular adenosine can result from either an increase in intracellular adenosine followed by its release into the extracellular space, or by the release of adenine nucleotides followed by their extracellular catabolism into adenosine [53]. Intracellularly, adenosine can be generated from the dephosphorylation of AMP by cytosolic 5'-nucleotidases [54]. Extracellularly, adenosine can be generated following the release and dephosphorylation

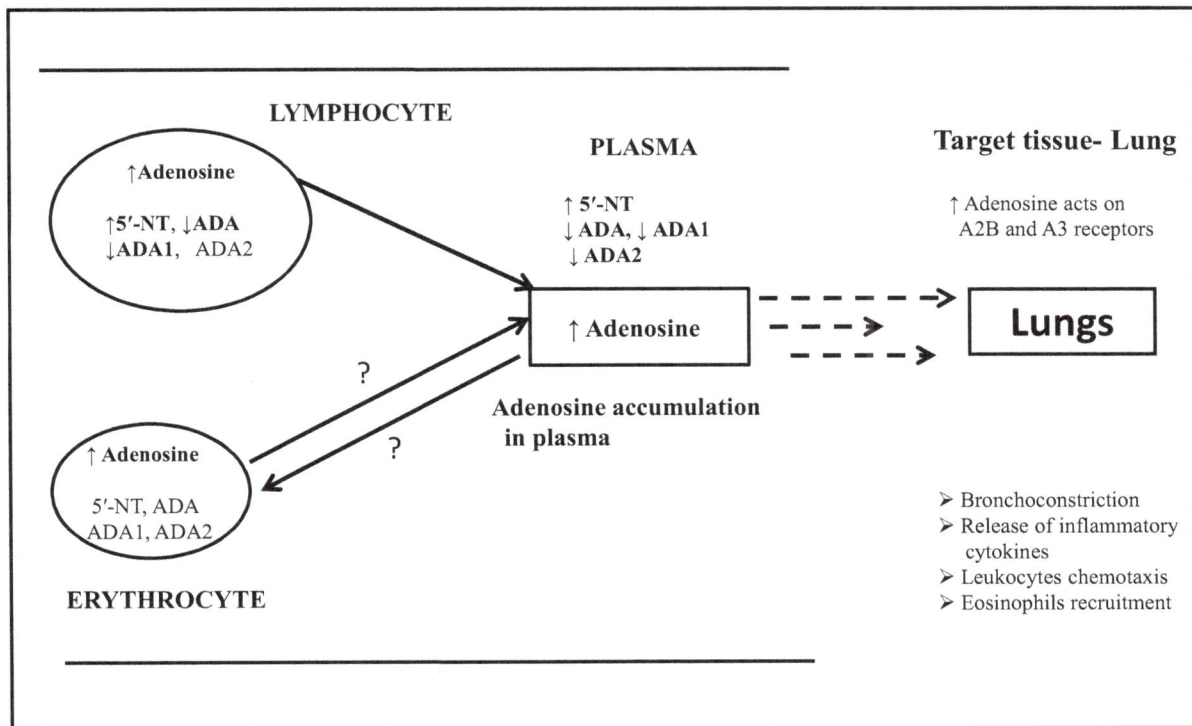

Figure 5. Adenosine metabolism in bronchial asthma. In asthma, elevated levels of adenosine in plasma are found due to (a) its increased synthesis extracellularly as a result of increased 5´-NT activity and decreased total ADA, ADA1 and ADA2 isoenzyme activity, (b) increased synthesis in lymphocytes (because of increased 5´-NT activity and decreased total ADA and ADA1 isoenzyme activity) followed by its release into plasma. In erythrocytes, adenosine levels were found to be raised but no change in 5´-NT and total ADA and its isoenzymes' activity were found. Thus, role of erythrocytes in adenosine release into plasma or adenosine uptake from plasma and storage is uncertain. Adenosine, thus accumulated in plasma may lead to its increased circulation in lungs, where it acts via its receptors to cause inflammatory changes.

of adenine nucleotides [53]. ATP and AMP are released from activated granulocytes [55] [56], upon degranulation [57]. Bronchial epithelium can release ATP under basal conditions [58] and upon perturbation of the plasma membrane [59]. Extracellular ATP and ADP can be converted into AMP and then into adenosine by ecto-5´-nucleotidase (CD73). In addition to the release of adenine nucleotides from cells, there is also evidence that adenosine itself can be released from inflammatory mast cells during the degranulation process [60]. This highlights the importance of inflammatory cells as a direct source of adenosine. It is still unclear which pathway and which enzymes are responsible for extracellular adenosine accumulations following tissue injury. But, from our study, it may be proposed that the increased level of adenosine in serum may be due to its leakage from airways or from lymphocytes and erythrocytes in asthma. Further, adenosine accumulation in the lung is not only a product of lung inflammation and damage, but can directly affect signalling pathway that lead to features of chronic lung disease [61]. Adenosine elevations in the lungs of patients with asthma suggest that this signalling molecule may regulate bronchoconstriction and the unique bronchial sensitivity of asthmatics to adenosine suggest a fundamental alteration in adenosine receptor signalling in the lungs of these patients. Adenosine, via engagement of the A2BR, increases the release of IL-6 and monocyte chemotactic protein-1 from bronchial smooth muscle cells [62] providing a mechanism whereby adenosine acts as a pro-inflammatory mediator in the airway. Recently, Ethier *et al.* found that the A1R mediates mobilization of calcium in human bronchial smooth muscle cells, suggesting that adenosine has direct effects on contractile signalling pathways [63], which may be one of the mechanisms for bronchoconstriction. Activation of the A2BR on human lung fibroblasts increases the release of IL-6 and induces differentiation into myofibroblasts suggesting that adenosine, via A2BR participates in the remodelling process occurring in chronic lung diseases [64]. Chunn *et al.* revealed that controlling adenosine levels with the use of exogenous ADA treatments may provide a significant approach to seize the progression or alter the features of pulmonary fibrosis in severe asthma [65].

5. Conclusion

The present study clearly demonstrates that the adenosine levels are raised in serum, lymphocytes and erythrocytes in bronchial asthma patients and correlation of this increase in adenosine with increase in airway obstruction provides evidence in favour of adenosine for its role as a crucial inflammatory mediator in asthma. It also confirms that adenosine levels tend to increase in serum, lymphocytes and erythrocytes with the severity of bronchial asthma. Next, increase in activity of 5'-nucleotidase and a concomitant decrease in activity of adenosine deaminase and its isoenzymes in serum and lymphocytes demonstrate the importance of these two enzymes in adenosine metabolism and suggest that the balance between these two enzymes determines the levels of adenosine in serum and lymphocytes which might act as potential inflammatory mediator in asthma. Further, increase in activity of 5'-nucleotidase and a corresponding decrease in adenosine deaminase activity with the worsening of asthma clearly emphasize that these two enzymes play a crucial role in accumulation of adenosine which may result in pathogenesis of bronchial asthma, or *vice versa*.

References

[1]   Asher, M.I., Montefort, S., Björkstén, B., Lai, C.K., Strachan, D.P., Weiland, S.K. and Williams, H. (2006) ISAAC Phase Three Study Group. Worldwide Time Trends in the Prevalence of Symptoms of Asthma, Allergic Rhinoconjunctivitis, and Eczema in Childhood: ISAAC Phases One and Three Repeat Multicountry Cross-Sectional Surveys. *Lancet*, **368**, 733-743. http://dx.doi.org/10.1016/S0140-6736(06)69283-0

[2]   Jindal, S.K. (2007) Bronchial Asthma the Indian Scene. *Current Opinion in Pulmonary Medicine*, **13**, 8-12. http://dx.doi.org/10.1097/MCP.0b013e32800ffd09

[3]   McFadden Jr., E.R., Kasper, D.L., Braunwald, E., Fauci, A.S., Longo, D.L., Hauser, S.L. and Jameson, J.L. (2005) Harrison's Principles of Internal Medicine. 16th Edition, McGraw Hill, New York, 1508-1516.

[4]   Busse, W.W. and Lemanske, R.F. (2001) Asthma. *New England Journal of Medicine*, **344**, 350-362. http://dx.doi.org/10.1056/NEJM200102013440507

[5]   Linssen, M.J., Wilhelms, O.H. and Timmerman, H. (1991) Animal Models for Testing Anti-Inflammatory Drugs for Treatment of Bronchial Hyperreactivity in Asthma. *Pharmaceutisch Weekblad* (*Scientific Edition*), **13**, 225-237. http://dx.doi.org/10.1007/BF02015576

[6]   Dunnill, M.S. (1960) The Pathology of Asthma, with Special Reference to Changes in the Bronchial Mucosa. *Journal of Clinical Pathology*, **13**, 27-33. http://dx.doi.org/10.1136/jcp.13.1.27

[7]   Winn, H.R., Rubio, R. and Berne, R.M. (1981) Brain Adenosine Concentrations during Hypoxia in Rats. *American Journal of Physiology*, **241**, 235-242.

[8]   Van, B.H., Goossens, F. and Wynants, J. (1987) Formation and Release of Purine Catabolites during Hypoperfusion, Anoxia, and Ischemia. *American Journal of Pathology*, **252**, 886-893.

[9]   Linden, J. (2001) Molecular Approach to Adenosine Receptors: Receptor-Mediated Mechanisms of Tissue Protection. *Annual Review of Pharmacology and Toxicology*, **41**, 775-787. http://dx.doi.org/10.1146/annurev.pharmtox.41.1.775

[10]   Newby, A.C. (1984) Adenosine and the Concept of Retaliatory Metabolites. *Trends in Biochemical Sciences*, **9**, 42-44. http://dx.doi.org/10.1016/0968-0004(84)90176-2

[11]   Cushley, M.J., Tattersfield, A.E. and Holgate, S.T. (1983) Inhaled Adenosine and Guanosine on Airway Resistance in Normal and Asthmatic Subjects. *British Journal of Clinical Pharmacology*, **15**, 161-165. http://dx.doi.org/10.1111/j.1365-2125.1983.tb01481.x

[12]   Church, M.K., Hughes, P.J. and Vardey, C.J. (1986) Studies on the Receptor Mediating Cyclic AMP-Independent Enhancement by Adenosine of IgE Dependent Mediator Release from Rat Mast Cells. *British Journal of Pharmacology*, **87**, 233-242. http://dx.doi.org/10.1111/j.1476-5381.1986.tb10176.x

[13]   Salvatore, C.A., Jacobson, M.A., Taylor, H.E., Linden, J. and Johnson, R.G. (1993) Molecular Cloning and Characterization of the Human A_3 Adenosine Receptor. *Proceedings of the National Academy of Sciences of the United States of America*, **90**, 10365-10369. http://dx.doi.org/10.1073/pnas.90.21.10365

[14]   Tigani, B., Hannon, J.P., Mazzoni, L. and Fozard, J.R. (2000) Effects of Wortmannin on Bronchoconstrictor Responses to Adenosine in Actively Sensitised Brown Norway Rats. *European Journal of Pharmacology*, **406**, 469-476. http://dx.doi.org/10.1016/S0014-2999(00)00705-6

[15]   Tilley, S.L., Wagoner, V.A., Salvatore, C.A., Jacobson, M.A. and Koller, B.H. (2000) Adenosine and Inosine Increase Cutaneous Vasopermeability by Activating A_3 Receptors on Mast Cells. *Journal of Clinical Investigation*, **105**, 361-367. http://dx.doi.org/10.1172/JCI8253

[16]   Young, H.W., Molina, J.G., Dimina, D., Zhong, H., Jacobson, M., Chan, L.N., Chan, T.S., Lee, J.J. and Blackburn,

M.R. (2004) A₃ Adenosine Receptor Signalling Contributes to Airway Inflammation and Mucus Production in Adenosine Deaminase-Deficient Mice. *The Journal of Immunology*, **173**, 1380-1389. http://dx.doi.org/10.4049/jimmunol.173.2.1380

[17] Koshiba, M., Rosin, D.L., Hayashi, N., Linden, J. and Sitkovsky, M.V. (1999) Patterns of A₂ₐ Extracellular Adenosine Receptor Expression in Different Functional Subsets of Human Peripheral T Cells. Flow Cytometry Studies with Anti-A₂ₐ Receptor Monoclonal Antibodies. *Molecular Pharmacology*, **55**, 614-624.

[18] Henttinen, T., Jalkanen, S. and Yegutkin, G.G. (2003) Adherent Leukocytes Prevent Adenosine Formation and Impair Endothelial Barrier Function by Ecto-5-Nucleotidase/CD73-Dependent Mechanism. *The Journal of Biological Chemistry*, **278**, 24888-24895. http://dx.doi.org/10.1074/jbc.M300779200

[19] Todriko, L.D. (1998) Changes in Morpho-Functional State of the Erythrocyte Membranes in Bronchial Asthma in Patients of Different Ages. *Lik Sparva*, **2**, 51-54.

[20] Masuev, A.M. and Masuev, K.A. (1991) Changes in the Lipid Composition of Cell Membranes in Patients with Bronchial Asthma after Glucocorticoid Therapy. *Kliniceskaia Meditsina*, **69**, 86-88.

[21] Driver, A.G., Kukoly, C.A., Ali, S. and Mustafa, S.J. (1993) Adenosine in Bronchoalveolar Lavage Fluid in Asthma. *The American Review of Respiratory Disease*, **148**, 91-97. http://dx.doi.org/10.1164/ajrccm/148.1.91

[22] Ali, S., Mustafa, S.J., Driver, A.G. and Metzger, W.J. (1991) Release of Adenosine in Bronchoalveolar Lavage Fluid Following Allergen Bronchial Provocation in Allergic Rabbits. *The American Review of Respiratory Disease*, **143**, 417-421.

[23] Mann, J.S., Holgate, S.T., Renwick, A.G. and Cushley, M.J. (1986) Airway Effects of Purine Nucleosides and Nucleotides and Release with Bronchial Provocation in Asthma. *Journal of Applied Physiology*, **61**, 1667-1676.

[24] Chunn, J.L., Young, H.W., Banerjee, S.K., Colasurdo, G.N. and Blackburn, M.R. (2001) Adenosine-Dependent Airway Inflammation and Hyperresponsiveness in Partially Adenosine Deaminase-Deficient Mice. *The Journal of Immunology*, **167**, 4676-4685. http://dx.doi.org/10.4049/jimmunol.167.8.4676

[25] Livingston, M., Heaney, L.G. and Ennis, M. (2004) Adenosine, Inflammation and Asthma—A Review. *Inflammation Research*, **53**, 171-178. http://dx.doi.org/10.1007/s00011-004-1248-2

[26] Hasko, G. and Cronstein, B.N. (2004) Adenosine an Endogenous Regulator of Innate Immunity. *Trends in Immunology*, **25**, 62-70. http://dx.doi.org/10.1016/j.it.2003.11.003

[27] Thompson, L.F. and Seegmiller, J.E. (1980) Adenosine Deaminase Deficiency and Severe Combined Immunodeficiency Disease. *Advances in Enzymology and Related Areas of Molecular Biology*, **51**, 167-210.

[28] Cirulea, F., Saura, C., Canela, E.I., Mallot, J., Lluis, C. and Franco, R. (1996) Adenosine Deaminase Affects Ligand-Induced Signalling by Interacting with Cell-Surface Adenosine Receptors. *FEBS Letters*, **380**, 219-223. http://dx.doi.org/10.1016/0014-5793(96)00023-3

[29] Herrara, C., Casado, V., Cirulea, F., Schofield, P., Mallol, J., Lluis, C. and Franco, R. (2001) Adenosine A₂ᴮ Receptors Behave as an Alternative Anchoring Protein for Cell Surface Adenosine Deaminase in Lymphocytes and Cultured Cells. *Molecular Pharmacology*, **59**, 127-134.

[30] Fredholm, B.B., Ijzerman, A.P., Jacobson, K.A., Klotz, K.N. and Linden, J. (2001) International Union of Pharmacology XXV: Nomenclature and Classification of Adenosine Receptors. *Pharmacological Reviews*, **53**, 352-527.

[31] Dunwiddie, T.V., Diao, L. and Proctor, W.R. (1997) Adenine Nucleotides Undergo Rapid, Quantitative Conversion to Adenosine in the Extracellular Space in Rat Hippocampus. *The Journal of Neuroscience*, **17**, 7673-7682.

[32] Polosa, R. (2002) Adenosine-Receptor Subtypes: Their Relevance to Adenosine Mediated Responses in Asthma and Chronic Obstructive Pulmonary Disease. *European Respiratory Journal*, **20**, 488-496. http://dx.doi.org/10.1183/09031936.02.01132002

[33] Andrew, J.H., Jaclyn, R., Stonebraker, C.A., Van, H., Eduardo, L., Richard, C.B. and Maryse, P. (2007) Adenosine Deaminase 1 and Concentrative Nucleoside Transporters 2 and 3 Regulate Adenosine on the Apical Surface of Human Airway Epithelia: Implications for Inflammatory Lung Diseases. *Biochemistry*, **46**, 10373-10383. http://dx.doi.org/10.1021/bi7009647

[34] Ratech, H., Thorbecke, G.J., Merdith, G. and Hirschhorn, R. (1981) Comparison and Possible Homology of Isoenzymes of Adenosine Deaminase in Aves and Humans. *Enzyme*, **26**, 74-84.

[35] (2007) National Asthma Education and Prevention Program Expert Panel Report 3. NIH Publication No. 08, 5846.

[36] Boyum, A. (1976) Isolation of Lymphocytes, Granulocytes and Macrophages. *Scandinavian Journal of Immunology*, **5**, 9-15. http://dx.doi.org/10.1111/j.1365-3083.1976.tb03851.x

[37] Bansal, S.K., Jha, A., Jaiswal, A.S. and Chhabra, S.K. (1997) Increased Levels of Protein Kinase C in Lymphocytes in Asthma: Possible Mechanism of Regulation. *European Respiratory Journal*, **10**, 308-313. http://dx.doi.org/10.1183/09031936.97.10020308

[38] Mollering, H. and Bergmeyer, H.U. (1974) Adenosine. In: Bergmeyer, H.U., Ed., *Methods of Enzymatic Analysis*, 2nd Edition, Academic Press, New York, 1919-1922.

[39] Gerlach, U. and Hiby, W. (1974) 5'-Nucleotidase. In: Bergmeyer, H.U., Ed., *Methods of Enzymatic Analysis*, 2nd Edition, Academic Press, New York, 871-875.

[40] Giusti, G. (1974) Adenosine Deaminase. In: Bergmeyer, H.U., Ed., *Methods of Enzymatic Analysis*, 2nd Edition, Academic Press, New York, 1092-1099.

[41] Goodarzi, M.T., Abdi, M., Tavilani, H., Nadi, E. and Rashidi, M. (2010) Adenosine Deaminase Activity in COPD Patients and Healthy Subjects. *Iranian Journal of Allergy, Asthma and Immunology*, **9**, 7-12.

[42] Hua, X., Chason, K.D., Patel, J.Y., Naselsky, W.C. and Tilley, S.L. (2011) IL-4 Amplifies the Pro-Inflammatory Effect of Adenosine in Human Mast Cells by Changing Expression Levels of Adenosine Receptors. *PLoS ONE*, **6**, e24947. http://dx.doi.org/10.1371/journal.pone.0024947

[43] Huszar, E., Vass, G., Vizi, E., Csoma, Z., Barat, E., Molnar, V.G., Herjavecz, I. and Horvath, I. (2002) Adenosine in Exhaled Breath Condensate in Healthy Volunteers and in Patients with Asthma. *European Respiratory Journal*, **20**, 1393-1398. http://dx.doi.org/10.1183/09031936.02.00005002

[44] Mann, J.S., Renwick, A.G. and Holgate, S.T. (1986) Release of Adenosine and Its Metabolites from Activated Human Leucocytes. *Clinical Science*, **70**, 461-468.

[45] Finney, M.J., Karlsson, J.A. and Persson, C.G. (1985) Effects of Bronchoconstrictors and Bronchodilators on a Novel Human Small Airway Preparation. *British Journal of Pharmacology*, **85**, 29-36. http://dx.doi.org/10.1111/j.1476-5381.1985.tb08827.x

[46] Volmer, J.B., Thompson, L.F. and Blackburn, M.R. (2006) Ecto-5'-Nucleotidase (CD73)-Mediated Adenosine Production Is Tissue Protective in a Model of Bleomycin Induced Lung Injury. *The Journal of Immunology*, **176**, 4449-4458. http://dx.doi.org/10.4049/jimmunol.176.7.4449

[47] Picher, M., Burch, L.H. and Boucher, R.C. (2004) Metabolism of P2 Receptor Agonists in Human Airways: Implications for Mucociliary Clearance and Cystic Fibrosis. *The Journal of Biological Chemistry*, **279**, 20234-20241. http://dx.doi.org/10.1074/jbc.M400305200

[48] Blackburn, M.R. and Kellems, R.E. (2005) Adenosine Deaminase Deficiency: Metabolic Basis of Immune Deficiency and Pulmonary Inflammation. *Advances in Immunology*, **86**, 1-41. http://dx.doi.org/10.1016/S0065-2776(04)86001-2

[49] Blackburn, M.R., Lee, C.G., Young, H.W., Zhu, Z., Chunn, J.L., Kang, M.J., Banerjee, S.K. and Elias, J.A. (2003) Adenosine Mediates IL-13-Induced Inflammation and Remodeling in the Lung and Interacts in an IL-13-Adenosine Amplification Pathway. *Journal of Clinical Investigation*, **112**, 332-344. http://dx.doi.org/10.1172/JCI200316815

[50] Ma, B., Blackburn, M.R., Lee, C.G., Homer, R.J., Liu, W., Flavell, R.A., Boyden, L., Lifton, R.P., Sun, C.X., Young, H.W. and Elias, J.A. (2006) Adenosine Metabolism and Murine Strain-Specific IL-4-Induced Inflammation, Emphysema, and Fibrosis. *Journal of Clinical Investigation*, **116**, 1274-1283. http://dx.doi.org/10.1172/JCI26372

[51] Eltzschig, H.K., Ibla, J.C., Furuta, G.T., Leonard, M.O., Jacobson, K.A., Enjyoji, K., Robson, S.C. and Colgan, S.P. (2003) Coordinated Adenine Nucleotide Phosphohydrolysis and Nucleoside Signaling in Posthypoxic Endothelium: Role of Ectonucleotidases and Adenosine A_{2B} Receptors. *The Journal of Experimental Medicine*, **198**, 783-796. http://dx.doi.org/10.1084/jem.20030891

[52] Volmer, J.B., Thompson, L.F. and Blackburn, M.R. (2006) Ecto-5-Nucleotidase (CD73)-Mediated Adenosine Production Is Tissue Protective in a Model of Bleomycin-Induced Lung Injury. *The Journal of Immunology*, **176**, 4449-4458. http://dx.doi.org/10.4049/jimmunol.176.7.4449

[53] Zimmermann, H. (2000) Extracellular Metabolism of ATP and Other Nucleotides. *Naunyn-Schmiedeberg's Archives of Pharmacology*, **362**, 299-309. http://dx.doi.org/10.1007/s002100000309

[54] Sala-Newby, G.B., Skladanowski, A.C. and Newby, A.C. (1999) The Mechanism of Adenosine Formation in Cells: Cloning of Cytosolic 5'-Nucleotidase. *The Journal of Biological Chemistry*, **274**, 17789-17793. http://dx.doi.org/10.1074/jbc.274.25.17789

[55] Madara, J.L., Patapoff, T.W., Gillece-Castro, B., Colgan, S.P., Parkos, C.A., Delp, C. and Mrsny, R.J. (1993) 5'-Adenosine Monophosphate Is the Paracrine Factor That Elicits Chloride Secretion from T84 Intestinal Epithelial Cell Monolayers. *Journal of Clinical Investigation*, **91**, 2320-2325. http://dx.doi.org/10.1172/JCI116462

[56] Resnick, M.B., Colgan, S.P., Patapoff, T.W., Mrsny, R.J., Awtrey, C.S., Delp, C., Weller, P.F. and Madara, J.L. (1993) Activated Eosinophils Evoke Chloride Secretion in Model Intestinal Epithelia Primarily via Regulated Release of 5'-AMP. *The Journal of Immunology*, **151**, 5716-5723.

[57] Cattaneo, M., Canciani, M.T., Lecchi, A., Kinlough-Rathbone, R.L., Packham, M.A., Mannucci, P.M. and Mustard, J.F. (1990) Released Adenosine Diphosphate Stabilizes Thrombin-Induced Human Platelet Aggregates. *Blood*, **75**, 1081-1086.

[58] Donaldson, S.H., Lazarowski, E.R., Picher, M., Knowles, M.R., Stutts, M.J. and Boucher, R.C. (2000) Basal Nucle-otide Levels, Release, and Metabolism in Normal and Cystic Fibrosis Airways. *Molecular Medicine*, **6**, 969-982.

[59] Felix, J.A., Woodruff, M.L. and Dirksen, E.R. (1996) Stretch Increases Inositol 1,4,5-Trisphosphate Concentration in Airway Epithelial Cells. *American Journal of Respiratory Cell and Molecular Biology*, **14**, 296-301. http://dx.doi.org/10.1165/ajrcmb.14.3.8845181

[60] Marquardt, D.L., Gruber, H.E. and Wasserman, S.I. (1984) Adenosine Release from Stimulated Mast Cells. *Proceedings of the National Academy of Sciences of the United States of America*, **81**, 6192-6196. http://dx.doi.org/10.1073/pnas.81.19.6192

[61] Blackburn, M.R. (2003) Too Much of a Good Thing: Adenosine Overload in Adenosine-Deaminase Deficient Mice. *Trends in Pharmacological Sciences*, **24**, 66-70. http://dx.doi.org/10.1016/S0165-6147(02)00045-7

[62] Zhong, H., Belardinelli, L., Maa, T., Feoktistov, I., Biaggioni, I. and Zeng, D. (2004) A_{2B} Adenosine Receptors Increase Cytokine Release by Bronchial Smooth Muscle Cells. *American Journal of Respiratory Cell and Molecular Biology*, **30**, 118-125. http://dx.doi.org/10.1165/rcmb.2003-0118OC

[63] Ethier, M.F. and Madison, J.M. (2006) Adenosine A_1 Receptors Mediate Mobilization of Calcium in Human Bronchial Smooth Muscle Cells. *American Journal of Respiratory Cell and Molecular Biology*, **35**, 496-502. http://dx.doi.org/10.1165/rcmb.2005-0290OC

[64] Zhong, H., Belardinelli, L., Maa, T. and Zeng, D. (2005) Synergy between A_{2B} Adenosine Receptors and Hypoxia in Activating Human Lung Fibroblasts. *American Journal of Respiratory Cell and Molecular Biology*, **32**, 2-8. http://dx.doi.org/10.1165/rcmb.2004-0103OC

[65] Chunn, J.L., Molina, J.G., Mi, T., Xia, Y., Kellems, R.E. and Blackburn, M.R. (2005) Adenosine Dependent Pulmonary Fibrosis in Adenosine Deaminase Deficient Mice. *The Journal of Immunology*, **175**, 1937-1946. http://dx.doi.org/10.4049/jimmunol.175.3.1937

14

The Action of Chronic Nicotine on the Effects of Ethanol on Anxiety, Locomotion and Metabolism and the Feeding and Drinking Behaviors of Rats

Valentina Bashkatova*, Sergey Sudakov, Galina Nazarova, Elena Alexeeva

P.K. Anokhin Research Institute of Normal Physiology, Moscow, Russia
Email: *v.bashkatova@nphys.ru

Abstract

The objective of these experiments was to study the effects of ethanol on the anxiety level, activity, metabolic rate, and feeding and drinking behaviors of rats that were chronically treated with nicotine. The chronic intake of nicotine changed the effects of the acute administration of ethanol. Thus, the nicotine-dependent rats demonstrated a significantly decreased anxiolytic-like effect in response to ethanol than did the control rats. This decrease may lead to a decrease in the sensitivity of animals to the positive reinforcing effects of ethanol and an increase in their consumption to achieve the desired effect. The negative action of ethanol on the metabolism, motor activity and drinking behavior of rats that chronically consumed nicotine was increased. Chronic nicotine intake can be assumed to lead to cross-tolerance of the effects of ethanol. On the contrary, the sensitivity to the action of ethanol increased.

Keywords

Nicotine, Ethanol, Metabolism, Drinking Behavior, Locomotion

1. Introduction

The joint use of nicotine and ethanol is widespread among humans. The episodic consumption of alcoholic beverages most often occurs against a background of chronic tobacco smoking [1]. Smoking tobacco is known to result in the action of nicotine on the nicotinic acetylcholine receptors in the brain. Receptors that are situated on

---

*Corresponding author.

dopamine-containing neurons in the mesocorticolimbic system are especially affected, which leads to an increased release of dopamine and produces various behavioral effects [2] [3]. The effects of ethanol on emotional and motivational processes also involve the release of dopamine in the extracellular space of the nucleus accumbens [4]. The chronic intake of nicotine induces changes in the density and affinity of acetylcholine receptors, which may change the effects of ethanol in such subjects [5] [6]. Chronic nicotine consumption was noted to lower the positive reinforcing effect of ethanol by suppressing ethanol-induced dopamine release in the nucleus accumbens [7] [8]. Chronic nicotine reduced the impact of ethanol on the locomotor activity of rats [6] [9], affected the NMDA current in the hippocampus [10] and decreased the heart rate and body temperature [11] [5]. Conversely, chronic nicotine administration increased the effect of ethanol on motor activity and dopamine turnover in the brain [12]. In addition, chronic nicotine intake increased ethanol self-administration behavior [13].

Ethanol and nicotine are known to significantly affect metabolic processes [14]-[16]. However, we did not find data that showed the mechanism by which ethanol affects the metabolism of animals that chronically receive nicotine.

Ethanol and nicotine cause positive reinforcing actions, which result in pleasant sensations. This effect includes anxiolytic effects. Unfortunately, we have not found data on the ethanol anxiolytic effect in animals that were chronically administered nicotine.

Ethanol and nicotine are well known to cause changes in feeding and drinking behaviors [15] [17] [18]. However, we have not discovered data on the effects of ethanol on the eating and drinking behaviors of animals that chronically consume nicotine.

Accordingly, the objective of these experiments was to study the effects of ethanol on the anxiety level, locomotor activity, metabolic rate and feeding and drinking behaviors of rats that were chronically treated with nicotine.

2. Materials and Methods

The experiments were performed on 32 male Wistar rats obtained from the Stolbovaja nursery (Russian Academy of Medical Sciences). The animals (basal weight 240 - 270 g) were housed in individually ventilated cages (4 rats per cage) under a 12:12-h light-dark cycle with free access to food and water. The experiment was conducted in accordance with the "Rules of Studies on Experimental Animals" (approved by the Ethics Committee of the P. K. Anokhin Institute of Normal Physiology; protocol No. 1, 3.09.2005), the requirements of the World Society for the Protection of Animals (WSPA) and the European Convention for the Protection of Experimental Animals.

All rats were divided into 4 groups (8 animals per group). Two groups of animals were subcutaneously (sc) treated twice per day with nicotine at dose of 2 mg/kg for 7 days, followed by 3 mg/kg nicotine for the next 14 days. Determination of PH values of nicotine solutions was measured using Orion Research digital ionalyzer/ 501Ph. The PH values of studied nicotine solutions (2 mg/kg or 3 mg/kg) were 3.45 - 3.50 in depend on concentration. Nicotine at dose 2 mg/kg or 3 mg/kg was injected to rats subcutaneously and the irritations after injections were not observed. The animals in the other two groups received equivalent amounts of sc saline twice per day for 21 days. On the day of the behavior experiment, the animals in group 1 (control, pretreated with saline for 21 days) received sc saline and a second dose of gastrically administered saline after 5 minutes. Group 2 (pretreated with nicotine for 21 days) received nicotine (3 mg/kg, sc) and a dose of gastrically administered saline after 5 minutes. Group 3 (pretreated with saline for 21 days) received saline and a 40% solution of ethanol (6 g/kg intragastrically) after 5 minutes. Group 4 (pretreated with nicotine for 21 days) received nicotine 3 mg/kg, sc) and a 40% solution ethanol (6 g/kg intragastrically) after 5 minutes. After 60 minutes, the rats were placed in an elevated plus maze (EPM, Columbus, USA) for 5 minutes, which recorded the time spent in the center, in the open arms and closed arms, the motor activity in different parts of the EPM and the duration of grooming [19]. Immediately thereafter, the animals were placed into the standard "home" cages designed by Phenomaster systems (TSE Instruments, Germany) for 24 hours. The metabolic rate was determined using indirect calorimetry, locomotor activity, water and food consumption, which we registered for every Phenomaster cage for 24 hours at intervals of 60 minutes.

The data obtained were subjected to statistical and analytical processing. A normal distribution was assumed for the data to derive indicators to evaluate statistically significant differences between the parameters obtained from experimental and control animals using ANOVA.

3. Results

Our study showed that the chronic administration of nicotine for 3 weeks did not significantly affect the level of anxiety. The time spent on the open arms of the EPM and locomotor activity in the open arms of the EPM was not significantly different between the animals treated with nicotine and the control group treated with saline. Nevertheless, the activity in other parts of the EPM was increased compared to the control (**Table 1**). During the first 8 hours after the administration of nicotine (light phase of the day), the rats did not demonstrate a significant effect on locomotor activity, metabolism, food and water intake, or the intensity of the movement in the cage center compared with the control animals. However, these animals showed decreased locomotor activity, inhibited drinking and eating and reduced activity in the center of the cage 8 h aver the last injection of nicotine, which coincided with the onset of the dark phase. These changes were observed after the end of the dark phase and persisted until the end of the experiment (**Figures 1-5**).

Table 1. The effect of nicotine and ethanol on the anxiety-like behavior of rats tested in the EPM.

	Time spent on the open arms (c)	Activity on the open arms (relative units)	Activity on the close arms (relative units)	Activity in the center (relative units)
S-S	5.1 ± 2.7	0.63 ± 0.15	1.87 ± 0.39	1.8 ± 0.43
S-E	$65.5 \pm 12.9^*$	$2.88 \pm 0.67^*$	$3.62 \pm 0.57^*$	$6.2^* \pm 0.75^*$
N-S	10.0 ± 2.2	1.13 ± 0.47	$3.75 \pm 0.73^*$	$3.8^* \pm 0.52^*$
N-E	$17.2 \pm 4.1^{*\#}$	$1.88 \pm 0.72^*$	$2.87 \pm 0.65^*$	$4.6^* \pm 0.81^*$

S-S: control group (rats chronically with saline and then once on the experiment day); S-E: a group of rats chronically treated with saline and one dose of ethanol on the experiment day; N-S: a group of rats that were chronically administered nicotine and one dose of saline on the experiment day; N-E: a group of rats chronically administered nicotine and one dose of ethanol on the experiment day; $^*P < 0.05$ compared to the group S-S; $^\#P < 0.05$ compared to the group of S-E.

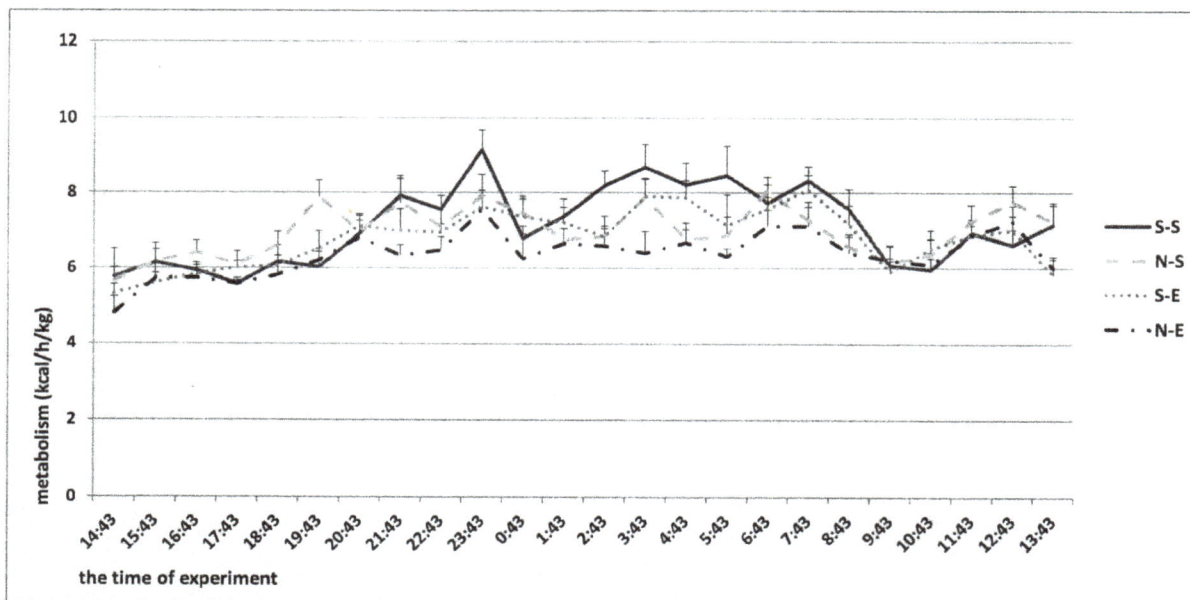

Figure 1. Effect of chronic nicotine on ethanol effects on dynamics of metabolism level (kcal/h/kg). S-S: control group—rats treated with saline chronically (21 day) and then saline once in experimental day. N-S: a group of rats that chronically administered nicotine (2 mg/kg subcutaneously (sc), twice per day, for 7 days, followed for next 14 days—nicotine 3 mg/kg) and once saline in experimental day. S-E: a group of rats chronically treated with saline during 21 days and once 40% solution ethanol (6 g/kg intragastrically) in experimental day. N-E: a group of rats chronically administered nicotine (2 mg/kg subcutaneously (sc), twice per day, for 7 days, followed for next 14 days—nicotine 3 mg/kg) and once 40% solution ethanol (6 g/kg intragastrically) in experimental day. On the horizontal axis: the time of the experiment (dark period from 20:00 to 08:00). For measurement of metabolism level the animals were placed into the standard cages of "Phenomaster system" for 24 hours. The metabolic rate determined using indirect calorimetry. Ethanol injected to nicotine-addicted rats decreased metabolic rate activity followed 7 h after administration of ethanol (which coincides with the beginning of the dark phase).

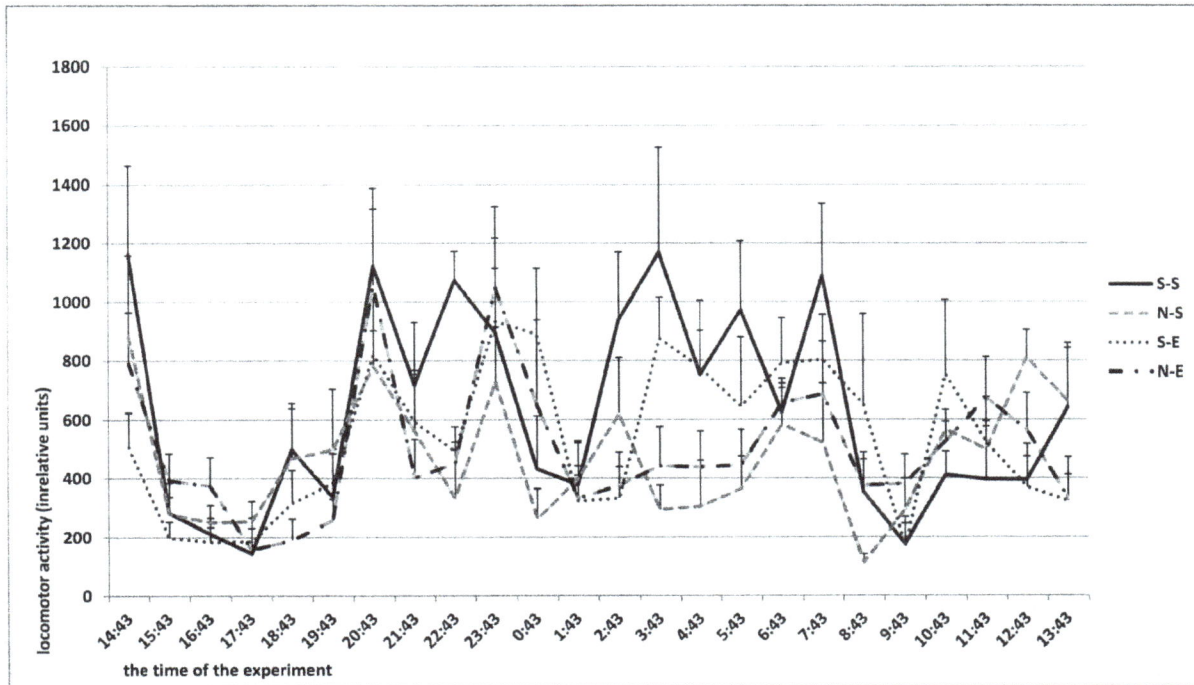

Figure 2. Effect of chronic nicotine on ethanol effects on dynamics of locomotor activity (in relative units). The other legends (groups of animals were) the same as in **Figure 1**. On the horizontal axis—the time of the experiment (dark period from 20:00 to 08:00). For measurement of dynamics of locomotor activity were placed into the standard cages of "Phenomaster system" for 24 hours. Ethanol injected to nicotine-treated rats produced decrease of locomotor activity with the beginning of the dark phase (5 - 7 h after administration of ethanol.

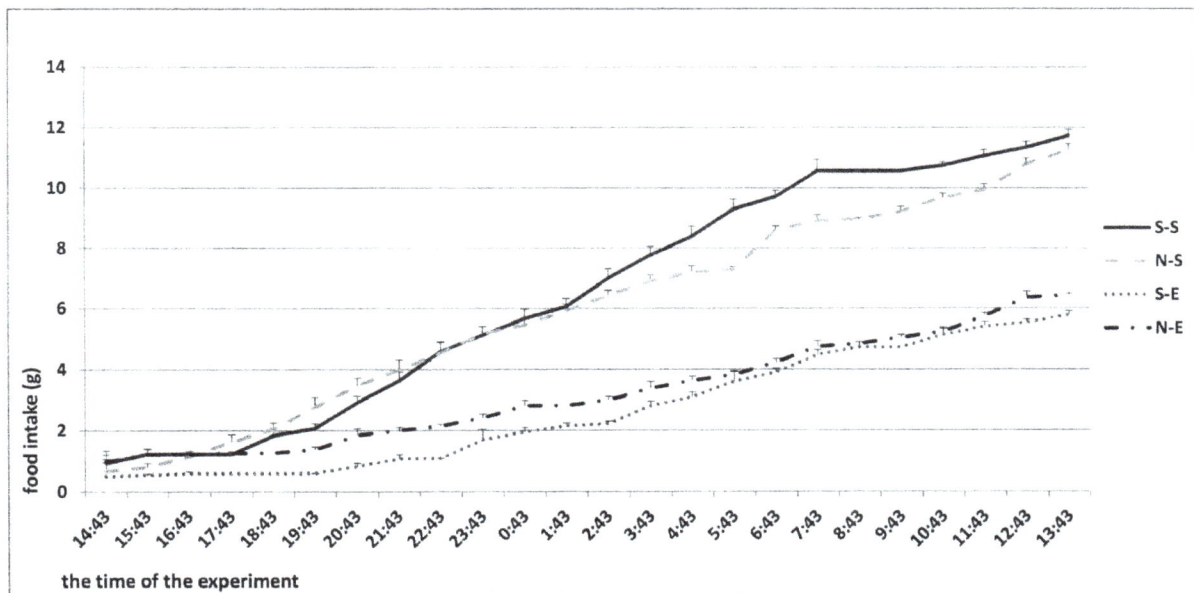

Figure 3. Effect of chronic nicotine on ethanol effects on dynamics of food intake (grams). The other legends (groups of animals were) the same as in **Figure 1**. On the horizontal axis—the time of the experiment (dark period from 20:00 to 08:00). On the ordinate axis—cumulative curve, where each value is added to the previous one. For measurement of dynamics of locomotor activity were placed into the standard cages of "Phenomaster system" for 24 hours. A suppression of feeding behavior was observed within 12 - 14 hours after administration of ethanol to nicotine treated rats as well as in saline treated animals.

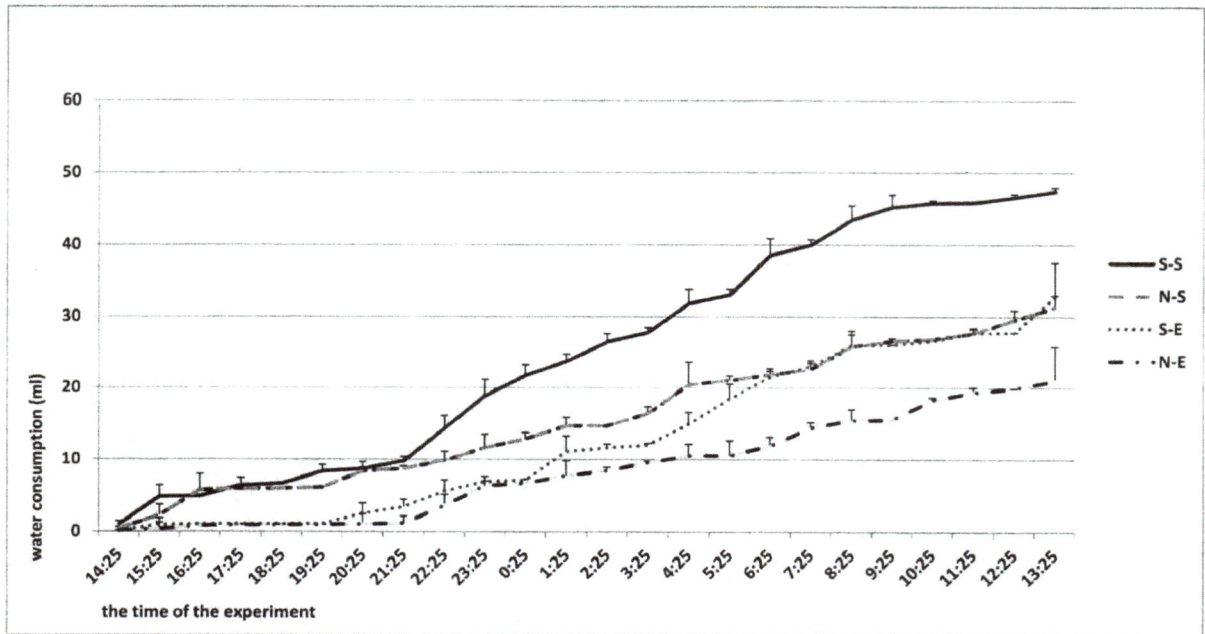

Figure 4. Effect of chronic nicotine on ethanol effects on dynamics of water consumption (ml). The other legends (groups of animals were) the same as in **Figure 1**. On the horizontal axis—the time of the experiment (dark period from 20:00 to 08:00). On the ordinate axis—cumulative curve, where each value is added to the previous one. For measurement of dynamics of locomotor activity were placed into the standard cages of "Phenomaster system" for 24 hours. Rats which received ethanol 13 h before placing them in the cages "Phenomaster" drank 2.5 times less than the control animals. For the rest time the water and food intake of these rats was also reduced.

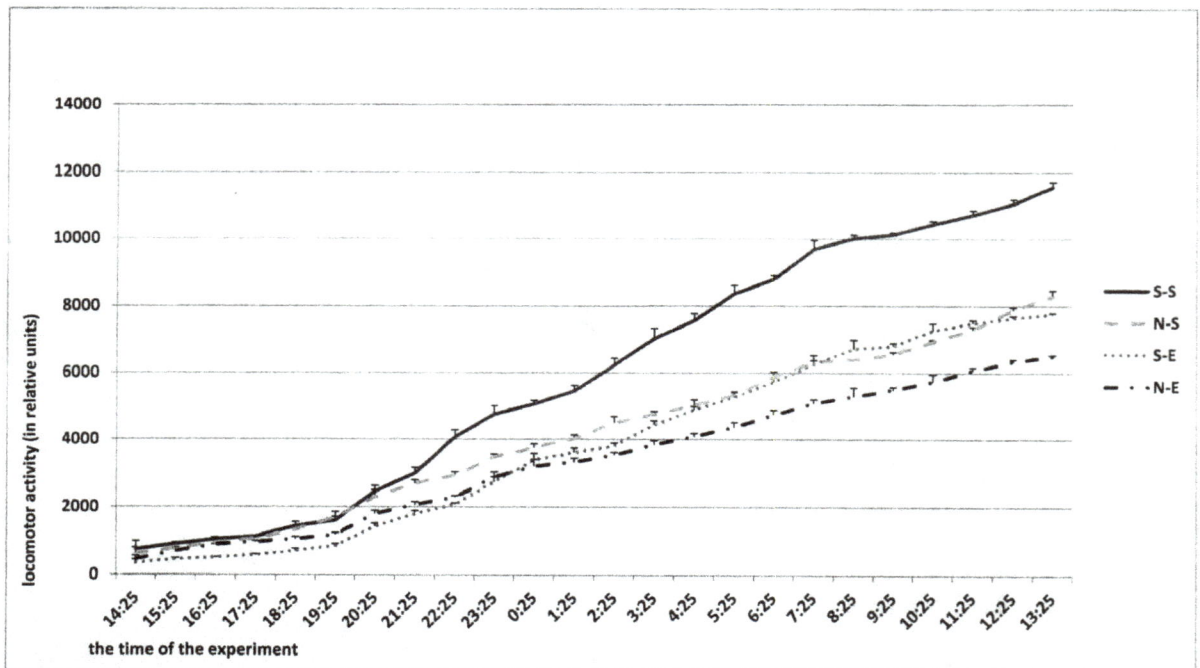

Figure 5. Effect of chronic nicotine on ethanol effects on dynamics of locomotor activity in the cage center (relative units) of the different experimental groups of rats. The other legends (groups of animals were) the same as in **Figure 1**. On the horizontal axis—the time of the experiment (dark period from 20:00 to 08:00). Animals received ethanol as compared with the control, significantly reduced motor activity in the center of cages "Phenomaster" during all the observation time (24 h).

The animals treated with chronic saline1 h after the intragastric administration of ethanol manifested a significant increase in the time spent in the open arms of the EPM. In addition, an increase in the motor activity in all parts of the EPM was also observed (**Table 1**). We did not find any significant changes in the level of metabolism or the locomotor activity in the center of the cage for 24 h after a single injection of ethanol (**Figure 1**, **Figure 2**). However, the eating and drinking behavior of the rats was significantly suppressed within 12 - 14 hours after ethanol administration. Rats that received ethanol 13 h before placing them in Phenomaster home cages ate in 3 times and drank 2.5 times less than the control animals. The water and food intake of these rats was also reduced during the rest time. The daily water intake of control animals was 47 ± 6.2 ml, while that of the animals treated with ethanol was 32.7 ± 5.8 ml. Control rats ate 11.7 ± 1.9 g for 24 h, and the animals treated with ethanol ate 5.7 ± 1.2 g (**Figure 3** and **Figure 4**). Animals that received ethanol showed significantly reduced motor activity in the center Phenomaster cages compared to the control during the entire observation time (24 h) (**Figure 5**).

The administration of the ethanol to animals chronically treated with nicotine led to a significantly reduced anxiolytic effect compared to the saline treated rats. The animals treated with ethanol demonstrated an almost 4-fold decrease in the time spent in the open arms of the EPM (**Table 1**). Ethanol injected into nicotine-addicted rats decreased the metabolic rate and locomotor activity 7 h after the administration of ethanol (which coincides with the beginning of the dark phase). A suppression of feeding and drinking behavior was observed within 12 - 14 hours after the administration of ethanol to nicotine-treated rats and saline-treated animals. Moreover, the inhibition of the drinking behavior of nicotine-dependent rats was more pronounced. The daily intake of water by nicotine-treated rats after ethanol administration was 20.97 ± 4.5 ml.

4. Discussion

The data indicate that the chronic intake of nicotine in rats does not change the registered physiological parameters, except for the psychostimulant-like effect, which was observed just after each regular injection of nicotine. On the contrary, a suppression of eating and drinking behavior was established 8 h after the injection of nicotine. Although the appearance of these indicated effects coincided with the onset of the dark phase of the day, these effects were connected to the waning of nicotine influence, which leads to withdrawal syndrome in nicotine-dependent animals.

Nicotine has been shown to affect anxiety and depression in both human and animal studies [20]-[22]. The data suggest that nicotinic acetylcholine receptors (nAChRs) can modulate the function of pathways involved in the stress response, anxiety and depression in the normal brain and that smoking can result in changes in the anxiety level and mood [23] [24]. However, the effects of nicotine are complex, and nicotine treatment can be either anxiolytic or anxiogenic depending on the anxiety model tested, the route of nicotine administration and the time course of administration. The paradoxical effects of nicotine on emotion are likely due to the broad expression of nAChRs throughout the brain, the large number of nAChR subtypes that have been identified and the ability of nicotine treatment to both activate and desensitize nAChRs [25]. A single injection of nicotine (0.1 - 0.5 mg/kg s.c.) reportedly decreased the percentage of time spent on the open arms of EPM, while nicotine injected for 7 days at the same dose increased this parameter, *i.e.*, produced an anxiolytic effect [20]. The individual sensitivity of animals is also very important for the anxiolitic/anxiogenic action of nicotine. Thus, nicotine was shown to act as an anxiolytic agent in transgenic mice that constitutively overexpressed AChE-R. This effect was not observed in wild type control mice [26].

Chronic treatment with nicotine alters the effects of the acute administration of ethanol. Thus, the administration of ethanol to nicotine-dependent rats, produced a significant increase of time spent in the open arms of the EPM than that of saline treated rats. However, the psychostimulant effect of ethanol was maintained. Thus, the chronic intake of nicotine may lead to selective cross-tolerance to the action of ethanol, which correlates with results of other studies [10] [27]. Nicotine-dependent animals showed a more pronounced response to the administration of ethanol when no longer under the influence of nicotine. Thus, they experienced a more significant depressive-like effect. This effect was accompanied by a more pronounced suppression of drinking behavior and anxiogenic effects as well as a suppressed metabolism, which was not observed in saline-treated rats. Nicotine pretreatment was shown to significantly enhance the ethanol-induced locomotor stimulation and elevation of dihydroxyphenylacetic acid/dopamine quotient in the brain [12]. These results suggest that neuronal mechanisms related to the locomotor stimulatory effects of ethanol may be sensitized by pre-exposure to nicotine.

Chronic nicotine treatment also produced cross-tolerance to the effects of ethanol on glutamatergic activity, which led to a potential increase in the use of these products [10].

5. Conclusion

In summary, the chronic administration of nicotine suppressed the sensitivity of animals to the anxiolytic effect of ethanol. This fact may stipulate a reduction of rat sensitivity to the positively reinforced, euphoric effect of ethanol and the increase of ethanol consumption in order to achieve the desired effect. In this case, the negative effect of ethanol on the metabolism, locomotor activity and drinking behavior in rats treated with nicotine chronically was exacerbated. It might be concluded that more studies including detailed monitoring of many physiological parameters are needed to draw attention to the gaps in our knowledge of combined administration of nicotine with alcohol and argues that neuroscience and clinical research efforts need to be combined with health policy options to reduce the harm associated with nicotine and alcohol abuse.

References

[1]   Miller, N.S. and Gold, M.S. (1998) Comorbid Cigarette and Alcohol Addiction: Epidemiology and Treatment. *Journal of Addictive Diseases*, **17**, 55-66. http://dx.doi.org/10.1300/J069v17n01_06

[2]   Alburges, M.E., Hoonakker, A.J. and Hanson, G.R. (2007) Nicotinic and Dopamine D2 Receptors Mediate Nicotine-Induced Changes in Ventral Tegmental Area Neurotensin System. *European Journal of Pharmacology*, **573**, 124-132. http://dx.doi.org/10.1016/j.ejphar.2007.06.063

[3]   Novak, G., Seeman, P. and Le Foll, B. (2010) Exposure to Nicotine Produces an Increase in Dopamine D2 (High) Receptors: A Possible Mechanism for Dopamine Hypersensitivity. *International Journal of Neuroscience*, **120**, 691-697. http://dx.doi.org/10.3109/00207454.2010.513462

[4]   Schier, C.J., Dilly, G.A. and Gonzales, R.A. (2013) Intravenous Ethanol Increases Extracellular Dopamine in the Medial Prefrontal Cortex of the Long-Evans rat. *Alcoholism: Clinical and Experimental Research*, **37**, 740-747. http://dx.doi.org/10.1111/acer.12042

[5]   Collins, A.C., Burch, J.B., de Fiebre, C.M. and Marks, M.J. (1988) Tolerance to and Cross Tolerance between Ethanol and Nicotine. *Pharmacology, Biochemistry and Behavior*, **29**, 365-373. http://dx.doi.org/10.1016/0091-3057(88)90170-0

[6]   Collins, A.C., Wilkins, L.H., Slobe, B.S., Cao, J.Z. and Bullock, A.E. (1996) Long-Term Ethanol and Nicotine Treatment Elicit Tolerance to Ethanol. *Alcoholism: Clinical and Experimental Research*, **6**, 990-999. http://dx.doi.org/10.1111/j.1530-0277.1996.tb01936.x

[7]   López-Moreno, J.A., Scherma, M., Rodríguez de Fonseca, F., González-Cuevas, G., Fratta, W. and Navarro, M. (2008) Changed Accumbal Responsiveness to Alcohol in Rats Pre-Treated with Nicotine or the Cannabinoid Receptor Agonist WIN 55,212-2. *Neuroscience Letters*, **433**, 1-5. http://dx.doi.org/10.1016/j.neulet.2007.11.074

[8]   Söderpalm, B., Ericson, M., Olausson, P., Blomqvist, O. and Engel, J.A. (2000) Nicotinic Mechanisms Involved in the Dopamine Activating and Reinforcing Properties of Ethanol. *Behavioural Brain Research*, **113**, 85-96. http://dx.doi.org/10.1016/S0166-4328(00)00203-5

[9]   Lallemand, F., Ward, R.J. and De Witte, P. (2009) The Influence of Chronic Nicotine Administration on Behavioral and Neurochemical Parameters of Male and Female Rats after Repeated Binge Drinking Exposure. *Alcohol Alcoholism*, **44**, 535-546. http://dx.doi.org/10.1093/alcalc/agp047

[10]   Proctor, W.R., Dobelis, P., Moritz, A.T. and Wu, P.H. (2011) Chronic Nicotine Treatment Differentially Modifies acute Nicotine and Alcoholactions on GABA(A) and Glutamate Receptors in Hippocampal Brain Slices. *British Journal of Pharmacology*, **162**, 1351-1363. http://dx.doi.org/10.1111/j.1476-5381.2010.01141.x

[11]   Burch, J.B., de Fiebre, C.M., Marks, M.J. and Collins, A.C. (1988) Chronic Ethanol or Nicotine Treatment Results in Partial Cross-Tolerance between These Agents. *Psychopharmacology*, **95**, 452-458. http://dx.doi.org/10.1007/BF00172954

[12]   Johnson, D.H., Blomqvist, O., Engel, J.A. and Söderpalm, B. (1995) Subchronic Intermittent Nicotine Treatment Enhances Ethanol-Induced Locomotor Stimulation and Dopamine Turnover in Mice. *Behavioural Pharmacology*, **6**, 203-207. http://dx.doi.org/10.1097/00008877-199503000-00013

[13]   Clark, A., Lindgren, S., Brooks, S.P., Watson, W.P. and Little, H.J. (2001) Chronic Infusion of Nicotine Can Increase Operant Self-Administration of Alcohol. *Neuropharmacology*, **41**, 108-117. http://dx.doi.org/10.1016/S0028-3908(01)00037-5

[14]   Leow, Y.H. and Maibach, H.I. (1998) Cigarette Smoking, Cutaneous Vasculature, and Tissue Oxygen. *Clinics in*

Dermatology, **16**, 579-584. http://dx.doi.org/10.1016/S0738-081X(98)00042-X

[15] Levin, E.D., Morgan, M.M., Galvez, C. and Ellison, G.D. (1987) Chronic Nicotine and Withdrawal Effects on Body Weight and Food and Water Consumption in Female Rats. *Physiology & Behavior*, **39**, 441-444. http://dx.doi.org/10.1016/0031-9384(87)90370-2

[16] Taylor, B.E., Brundage, C.M. and McLane, L.H. (2013) Chronic Nicotine and Ethanol Exposure Both Disrupt Central Ventilatory Responses to Hypoxia in Bullfrog Tadpoles. *Respiratory Physiology & Neurobiology*, **187**, 234-243. http://dx.doi.org/10.1016/j.resp.2013.04.004

[17] Essig, C.F. (1968) Increased Water Consumption Following Forced Drinking of Alcohol in Rats. *Psychopharmacologia*, **12**, 333-337. http://dx.doi.org/10.1007/BF00401411

[18] Wager-Srdar, S.A., Levine, A.S., Morley, J.E., Hoidal, J.R. and Niewoehner, D.E. (1984) Effects of Cigarette Smoke and Nicotine on Feeding and Energy. *Physiology & Behavior*, **32**, 389-395. http://dx.doi.org/10.1016/0031-9384(84)90252-X

[19] Pellow, S., Chopin, P., File, S.E. and Briley, M. (1985) Validation of Open: Closed Arm Entries in an Elevated Plus-Maze as a Measure of Anxiety in the Rat. *Journal of Neuroscience Methods*, **14**, 149-167. http://dx.doi.org/10.1016/0165-0270(85)90031-7

[20] Biala, G. and Budzynska, B. (2006) Effects of Acute and Chronic Nicotine on Elevated Plus Maze in Mice: Involvement of Calcium Channel. *Life Sciences*, **79**, 81-88. http://dx.doi.org/10.1016/j.lfs.2005.12.043

[21] Tizabi, Y., Hauser, S.R., Tyler, K.Y., Getachew, B., Madani, R., Sharma, Y. and Manaye, K.F. (2010) Effects of Nicotine on Depressive-Like Behavior and Hippocampal Volume of Female WKY Rats. *Progress in Neuro-Psychopharmacology and Biological Psychiatry*, **34**, 62-69. http://dx.doi.org/10.1016/j.pnpbp.2009.09.024

[22] Turner, J.R., Castellano, L.M. and Blendy, J.A. (2011) Parallel Anxiolytic-Like Effects and Upregulation of Neuronal Nicotinic Acetylcholine Receptors Following Chronic Nicotine and Varenicline. *Nicotine & Tobacco Research*, **13**, 41-46. http://dx.doi.org/10.1093/ntr/ntq206

[23] Gotti, C., Clementi, F., Fornari, A., Gaimarri, A., Guiducci, S., Manfredi, I., Moretti, M., Pedrazzi, P., Pucci, L. and Zoli, M. (2009) Structural and Functional Diversity of Native Brain Neuronal Nicotinic Receptors. *Biochemical Pharmacology*, **78**, 703-711. http://dx.doi.org/10.1016/j.bcp.2009.05.024

[24] Sajja, R.K. and Rahman, S. (2012) Neuronal Nicotinic Receptor Ligands Modulate Chronic Nicotine-Induced Ethanol Consumption in C57BL/6J Mice. *Pharmacology Biochemistry and Behavior*, **102**, 36-43. http://dx.doi.org/10.1016/j.pbb.2012.03.017

[25] Picciotto, M.R., Brunzell, D.H. and Caldarone, B.J. (2002) Effect of Nicotine and Nicotinic Receptors on Anxiety and Depression. *Neuroreport*, **13**, 1097-1106. http://dx.doi.org/10.1097/00001756-200207020-00006

[26] Salas, R., Main, A., Gangitano, D.A., Zimmerman, G., Ben-Ari, S., Soreq, H. and De Biasi, M. (2008) Nicotine Relieves Anxiogenic-Like Behavior in Mice that Overexpress the Read-Through Variant of Acetylcholinesterase but Not in Wild-Type Mice. *Molecular Pharmacology*, **74**, 1641-1648. http://dx.doi.org/10.1124/mol.108.048454

[27] Gulick, D. and Gould, T.J. (2008) Interactive Effects of Ethanol and Nicotine on Learning in C57BL/6J Mice Depend on both Dose and Duration of Treatment. *Psychopharmacology*, **196**, 483-495. http://dx.doi.org/10.1007/s00213-007-0982-x

15

Leptin Causes the Early Inhibition of Glycolysis- and TCA Cycle-Related Genes in the Brain of Ob/Ob Mice to Restore Fertility

Carlos Fernandes Baptista[1,2], Samuel Marcos Ribeiro de Noronha[3],
Maria de Nazareth Gamboa Ritto[1,2], Eduardo Henrique da Silva Freitas[1,4],
Melquíades Pereira Júnior[1], Mauro Abi Haidar[1], Ismael Dale Cotrim Guerreiro da Silva[1],
Silvana Aparecida Alves Corrêa de Noronha[3], Marisa Teresinha Patriarca[1]

[1]Gynecology Department, Escola Paulista de Medicina/Universidade Federal de São Paulo (EPM-UNIFESP),
São Paulo, Brazil
[2]Departamento de Cirurgia Geral e Especializada, Universidade Federal do Rio de Janeiro (UNIRIO),
Rio de Janeiro, Brazil
[3]Surgery Department, Escola Paulista de Medicina/Universidade Federal de São Paulo (EPM-UNIFESP),
São Paulo, Brazil
[4]Departamento de Medicina Geral, Universidade Federal do Rio de Janeiro (UNIRIO), Rio de Janeiro, Brazil
Email: labgineco@globo.com

Abstract

Introduction: Polycystic ovarian syndrome (PCOS) is undoubtedly the commonest androgen disorder in woman's fertile period and certainly one of the most prevalent causes of anovulation. The syndrome has an estimated prevalence of 4% - 10% among women of childbearing age. Previously, our group demonstrated the effect of gonadal white adipose tissue transplantation from wild-type lean and fertile female mice to isogenic obese anovulatory ob/ob mice. These complex metabolic interrelationships between obesity and PCOS have yet to be fully understood. The aim of this study was to evaluate the effect of gonadal white adipose tissue (WAT) transplantation from the wild-type lean and fertile female mice to isogenic obese, anovulatory mice (Lep ob/Lep ob) on the expression of glycolysis- and TCA cycle-related genes and obtain a general view of the glucose metabolism in the brain of these animals. Methods: Fifteen ob/ob mice ranging from 2 to 3 months of age were divided into 3 experimental groups: control normal weight (n = 5), obese control (n = 5) and obese 7 days leptin treated (n = 5). The whole brains of the mice were processed for RNA extraction. The samples from each group were used to perform PCR assays using an array plate containing 84 primers to study the glucose metabolism-related genes. Results: The glycolysis- and TCA cycle-related genes were significantly downregulated. The most significantly affected genes were as follows: for glycolysis (fold regulation with $p < 0.05$): *Pgm*1, *Bpgm*, *Aldob*, and *Eno*3 (119, 45, 18, and 28 times less, respectively); and for the TCA cycle (fold regulation with $p < 0.05$): *Cs*, *Idh*3*b*, and *Mdh*2 (84, 27, and 37 times less, respectively). Conclusion: The seven-day leptin treated mice show a decrease in the glucose metabolism. These results confirm the ability of the adipose tissue-derived hormone leptin to regulate early crucial genes that are related to glycolysis mechanisms and to the TCA cycle. This hormone seems to revert early the central physiological conditions that are associated with PCOS; however, the morphological alterations can only be observed within a 45-day treatment.

Keywords

PCOS, Obesity, Leptin, Glycolysis, TCA Cycle, Gene Expression

---

1. Introduction

Polycystic ovarian syndrome (PCOS) is undoubtedly the commonest androgen disorder during a woman's fertile period and certainly one of the most prevalent causes of anovulation [1]-[4]. PCOS is the classic example of the loss of functional cyclicity rhythm associated with anomalous feed-back or, as it is also known as inappropriate feed-back [5]. In this case, the excessive production of androgens and their subsequent extra glandular conversion into estrogens form the pathophysiological basis for chronic anovulation [6]-[9]. Additionally, the excessive androgen production can be explained by extra- and intra-ovarian factors [10]. This syndrome has an estimated prevalence of 4% - 10% among women of childbearing age [11]-[14] and is remarkable for the heterogeneity of its symptoms, reflected by the presence or by the absence of insulin resistance (IR) among these women, as well as, by individual differences regarding the magnitude of the symptoms that are observed in women that are affected by the syndrome [14]-[16].

The clinical manifestations of PCOS include classic menstrual disorders, obesity, adrenal enzyme deficiencies, hirsutism, metabolic syndrome, diabetes, infertility, and hyperandrogenism, which may also be associated with insulin resistance [13] [17]-[19]. A significant number of women with PCOS have an abnormally high IR when compared to those of matched controls. Moreover, PCOS can be considered the initial manifestation of metabolic syndrome [20].

In fact, PCOS is often associated with obesity in women. Obesity is a worldwide problem that threatens the lives of adults, adolescents and children. Obesity has many associated comorbidities, such as the well-known components of metabolic syndrome (MetS), which harms the health of men and women [21].

Obesity is associated with several metabolic disorders and has reproductive consequences that are complex and not well understood [22]. Adipose tissue produces leptin, which has dominated the literature on female fertility complications, but other adipokines, such as adiponectin and resistin, seem to be important as well, as our understanding of their biological functions improves. Leptin influences the developing embryo and the functioning of the ovary and of the endometrium and modulates the release and the activity of gonadotropins and of the hormones that control their synthesis (inhibin, GnRH and kisspeptins). The biological actions and the potential roles of the adipokines leptin, adiponectin and resistin are frequently studied in the context of female fertility and its interplay with the complexity of the obese metabolic state [23].

Until recently, PCOS has been recognized as a hyperandrogenic disorder originating from hypothalamic pituitary gonadotropin secretion or ovarian dysfunction [24]. Lately, however, at least some cases of PCOS have been regarded as disorders of metabolic origin that impair reproduction [24]. Because obesity, particularly in the abdominal region, is found in approximately 50% of women with PCOS and appears in mid-childhood and increases during puberty [25], excess adiposity has generated a great deal of attention. Furthermore, the clinical phenotype and the development of PCOS are thought to be reinforced by obesity. Additionally, PCOS also has a genetic component, and different genetic polymorphisms have also been linked to the syndrome or its associated disorders [26]. Altogether, these associations highlight the importance of disentangling the relationship between obesity and PCOS and in particular their common metabolic disorders.

Leptin, which is a product of the ob gene, is a major hormone that is secreted by white adipose tissue (WAT) and is involved in the regulation of body weight, glucose metabolism, and fertility. Leptin null mice (Lep ob/

Lep ob) are obese, hyperphagic, insulin resistant, and sterile. In addition, ob/ob females are invariably sterile, and few ob/ob males have been reported to occasionally reproduce. These ob/ob mice develop many pathological features that are common to human obesity, which is also marked by disturbances of reproductive function [27].

Therefore, the complex metabolic interrelationships between obesity and PCOS have yet to be fully understood. The action of leptin in the brains of ob/ob mice seems to regulate early two key metabolic biological processes, glycolysis and the TCA cycle, especially in those nervous cells that express leptin receptors. Curiously, these receptors are not expressed by GnRH-releasing neurons. Leptin controls GnRH release by acting in other hypothalamic nuclei. Leptin regulates kiss1 neurons, making of these neurons probable targets for the hormonal control of the interaction between nutrition and reproduction [28]. Aiming to better understand these complex neuronal networks, the aim of this study was to evaluate the effect of gonadal WAT transplantation from wild-type lean and fertile female mice to isogenic obese, anovulatory mice (ob/ob) on the expression of glycolysis- and TCA cycle-related genes and to obtain a general view of glucose metabolism in the brains of these animals.

2. Methodologies

2.1. Experimental Animals and Surgical Procedure

In this study, ten transgenic obese and anovulatory leptin-deficient mice (B6.V-Lep ob/J, designated as ob/ob mice) and five isogenic lean ovulatory littermates (wild-type) were obtained from the Center for the Development of Experimental Models, Federal University of São Paulo, Brazil (CEDEME). These animals were maintained in a temperature-controlled environment at approximately 24°C under a 12/12-h light-dark cycle and were handled at least once a week. Five ob/ob mice received a white adipose tissue (WAT) transplant as described by Gavrilova and Marcus-Samuels et al. (2000) [29] and Pereira et al. (2011) [9]: the adipose gonad tissue samples that were obtained from the wild-type mice were placed in phosphate buffer solution (PBS) and fragmented into small pieces. The WAT grafts were implanted in the subcutaneous tissue through small, shaved skin incisions on the dorsal region of the animal, which was anesthetized with isoflurane. The brains of all of the animals were removed by the reported procedure and kept in liquid nitrogen until use.

2.2. Experimental Groups

The animals that were described in the previous section were divided into three experimental groups as follows:

2.2.1. Control Group (CG)
Five (5) normal-weight B6.V-Lep ob/J mice at two to three months of age and ovulatory cycles.

2.2.2. Obese Group (OG)
Five (5) ob/ob mice at two to three months of age and anovulatory cycles.

2.2.3. 7-Day Transplanted Mice Group (7dTM)
Five (5) ob/ob mice at two to three months of age and anovulatory cycles were implanted with adipose gonadal tissue from mice with ovulatory cycles. These animals were sacrificed seven (7) days after the surgical procedure.The template is used to format your paper and style the text. All margins, column widths, line spaces, and text fonts are prescribed; please do not alter them. You may note peculiarities. For example, the head margin in this template measures proportionately more than is customary. This measurement and others are deliberate, using specifications that anticipate your paper as one part of the entire journals, and not as an independent document. Please do not revise any of the current designations.

2.3. RNA Extraction

After using liquid nitrogen for cryogenic soaking, the tissues were homogenized in Trizol™ reagent (Invitrogen, Carlsbad, CA, USA) following the manufacturer's instructions. After the complete dissociation of the nucleoprotein complexes, phase separation was achieved with chloroform and centrifugation. The precipitated RNA from the aqueous phase was washed with 75% ethanol. The RNA was dried and dissolved in RNase-free water. The total RNA was then purified with the Qiagen RNeasy Mini Kit (Qiagen, Valencia, CA) and submitted to

DNase treatment. The amount and quality of the extracted RNA were assessed by spectrophotometry using NanoDrop v3.3.0 (NanoDrop Technologies Inc., Rockland, DE).

2.4. QPCR

The total RNA (1.0 µg) per plate/array from each experimental group pool was used to synthesize the cDNA. The samples were treated with buffers from the kit, and reverse transcription reactions were performed using the RT2 First Strand Kit from SA Biosciences (Qiagen Company) according to the manufacturer's protocol. The qPCR array was performed using the RT2 Profiler™ PCR array of SA Biosciences (http://www.sabiosciences.com/ArrayList.php). For each experimental group, 51 genes (29 for the TCA cycle- and 22 for the glycolysis-related genes) were examined in triplicate (PAHS-006). The amplification, data acquisition and analysis curves were performed on an ABI Prism 7500 Fast Sequence Detection System (Applied Biosystems, Foster City, CA). In turn, each gene was checked for the efficiency and the minimum and maximum threshold curve pattern. To ensure accurate comparisons between the curves, the same threshold was established for every gene. Three genes were used for normalization (*Hsp90ab1*, *Gapdh* and *Actb*), and the average qC values were used to standardize the gene expression (2-CT change table) and to determine the difference between the groups. To consider a gene differentially expressed, we used a differential cut-off of two-fold (up or downregulated).

2.5. Histology

For the histological evaluation of all of the study groups, the uteri were obtained and processed immediately after euthanasia. The tissues were fixed in 4% formalin in saline, embedded in paraffin, and cut to a thickness of 5 mm. The sections were deparaffinized, rehydrated, stained with hematoxylin/eosin (H.E.), and evaluated under light microscopy.

2.6. Statistical Analysis

The p values were calculated based on Student's t-test of the three replicate $2^{(-\Delta ct)}$ values for each gene in the control and treatment groups, and p values less than 0.05 were considered significant. The qPCR reactions were processed through the online software RT2 Profiler™ PCR Array Data Analysis (SA Biosciences).

2.7. Ethics

The procedures were performed in accordance with the ethical standards of the institution and national guidelines for the care and use of laboratory animals. The study protocol for the use of laboratory animals in research was approved by the local ethics committee (CEP/UNIFESP, number 0017/12).

3. Results

In general, we observed a marked downregulation of the glycolysis- and TCA cycle-related genes in the brain of 7dTM mice compared to those of the CG mice and a marked upregulation of these same groups of genes in the brains of the non-treated ob/ob mice (OG) compared to those of the CG mice. In the brains of the 7dTM mice, the most significantly downregulated genes were *Pgm*1, *Bpgm*, *Aldob* and *Eno*3, which were downregulated 119, 45, 18, and 28 times, respectively, for the glycolysis-related genes (fold regulation with p < 0.05), and *Cs*, *Idh3b*, and *Mdh*2, which were 84, 27, and 37 times, respectively, for the TCA cycle-related genes (fold regulation with p < 0.05). Curiously, *Pcx* was the only upregulated gene and was upregulated 27 times (fold regulation with p < 0.05). In contrast, the endometrial and ovarian morphologies could only be observed after a 45-day period.

To better describe the gene expression profiles that were obtained for each functional group of genes (glycolysis and TCA cycle) and in each experimental group comparison (7dTM with CG and OG with CG), the glycolysis- and TCA cycle-related genes are discussed separately in the following two distinct subsections.

3.1. 7dTM versus CG

Glycolysis—Seventeen out of the twenty-two (77%) glycolysis-related genes were differentially expressed in the 7dTM group, using the CG group as a calibrator. All of these seventeen genes were downregulated, and none were upregulated. The downregulated genes included *aldolases* a, b and c; *Bpgm*; *Enolases* 1, 2 and 3; *Gpi*1; *Pfkl*; *Pgam*2; *Pgk*1; *Pgms*1, 2 and 3; *Pklr*; and *Tpi*1. Among the non-differentially expressed genes, *Gapdhs* and *Hk3* were detected in both of the groups (7dTM and CG), while *Gck* and *Hk2* were only detected in the CG group, and *Pgk*2 could not be detected in any of the groups. The fold-regulation values of each assessed glycolysis-related gene can be observed in **Table 1**.

Table 1. Fold-regulation values that were obtained for the glycolysis- and TCA cycle-related genes in two different comparisons, 7dTM and OG, using the CG group as a calibrator. The data were processed with the online program Data Assist[TM] SA Biosciences (Qiagen Company). nde = non-differentially expressed.

Gene Symbol	Gene Name	Refseq	7dTM × CG		OG × CG	
			Fold regulation	p value	Fold regulation	p value
*Pgm*1	Phosphoglucomutase 1	NM_025700	−119.57	0.000312	nde	
Bpgm	2,3-bisphosphoglycerate mutase	NM_007563	−44.68	0.000517	2.02	0.006556
*Eno*3	Enolase 3, beta muscle	NM_007933	−27.95	0.000051	2.23	0.020764
Aldob	Aldolase B, fructose-bisphosphate	NM_144903	−17.94	0.000004	2.04	0.000378
*Tpi*1	Triosephosphate isomerase 1	NM_009415	−15.55	0.0000	2.26	0.000281
*Eno*1	Enolase 1, alpha non-neuron	NM_023119	−12.89	0.000003	2.47	0.000001
Aldoc	Aldolase C, fructose-bisphosphate	NM_009657	−12.51	0.000001	2.58	0.000007
*Pgk*1	Phosphoglycerate kinase 1	NM_008828	−9.57	0.0000	2.08	0.000001
*Eno*2	Enolase 2, gamma neuronal	NM_018870	−7.04	0.000151	2.52	0.002822
Pfkl	Phosphofructokinase, liver, B-type	NM_028352	−6.36	0.019107	3.19	0.000051
*Pgam*2	Phosphoglycerate mutase 2	NM_1177307	−6.08	0.000001	3.54	0.000187
*Pgm*3	Phosphoglucomutase 3	NM_028352	−5.33	0.000191	2.88	0.000009
Aldoa	Aldolase A, fructose-bisphosphate	NM_1177307	−5.31	0.000002	nde	
*Gpi*1	Glucose phosphate isomerase 1	NM_008155	−5.18	0.000355	2.76	0.000129
*Pgm*2	Phosphoglucomutase 2	NM_028132	−4.59	0.000001	2.04	0.000444
Galm	Galactose mutarotase	NM_176963	−2.58	0.000261	nde	
Pklr	Pyruvate kinase liver and red blood cell	NM_013631	−2.18	0.007846	nde	
Gck	Glucokinase	NM_010292	nde		3.54	0.00246
Hk2	Hexokinase 2	NM_013820	nde		2.36	0.00001
Hk3	Hexokinase 3	NM_1033245	nde		2.45	0.001786
Cs	Citrate synthase	NM_026444	−84.16	0.0000	2.43	0.000067
Pcx	Pyruvate carboxylase	NM_008797	26.75	0.000456	nde	
*Mdh*2	Malate dehydrogenase 2, NAD (mitochondrial)	NM_008617	−37.40	0.000244	2.03	0.001091
Idh3b	Isocitrate dehydrogenase 3 (NAD+) beta	NM_130884	−27.32	0.000024	2.05	0.000005
Mdh1b	Malate dehydrogenase 1B, NAD (soluble)	NM_029696	−23.73	0.0000	2.41	0.00011
Dlat	pyruvate dehydrogenase complex)	NM_145614	−19.32	0.000096	nde	
Dlst	oxo-glutarate complex)	NM_030225	−8.49	0.0000	3.05	0.000647
*Sucla*2	Succinate-Coenzyme A ligase, ADP-forming, beta subunit	NM_011506	−6.85	0.0000	2.24	0.000012
*Pck*1	Phosphoenolpyruvate carboxykinase 1, cytosolic	NM_011044	−6.77	0.000039	nde	

GLYCOLYSIS (rows Pgm1 through Pklr); TCA CYCLE (rows Cs through Pck1)

Continued

	Dld	Dihydrolipoamide dehydrogenase	NM_007861	−6.36	0.000001	nde	
	Sdha	Succinate dehydrogenase complex, subunit A, flavoprotein (Fp)	NM_023281	−5.73	0.0000	2.85	0.000006
	*Suclg*1	Succinate-CoA ligase, GDP-forming, alpha subunit	NM_019879	−5.22	0.000342	nde	
	Sdhb	Succinate dehydrogenase complex, subunit B, iron sulfur (Ip)	NM_023374	−4.94	0.000088	4.24	0.00075
	*Mdh*1	Malate dehydrogenase 1, NAD (soluble)	NM_008618	−4.81	0.000001	nde	
	Ogdh	Oxoglutarate dehydrogenase (lipoamide)	NM_010956	−4.26	0.0000	nde	
	Idh3g	Isocitrate dehydrogenase 3 (NAD+), gamma	NM_008323	−3.70	0.0000	nde	
TCA CYCLE	*Sdhc*	Succinate dehydrogenase complex, subunit C, integral membrane protein	NM_025321	−3.46	0.000001	nde	
	*Aco*1	Aconitase 1	NM_007386	−3.32	0.000006	2.80	0.000044
	Idh3a	Isocitrate dehydrogenase 3 (NAD+) alpha	NM_029573	−3.00	0.000091	3.21	0.00018
	Pdhb	Pyruvate dehydrogenase (lipoamide) beta	NM_024221	−2.30	0.000115	2.30	0.000196
	Acly	ATP citrate lyase	NM_134037	nde		2.68	0.000029
	*Aco*2	Aconitase 2, mitochondrial	NM_080633	nde		2.28	0.006074
	*Fh*1	Fumarate hydratase 1	NM_010209	nde		2.55	0.001199
	*Idh*1	Isocitrate dehydrogenase 1 (NADP+)	NM_010497	nde		2.31	0.000025
	*Pck*2	Phosphoenolpyruvate carboxykinase2	NM_028994	nde		2.17	0.036288
	*Pdha*1	Pyruvate dehydrogenase E1, alpha	NM_008810	nde		2.26	0.000247
	*Suclg*2	Succinate-Coenzyme A ligase, beta	NM_011507	nde		2.53	0.000292

TCA Cycle—Twenty out of the twenty-nine (67%) TCA cycle-related genes were differentially expressed in the 7dTM group, using the CG group as a calibrator. Nineteen of these genes were downregulated, and only one was upregulated. The downregulated genes included *Aco*1; *Cs*; *Dlat*; *Dld*; *Dlst*; *Idh3a*; *Idhg*; *Mdh*s 1, 1*b* and 2; *Suclg*1; *Ogdh*; *Pck*s 1 and 2; *Pdhb*; *Sdh*s *a*, *b* and *c*; *Sucla*2; and *Suclg*1. As mentioned earlier, *Pcx* was the only upregulated gene. Among the nine non-differentially expressed genes, *Acly*; *Aco*2; *Idh*s 1, 2 and 3*b*; *Pdha*1; *Sdhd*; and *Suclg*2 were detected in both of the groups (7dTM and CG), while *Fh1* could only be detected in the CG. The fold-regulation values of each assessed TCA cycle-related gene can be observed in **Table 1**.

3.2. OG versus CG

Glycolysis—Sixteen out of the twenty-two (72%) glycolysis-related genes were differentially expressed in the OG group, using the CG group as a calibrator. All of these sixteen genes were upregulated, and none were downregulated. The upregulated genes included aldolases b and c; *Bpgm*; Enolases 1, 2 and 3; *Gck*; *Gpi*1; hexokinases 2 and 3; *Pfkl*; *Pgam*2; *Pgk*1; *Pgms*2 and 3; and *Tpi*1. Among the non-differentially expressed genes, *Aldoa, Galm, Gapdhs, Pgm*1 and *Pklr* were detected in both of the groups (OG and CG), while *Pgk*2 could not be detected in any of these groups. The fold-regulation values of each assessed glycolysis-related gene can be observed in **Table 1**.

TCA Cycle—Eighteen out of the twenty-nine (62%) TCA cycle-related genes were differentially expressed in the OG group, using the CG group as a calibrator. All of these eighteen genes were upregulated, and none were downregulated. The upregulated genes included *Acly*; *Aco*1; *Aco*2; *Cs*; *Dlst*; *Fh*1; *Idh*1; *Idh3a*; *Idh3b*; *Mdh*s 1*b* and 2; *Pck*2; *Pdha*1; *Pdhb*; *Sdh*s *a* and *b*; *Sucla2*; and *Suclg2*. All of the eleven non-differentially expressed genes (*Dlat*; *Dld*; *Idh*s 2 and 3g; *Mdh*1; *Ogdh*; *Pck*1; *Pcx*; *Sdhc*; *Sdhd*; and *Suclg*1) were detected in both of the groups (OG and CG). The fold-regulation values of each assessed TCA cycle-related gene can be observed in **Table 1**.

3.3. Histomorphology of the Uterus

With respect to the histology of the uteri, after a 7-day treatment period, the endometrium was similar to that of the OG group, with an absence of glandular tissue (**Figure 1**). However, Pereira *et al.*, 2011 demonstrated that after a 45-day treatment period, these mice presented an endometrium similar to that of the CG group, with the presence of numerous leukocytes in the endometrium, signaling the restoration of hormonal control and the surface epithelial renewal that are typical of the estrous phase (**Figure 1**).

4. Discussion

We believe that investigating the molecular changes underlying the fertility restoration of leptin-treated ob/ob mice is crucial to better understanding the intracellular pathways controlling the interplay between metabolism and the female sexual cycle. With this in mind, we observed a lack of studies on glucose-related gene alterations in the brain of leptin-induced fertile ob/ob mice and decided to assess the expression of glycolysis- and TCA cycle-related genes in these animals.

It is largely known that leptin plays a primary role in regulating homeostasis, obesity and fertility [23] [28]. Moreover, in a previous work, Pereira *et al.* (2009) clearly demonstrated that WAT transplantation decreases insulin resistance and restores fertility in female ob/ob mice [9]. Behind these physiological and morphological changes lay complex molecular interactions that deserve to be better understood.

As such, the aim of this work was to investigate the central effects of leptin on glucose metabolism accompanying neuropeptide Y inhibition and the restoration of fertility in the same animal model that was used by Pereira *et al.* [9]. Additionally, this work seems to be a pioneer in presenting an overall profile of glycollysis- and TCA cycle-related gene expression in the brains of leptin-treated ob/ob mice.

Indicating the weak points, the results shown herein are restricted to mRNA quantifications and whole brain extracts, instead of specific brain nuclei, and were used to assess early central actions of leptin. However, as mentioned earlier, there is a lack of studies of these genes in the brains of leptin-treated ob/ob mice. In addition, we believe that differential gene expression will reflect specific adipokine hormone actions in leptin receptor-expressing cells, such as kiss1 neurons.

Leptin deficiency, which was observed in the ob/ob mice, caused obesity and led these animals to develop metabolic disorders such as insulin resistance and type II diabetes, as well as hypertension and infertility [27]-[29]. We do not know exactly in which cells in the brains of these 7-day leptin-treated mice have altered metabolic processes, but our results demonstrate an important early downregulation of glycolysis- and TCA cy-

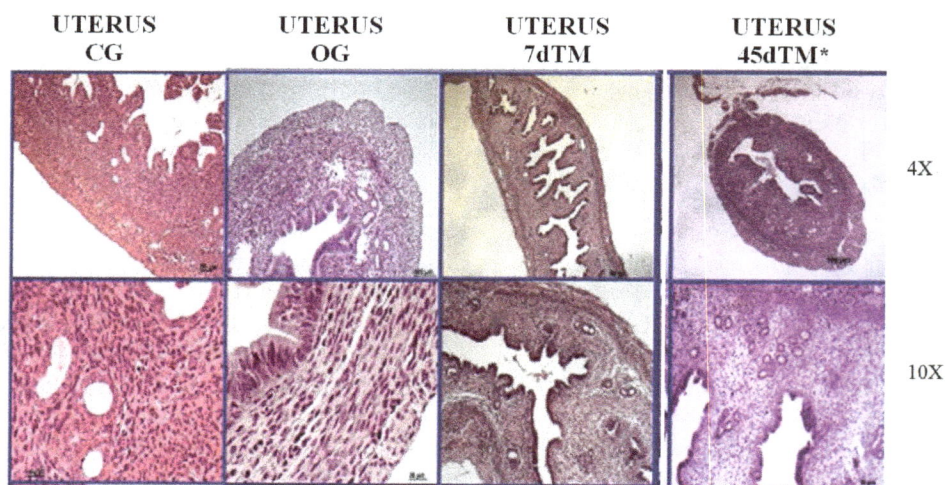

Figure 1. Histomorphological features of the uterus of animals from each experimental group at two different magnifications (4× and 10×). The 45dTM mice were obtained by Pereira *et al.* (2011) [9].

cle-related genesin the brains of ob/ob mice caused by this adipokine.

Khan *et al.*, 1998 have demonstrated through biochemical assays (glucose-6-phosphatase activity) that glucose cycling is increased in the brains of ob/ob mice [30]. Our gene expression results show the same, that is, except for *Pcx*, all of the other glycolysis-related genes assessed herein are upregulated in these mice, in contrast to the 7dTM and OG mice. Therefore, after 1 week of leptin treatment, there seems to be a marked reduction in the activity of these genes. We believe that among the early central neuronal circuitary changes caused by leptin and that will eventually lead to fertility restoration after a 45-day treatment, glucose cycling reduction, most likely in the hypothalamus, seems to be critical.

In general, similar to the profile that was observed for the glycolysis-related genes, the TCA cycle-related genes displayed a general downregulation in the 7dTM group compared to those of the CG group. However, these genes are upregulated in the brains of the OG mice compared to those in the CG mice. This profile matches previous reports, in which untreated ob/ob mice exhibited increased hepatic and central B-oxidation [31] [32], especially in the hypothalamic Arcuate and Ventromedial nuclei [33].

5. Conclusion

Overall, the data presented here indicate an early decrease in the central glucose metabolism after leptin treatment. These results confirm the ability of the adipose tissue-derived hormone leptin to regulate crucial genes that are related to glycolysis mechanisms and to the TCA cycle. In summary, this hormone seems to revert early the central physiological conditions that are associated with PCOS in the central nervous system; however, the morphological alterations that are associated with fertility in the peripheral tissues can only be observed within a 45-day treatment. The extrapolation of these results to patients with metabolic syndrome must await further investigation.

References

[1]   Edman, C.D., Aiman, E.J., Porter, J.C. and MacDonald, P.C. (1978) Identification of the Estrogen Product of Extraglandular Aromatization of Plasma Androstenedione. *American Journal of Obstetrics and Gynecology*, **130**, 439-447.

[2]   Edman, C.D. and MacDonald, P.C. (1978) Effect of Obesity on Conversion of Plasma Androstenedione to Estrone in Ovulatory and Anovulator Young Women. *American Journal of Obstetrics and Gynecology*, **130**, 456-461.

[3]   Ehrmann, D.A. (2005) Polycystic Ovary Syndrome. *The New England Journal of Medicine*, **352**, 1223-1236. http://dx.doi.org/10.1056/NEJMra041536

[4]   Pasquali, R. and Gambineri, A. (2006) Polycystic Ovary Syndrome: A Multifaceted Disease from Adolescence to Adult Age. *The New York Academy of Sciences*, **1092**, 158-174. http://dx.doi.org/10.1196/annals.1365.014

[5]   Goldzieher, J.W. and Green, J.A. (1962) The Polycystic Ovary. I. Clinical and Histologic Features. *The Journal of Clinical Endocrinology and Metabolism*, **22**, 325-338. http://dx.doi.org/10.1210/jcem-22-3-325

[6]   Vigil, P., Contreras, P., Alvarado, J.L., Godoy, A., Salgado, A.M. and Cortes, M.E. (2007) Evidence of Subpopulations with Different Levels of Insulin Resistance in Women with Polycystic Ovary Syndrome. *Human Reproduction*, **22**, 2974-2980. http://dx.doi.org/10.1093/humrep/dem302

[7]   Ingalls, A.M., Dickie, M.M. and Snell, G.D. (1950) Obese, a New Mutation in the House Mouse. *Journal of Heredity*, **41**, 317-318.

[8]   Jones, N. and Harrison, G.A. (1957) Genetically Determined Obesity and Sterility in the Mouse. In: Harrison, R.G., Ed., *Studies on Fertility*, Blackwell Scientific, Oxford, 51-64.

[9]   Pereira Jr., M., Vidotti, D.B., Borra, R.C., Simões Mde, J., Da Silva, I.D. and Haidar, M.A. (2011) Involvement of GDF-9, Leptin, and IGF1 Receptors Associated with Adipose Tissue Transplantation on Fertility Restoration in Obese Anovulatory Mice. *Gynecological Endocrinology*, **27**, 759-766. http://dx.doi.org/10.3109/09513590.2010.534330

[10]   Vilmann, L.S., Thisted, E., Baker, J.L. and Holm, J.C. (2012) Development of Obesity and Polycystic Ovary Syndrome in Adolescents. *Hormone Research in Paediatrics*, **78**, 269-278. http://dx.doi.org/10.1159/000345310

[11]   Buggs, C. and Rosenfield, R. (2005) Polycystic Ovary Syndrome in Adolescence. *Endocrinology and Metabolism Clinics of North America*, **34**, 677-705. http://dx.doi.org/10.1016/j.ecl.2005.04.005

[12]   Yildiz, B.O. and Azziz, R. (2010) Ovarian and Adipose Tissue Dysfunction in Polycystic Ovary Syndrome: Report of the 4th Special Scientific Meeting of the Androgen Excess and PCOS Society. *Fertility and Sterility*, **94**, 690-693. http://dx.doi.org/10.1016/j.fertnstert.2009.03.058

[13]   Azziz, R., Woods, K.S., Reyna, R., Key, T.J., Knochenhauer, E.S. and Yildiz, B.O. (2004) The Prevalence and Fea-

tures of the Polycystic Ovary Syndrome in an Unselected Population. *The Journal of Clinical Endocrinology and Metabolism*, **89**, 2745-2749. http://dx.doi.org/10.1210/jc.2003-032046

[14]   Lecke, S.B., Mattei, F., Morsch, D.M. and Spritzer, P.M. (2011) Abdominal Subcutaneous Fat Gene Expression and Circulating Levels of Leptin and Adiponectin in Polycystic Ovary Syndrome. *Fertility and Sterility*, **95**, 2044-2049. http://dx.doi.org/10.1016/j.fertnstert.2011.02.041

[15]   Glueck, C.J., Morrison, J.A., Daniels, S., Wang, P. and Stroop, D. (2011) Sex Hormone-Binding Globulin, Oligomenorrhea, Polycystic Ovary Syndrome, and Childhood Insulin at Age 14 Years Predict Metabolic Syndrome and Class III Obesity at Age 24 Years. *The Journal of Pediatrics*, **159**, 308-313.

[16]   Nair, M.K., Pappachan, P., Balakrishnan, S., Leena, M.L., George, B. and Russell, P.S. (2012) Menstrual Irregularity and Poly Cystic Ovarian Syndrome among Adolescent Girls—A 2 Year Follow-Up Study. *The Indian Journal of Pediatrics*, **79**, S69-S73.

[17]   de Zegher, F., Lopez-Bermejo, A. and Ibáñez, L. (2009) Adipose Tissue Expandability and the Early Origins of PCOS. *Trends in Endocrinology Metaboilism*, **20**, 418-423. http://dx.doi.org/10.1016/j.tem.2009.06.003

[18]   Hickey, M., Doherty, D.A., Atkinson, H., Sloboda, D.M., Franks, S., Norman, R.J., *et al.* (2011) Clinical, Ultrasound and Biochemical Features of Polycystic Ovary Syndrome in Adolescents: Implications for Diagnosis. *Human Reproduction*, **26**, 1469-1477. http://dx.doi.org/10.1016/j.tem.2009.06.003

[19]   Reinehr, T., de Sousa, G., Roth, C.L. and Andler, W. (2005) Androgens before and after Weight Loss in Obese Children. *The Journal of Clinical Endocrinology & Metabolism*, **90**, 5588-5595. http://dx.doi.org/10.1210/jc.2005-0438

[20]   Zhang, Y., Proenca, R., Maffei, M., Barone, M., Leopold, L. and Friedman, J.M. (1994) Positional Cloning of the Mouse Obese Gene and Its Human Homologue. *Nature*, **372**, 425-432. http://dx.doi.org/10.1038/372425a0

[21]   Mantzoros, C.S. (2001) The Role of Leptin and Hypothalamic Neuropeptides in Energy Homeostasis: Update on Leptin in Obesity. *Growth Hormone and IGF Research*, **11**, S85-S89. http://dx.doi.org/10.1016/S1096-6374(01)80014-9

[22]   Ceddia, R.B., Koistinen, H.A., Zierath, J.R. and Sweeney, G. (2002) Analysis of Paradoxical Observations on the Association between Leptin and Insulin Resistance. *The FASEB Journal*, **16**, 1163-1176. http://dx.doi.org/10.1096/fj.02-0158rev

[23]   Moschos, S., Chan, J.L. and Mantzoros, C.S. (2002) Leptin and Reproduction: A Review. *Fertility and Sterility*, **77**, 433-444. http://dx.doi.org/10.1016/S0015-0282(01)03010-2

[24]   Coleman, D.L. (1978) Obese and Diabetes: Two Mutant Genes Causing Diabetes-Obesity Syndromes in Mice. *Diabetologia*, **14**, 141-148. http://dx.doi.org/10.1007/BF00429772

[25]   Hummel, K.P., Dickie, M.M. and Coleman, D.L. (1966) Diabetes, a New Mutation in the Mouse. *Science*, **153**, 1127-1128. http://dx.doi.org/10.1126/science.153.3740.1127

[26]   Kashima, K., Yahata, T., Fujita, K. and Tanaka, K. (2013) Polycystic Ovary Syndrome: Association of a C/T Single Nucleotide Polymorphism at Tyrosine Kinase Domain of Insulin Receptor Gene with Pathogenesis among Lean Japanese Women. *Journal of Reproductive Medicine*, **58**, 491-496.

[27]   Burcelin, R., Thorens, B., Glauser, M., Gaillard, R.C. and Pralong, F.P. (2003) FP Gonadotropin-Releasing Hormone Secretion from Hypothalamic Neurons: Stimulation by Insulin and Potentiation by Leptin. *Endocrinology*, **144**, 4484-4491. http://dx.doi.org/10.1210/en.2003-0457

[28]   Lake, J.K., Power, C. and Cole, T.J. (1997) Women's Reproductive Health: The Role of Body Mass Index in Early and Adult Life. *International Journal of Obesity and Related Metabolic Disorders*, **21**, 432-438. http://dx.doi.org/10.1038/sj.ijo.0800424

[29]   Gavrilova, O., Marcus-Samuels, B., Graham, D., Kim, J.K., Shulman, G.I., Castle, A.L., Vinson, C., Eckhaus, M., Reitman, M.L. (2000) Surgical Implantation of Adipose Tissue Reverses Diabetes in Lipoatrophic Mice. *Journal of Clinical Investigation*, **105**, 271-278.

[30]   Khan, A., Zong-Chao, L., Efendic, S. and Landau, B.R. (1998) Glucose-6-Phosphatase Activity in the Hypothalamus of *ob/ob* Mice. *Metabolism, Clinical and Experimental*, **47**, 627-629.

[31]   Hartz, A.J., Barboriak, P.N, Wong, A., Katayama, K.P. and Rimm, A.A. (1979) The Association of Obesity with Infertility and Related Menstural Abnormalities in Women. *International Journal of Obesity*, **3**, 57-73.

[32]   Brady, L.J., Silverstein, L.J., Hoppel, C.L. and Brady, P.S. (1985) Hepatic Mitochondrial Inner Membrane Properties and Carnitine Palmitoyltransferase A and B. Effect of Diabetes and Starvation. *Biochemical Journal*, **232**, 445-450.

[33]   Delgado, T.C., Violante, I.R., Nieto-Charques, L. and Cerdan, S. (2011) Neuroglial Metabolic Compartmentation Underlying Leptin Deficiency in the Obese *ob/ob* Mice as Detected by Magnetic Resonance Imaging and Spectroscopy Methods. *Journal of Cerebral Blood Flow & Metabolism*, **31**, 2257-2266. http://dx.doi.org/10.1038/jcbfm.2011.134

16

Enzyme Kinetic Equations of Irreversible and Reversible Reactions in Metabolism

Santiago Imperial, Josep J. Centelles

Departament de Bioquímica i Biologia Molecular (Biologia), Facultat de Biologia, Universitat de Barcelona, Barcelona, Spain
Email: josepcentelles@ub.edu

Abstract

This paper compares the irreversible and reversible rate equations from several uni-uni kinetic mechanisms (Michaelis-Menten, Hill and Adair equations) and bi-bi mechanisms (single- and double-displacement equations). In reversible reactions, Haldane relationship is considered to be identical for all mechanisms considered and reversible equations can be also obtained from this relationship. Some reversible reactions of the metabolism are also presented, with their equilibrium constant.

Keywords

Adair Equation, Enzyme Kinetics, Equilibrium Constant, Haldane Relationship, Hill Equation, Metabolism, Michaelis Menten Equation, Reversible Reactions

1. Introduction

Thermodinamical considerations in a metabolic pathway include different aspects like kinetic analysis, and identification of reversible steps in this pathway [1]. Although most of the reactions are reversible, it is usual in general Biochemistry textbooks to present to students kinetic irreversible equations. For instance, the irreversible Michaelis-Menten equation is a well-known example and it is presented in this way in general Biochemistry books (either to simplify the mechanism, or because this reaction is used for an *in vitro* study in absence of the product of the reaction). Nevertheless, when performing an *in vivo* study, or when using a biochemical mathematical model presenting several reactions of a metabolic pathway, reversible equations should be considered. In this paper, we present several reversible equations and we compare them with the irreversible ones.

Haldane relationship, an equation which can only be used for reversible reactions, connects biochemical thermodynamics and biochemical kinetics. Thus, for a reversible uni-uni reaction $A = P$, Haldane relationship connects equilibrium constant K_{eq} with kinetic parameters for both irreversible reactions, $A \rightarrow P$ (V_f and K_{mA}) and $P \rightarrow A$ (V_r and K_{mP}). Haldane relationship is in this case: $K_{eq} = V_f K_{mP}/V_r K_{mA}$. This is a general relationship that is also valid for several other mechanisms, including Hill equation (although $[P]_{0.5}$ and $[S]_{0.5}$ should replace the values of K_{mP} and K_{mA}, respectively). Several reversible equations are obtained from the Haldane relationship considering that in equilibrium total velocity should be zero, and that $v = v_{A \rightarrow P} - v_{P \rightarrow A}$. Nevertheless, this relationship is not considered universal, as when considering a bi-bi reaction with two reactions: $A = Q$, followed by B = P, Haldane relationship will be the product of the two equilibrium constants:

$K_{eq} = K_{eq(1)} K_{eq(2)} = (V_f K_{mQ}/V_r K_{mA})(V_f K_{mP}/V_r K_{mB}) = V_f^2 K_{mP} K_{mQ}/V_r^2 K_{mA} K_{mB}.$

In general, Haldane relationship for a bi-bi mechanism is an equation more similar to the uni-uni equation:

$K_{eq} = V_f K_{mP} K_{mQ}/V_r K_{mA} K_{mB}.$

2. Kinetic Equations of Reversible Reactions

2.1. Uni-Uni Mechanisms

The easiest mechanism for uni-uni enzyme kinetics is the Michaelis-Menten mechanism. The best known equation is the irreversible equation, which is used for a reaction with one substrate, independently on if the obtained products are one, two, or several. For a uni-uni mechanism, it can be observed a competitive inhibition by the product, as both the substrate and the product bind to the active site. This is the reason for the presence of a term depending on [P] at the denominator of the reversible equation, which is not considered for an irreversible equation, as [P] = 0.

Figure 1 shows the different kinetic equations obtained for several uni-uni mechanisms. Reversible Michaelis-Menten equation is considered as a uni-uni reaction, where α and π are the relative concentrations for the substrate and the product respectively: $\alpha = [A]/K_{mA}$ and $\pi = [P]/K_{mP}$.

Although irreversible Hill equation is presented as a general equation (where h is the Hill coefficient), the Adair irreversible equation is presented only for an enzyme with two active centers. **Figure 1** also shows the equation obtained for two enzymes (with different kinetic parameters) acting in the same reaction. This could be the case of two isoenzymes. This equation for two enzymes is the same as Adair equation for two sites, as two enzymes have also two active sites. Reversible Hill equation is very similar to Adair equation [2], as it can be calculated from **Figure 1** for $h = 2$.

It should be noted that the reversible equations should be always converted into irreversible equations considering zero the products concentrations. Thus, Michaelis-Menten and Hill irreversible equations are obtained from the reversible equations on **Figure 1** considering $\pi = 0$, and Adair irreversible equation is obtained from

A ⟶ P	Irreversible	Reversible		
Michaelis-Menten	$v = \dfrac{V_f \cdot \alpha}{1 + \alpha}$	$v = \dfrac{V_f \cdot \alpha - V_r \cdot \pi}{1 + \alpha + \pi}$	$\alpha = \dfrac{[A]}{K_{m(A)}}$	$\pi = \dfrac{[P]}{K_{m(P)}}$
Hill	$v = \dfrac{V_f \cdot \alpha^h}{1 + \alpha^h}$	$v = \dfrac{(V_f \cdot \alpha - V_r \cdot \pi)(\alpha + \pi)^{h-1}}{1 + (\alpha + \pi)^h}$	$\alpha = \dfrac{[A]}{[A]_{0.5}}$	$\pi = \dfrac{[P]}{[P]_{0.5}}$
Adair	$v = \dfrac{N_1 [A] + N_2 [A]^2}{1 + D_1 [A] + D_2 [A]^2}$	$v = \dfrac{N_1 [A] + N_2 [A]^2 + N_3 [A][P] - N_4 [P] - N_5 [P]^2}{1 + D_1 [A] + D_2 [A]^2 + D_3 [A][P] + D_4 [P] + D_5 [P]^2}$		

$$N_1 = \dfrac{V_{f1} \cdot K_{m(A)2} + V_{f2} \cdot K_{m(A)1}}{K_{m(A)1} \cdot K_{m(A)2}} \qquad N_2 = \dfrac{V_{f1} + V_{f2}}{K_{m(A)1} \cdot K_{m(A)2}}$$

$$N_3 = \dfrac{(V_{f1} - V_{r2}) \cdot K_{m(A)2} \cdot K_{m(P)1} + (V_{f2} - V_{r1}) \cdot K_{m(A)1} \cdot K_{m(P)2}}{K_{m(A)1} \cdot K_{m(A)2} \cdot K_{m(P)1} \cdot K_{m(P)2}} \qquad N_4 = \dfrac{V_{r1} \cdot K_{m(P)2} + V_{r2} \cdot K_{m(P)1}}{K_{m(P)1} \cdot K_{m(P)2}} \qquad N_5 = \dfrac{V_{r1} + V_{r2}}{K_{m(P)1} \cdot K_{m(P)2}}$$

$$D_1 = \dfrac{K_{m(A)1} + K_{m(A)2}}{K_{m(A)1} \cdot K_{m(A)2}} \qquad D_2 = \dfrac{1}{K_{m(A)1} \cdot K_{m(A)2}}$$

$$D_3 = \dfrac{K_{m(A)1} \cdot K_{m(P)2} + K_{m(A)2} \cdot K_{m(P)1}}{K_{m(A)1} \cdot K_{m(A)2} \cdot K_{m(P)1} \cdot K_{m(P)2}} \qquad D_4 = \dfrac{K_{m(P)1} + K_{m(P)2}}{K_{m(P)1} \cdot K_{m(P)2}} \qquad D_5 = \dfrac{1}{K_{m(P)1} \cdot K_{m(P)2}}$$

Two michaelian enzymes

$$v = \dfrac{V_{f1} \cdot \alpha}{1 + \alpha} + \dfrac{V_{f2} \cdot \alpha'}{1 + \alpha'} \qquad v = \dfrac{V_{f1} \cdot \alpha - V_{r1} \cdot \pi}{1 + \alpha + \pi} + \dfrac{V_{f2} \cdot \alpha' - V_{r2} \cdot \pi'}{1 + \alpha' + \pi'}$$

$$\alpha = \dfrac{[A]}{K_{m(A)1}} \qquad \alpha' = \dfrac{[A]}{K_{m(A)2}}$$

$$\pi = \dfrac{[P]}{K_{m(P)1}} \qquad \pi' = \dfrac{[P]}{K_{m(P)2}}$$

Figure 1. Comparison between the reversible and the irreversible kinetic equations of an uni-uni reaction.

the reversible equation by considering [P] = 0.

Similar equations should be also obtained for the inverse irreversible reaction (P $\rightarrow$ A) by considering [A] = 0 (or α = 0) although in these cases a negative equation is obtained, as the velocity is considered in the inverse sense.

Haldane relationship from these reversible equations can be solved by considering that equilibrium concentrations would led to v = 0 (for Michaelis-Menten and Hill equations, $V_f \alpha_{eq} = V_r \pi_{eq}$), and $K_{eq} = [P]_{eq}/[A]_{eq}$. Thus, resulting Haldane relationship to be: $K_{eq} = V_f K_{mP}/V_r K_{mA}$.

2.2. Bi-Bi Mechanisms

Although there are several possible mechanisms, the most common bi-bi mechanisms include the ternary complex mechanism (random or ordered bi-bi) and the substituted-enzyme mechanism (ping-pong bi-bi). As it can be seen in **Figure 2**, the main difference between both mechanisms is the independent term present in the denominator of the ternary complex mechanism. This independent term is present either for the irreversible or the reversible equation.

These equations are more complex than those for the uni-uni mechanism, but it should be observed that both irreversible equations can be simplified to a Michaelis-Menten uni-uni equation by considering saturated the concentration of one of the substrates. For example, for a high β, v = $V_f \alpha\beta/(\beta + \alpha\beta)$, and simplifying, v = $V_f \alpha/(1 + \alpha)$. Similarly, for a high α, the equation obtained would be v = $V_f \beta/(1 + \beta)$.

The reversible equation, when considering high β, is transformed to an irreversible Michaelis-Menten equation, with inhibitions of products (P and Q). These inhibitions depend on the bi-bi mechanism considered, and they follow the Cleland laws.

Haldane relationship from these equations can be solved by considering that equilibrium concentrations would led to v = 0 (in both cases, $V_f \alpha_{eq} \beta_{eq} = V_r \pi_{eq} \rho_{eq}$), and $K_{eq} = [P]_{eq}[Q]_{eq}/[A]_{eq}[B]_{eq}$. Thus, resulting Haldane relationship would be: $K_{eq} = V_f K_{mP} K_{mQ}/V_r K_{mA} K_{mB}$.

2.3. Multisubstrate Mechanisms

We have considered until now uni-uni and bi-bi mechanism. Nevertheless, some reactions can be also uni-bi, or bi-uni. Irreversible equations from uni-uni and from uni-bi are identical, as both consider only one substrate. But reversible reactions present other factors in the numerators, as it can be seen in **Figure 1** and **Figure 2**. Thus, for uni-bi reactions, numerators of the equations can be easily corrected by using the uni positive factor and the bi negative factor in the numerator: $V_f \alpha - V_r \pi \rho$. And in the same way, the bi-uni equation should have the following factor as numerator: $V_f \alpha \beta - V_r \pi$. In general, numerators can be deduced from the previous Figures. In fact, if the reaction mechanism is known, the King and Altman method [3] can be used to deduce the enzymatic equation. This method can be easily performed from the web page http://biokin.com/king-altman/index.html .

3. Some Examples of Reversible Reactions in Metabolism

Equilibrium constant can be used to calculate kinetic parameters by using Haldane relationship. For this reason, we present in **Table 1** a brief summary of some reversible reactions extracted from Barman [4]. Equilibrium constants from the table are not taken all in the same conditions of pH and temperature, and the substrate or products concentrations in the cell would indicate whether the reaction is far or near equilibrium. Reversible

A + B $\longrightarrow$ P + Q	Irreversible	Reversible
Ternary complex mechanism	$v = \dfrac{V_f \cdot \alpha\beta}{1 + \alpha + \beta + \alpha\beta}$	$v = \dfrac{V_f \cdot \alpha\beta - V_r \cdot \pi\rho}{1 + \alpha + \beta + \pi + \rho + \alpha\beta + \alpha\pi + \beta\rho + \pi\rho + \alpha\beta\pi + \beta\pi\rho}$
Substituted-enzyme mechanism	$v = \dfrac{V_f \cdot \alpha\beta}{\alpha + \beta + \alpha\beta}$	$v = \dfrac{V_f \cdot \alpha\beta - V_r \cdot \pi\rho}{\alpha + \beta + \pi + \rho + \alpha\beta + \alpha\pi + \beta\rho + \pi\rho}$

$$\alpha = \frac{[A]}{K_{m(A)}} \qquad \beta = \frac{[B]}{K_{m(B)}} \qquad \pi = \frac{[P]}{K_{m(P)}} \qquad \rho = \frac{[Q]}{K_{m(Q)}}$$

Figure 2. Comparison between the reversible and irreversible kinetic equations of a bi-bi reaction.

Table 1. Some reversible reactions of the most common pathways in metabolism (extracted from [4]).

Enzyme (E.C. number)	Reaction	K_{eq}
Alcohol dehydrogenase (EC 1.1.1.1.)	alcohol + NAD = aldehyde or ketone + reduced NAD	8.0×10^{-12}
Glycerol-3-phosphate dehydrogenase (EC 1.1.1.8.)	L-glycerol-3-P + NAD = dihydroxyacetone phosphate + reduced NAD	$1.0\ 10^{-12}$
Lactate dehydrogenase (EC 1.1.1.27.)	L-lactate + NAD = pyruvate + reduced NAD	2.76×10^{-6}
Malate dehydrogenase (EC 1.1.1.37.)	L-malate + NAD = oxaloacetate + reduced NAD	6.4×10^{-13}
Glucose 6-phosphate dehydrogenase (EC 1.1.1.49.)	D-glucose 6-phosphate + NADP = D-glucono-δ-lactone 6-phosphate + reduced NADP	6.0×10^{-7}
Glyceraldehyde-phosphate dehydrogenase (EC 1.2.1.12.)	D-glyceraldehyde-3-phosphate + Pi + NAD = 1,3-diphospho-D-glycerate + reduced NAD	0.5
Butyryl-CoA dehydrogenase (EC 1.3.99.2.)	butyryl-CoA + FAD = crotonoyl-CoA + $FADH_2$	0.22
Alanine dehydrogenase (EC 1.4.1.1.)	L-alanine + H_2O + NAD = pyruvate + NH_3 + reduced NAD	6.98×10^{-14}
Glutamate dehydrogenase (EC 1.4.1.2.)	L-glutamate + H_2O + NAD = 2-oxoglutarate + NH_3 + reduced NAD	4.5×10^{-14}
Tetrahydrofolate dehydrogenase (EC 1.5.1.3.)	5,6,7,8-tetrahydrofolate + NADP = 7,8-dihydrofolate + reduced NADP	$1.79\ 10^{-12}$
NAD(P) transhydrogenase (EC 1.6.1.1.)	reduced NADP + NAD = NADP + reduced NAD	1.43
Glutathione reductase (EC 1.6.4.2.)	reduced NAD(P) + oxidized glutathione = NAD(P) + 2 glutathione	9.8×10^{-6}
Serine hydroxymethyltransferase (EC 2.1.2.1.)	L-serine + tetrahydrofolate = glycine + 5,10-methylenetetrahydrofolate	10.2
Methylmalonyl-CoA carboxyltransferase (EC 2.1.3.1.)	methylmalonyl-CoA + pyruvate = propionyl-CoA + oxaloacetate	0.526
Ornithine carbamoyltransferase (EC 2.1.3.3.)	carbamoylphosphate + L-ornithine = Pi + L-citrulline	1×10^5
Transketolase (EC 2.2.1.1.)	sedoheptulose 7-P + D-glyceraldehyde 3-P = D-ribose 5-P + D-xylulose 5-P	0.95
Transaldolase (EC 2.2.1.2.)	sedoheptulose 7-P + D-glyceraldehyde 3-P = D-erythrose 4-P + D-fructose 6-P	1.05
Choline acetyltransferase (EC 2.3.1.6)	acetyl-CoA + choline = CoA + acetylcholine	5.1×10^3
Carnitine acyltransferase (EC 2.3.1.7.)	acetyl-CoA + carnitine = CoA + acetylcarnitine	1.67
Phosphate acyltransferase (EC 2.3.1.8.)	acetyl-CoA + P_i = CoA + acetylphosphate	1.35×10^{-2}
Acetyl-CoA acetyltransferase (EC 2.3.1.9.)	2 acetyl-CoA = CoA + acetoacetyl-CoA	$\sim 2 \times 10^{-5}$
Adenine phosphoribosyltransferase (EC 2.4.2.7.)	AMP + pyrophosphate = adenine + 5-phospho-α-ribosyl-pyrophosphate	0.1
Aspartate aminotransferase (EC 2.6.1.1.)	L-aspartate + 2-oxoglutarate = oxaloacetate + L-glutamate	0.16 - 0.17
Alanine aminotransferase (EC 2.6.1.2.)	L-alanine + 2-oxoglutarate = pyruvate + L-glutamate	2.2
Glucokinase (EC 2.7.1.2.)	ATP + D-glucose = ADP + D-glucose-6-phosphate	3.86×10^2

Continued

Galactokinase (EC 2.7.1.6.)	ATP + D-galactose = ADP + D-galactose-1-phosphate	26
Pyruvate kinase (EC 2.7.1.40.)	ATP + pyruvate = ADP + phosphoenolpyruvate	1.55×10^{-4}
Acetate kinase (EC 2.7.2.1.)	ATP + acetate = ADP + acetylphosphate	$\sim 8 \times 10^{-3}$
Carbamate kinase (EC 2.7.2.2.)	ATP + NH_3 + CO_2 = ADP + carbamoylphosphate	$4 \, 10^{-2}$
Phosphoglycerate kinase (EC 2.7.2.3.)	ATP + 3-phospho-D-glycerate = ADP + 1,3-diphospho-D-glycerate	2.9×10^{-4}
Creatine kinase (EC 2.7.3.2.)	ATP + creatine = ADP + phosphocreatine	7.2×10^{-9}
Adenylate kinase (EC 2.7.4.3.)	ATP + AMP = 2 ADP	2.26
Glutaminase (EC 3.5.1.2.)	L-glutamine + H_2O = L-glutamate + NH_3	320
Dihydropyrimidinase (EC 3.5.2.2.)	4,5-dihydrouracil + H_2O = 3-ureidopropionate	0.67
Dihydro-orotase (EC 3.5.2.3.)	L-4,5-dihydro-orotate + H_2O = N-carbamoyl-L-aspartate	1.9
Methenyltetrahydrofolate cyclohydrolase (EC 3.5.4.9.)	5,10-methyltetrahydrofolate + H_2O = 10-formyltetrahydrofolate	2.4×10^{-8}
Phosphopyruvate carboxylase (EC 4.1.1.32.)	GTP + oxaloacetate = GDP + phosphoenolpyruvate + CO_2	0.372
Fructosediphosphate aldolase (EC 4.1.2.13.)	fructose-1,6-diphosphate = dihydroxyacetone-P + D-glyceraldehyde-3-P	8.1×10^{-5}
Citrate lyase (EC 4.1.3.6.)	citrate = acetate + oxaloacetate	0.325
Citrate synthase (EC 4.1.3.7.)	citrate + CoA = acetyl-CoA + H_2O + oxaloacetate	1.2×10^{-4}
ATP citrate lyase (EC 4.1.3.8.)	ATP + citrate + CoA = ADP + P_i + acetyl-CoA + oxaloacetate	1.0 - 1.5
Carbonic anhydrase (EC 4.2.1.1.)	H_2CO_3 = CO_2 + H_2O	2.51×10^6
Fumarate hydratase (EC 4.2.1.2.)	L-malate = fumarate + H_2O	0.23
Enoyl-CoA hydratase (EC 4.2.1.1.7)	L-3-hydroxyacil-Coa = crotonoyl-CoA + H_2O	16.2
Argininosuccinate lyase (EC 4.3.2.1.)	L-argininosuccinate = fumarate + L-arginine	1.14×10^{-2}
Adenylosuccinate lyase (EC 4.3.2.2.)	adenylosuccinate = fumarate + AMP	6.8×10^{-3}
Glutamate racemase (EC 5.1.1.3.)	L-glutamate = D-glutamate	~ 1
Hydroxyproline epimerase (EC 5.1.1.8.)	L-hydroxyproline = D-allohydroxyproline	0.99
Ribulosephosphate 3-epimerase (EC 5.1.3.1.)	D-ribulose 5-phosphate = D-xylulose 5-phosphate	1.5 - 3.0
UDP-glucose epimerase (EC 5.1.3.2.)	UDP-glucose = UDP-galactose	0.284
Ribulosephosphate 4-epimerase (EC 5.1.3.4.)	L-ribulose 5-phosphate = D-xylulose 5-phosphate	1.86
Methylmalonyl-CoA racemase (EC 5.1.99.1.)	D-methylmalonyl-CoA = L-methylmalonyl-CoA	1.0
Triose phosphate isomerase (EC 5.3.1.1.)	D-glyceraldehyde 3-phosphate = dihydroxyacetone phosphate	22
Arabinose isomerase (EC 5.3.1.3.)	D-arabinose = D-ribulose	0.179
L-arabinose isomerase (EC 5.3.1.4.)	L-arabinose = L-ribulose	~ 0.11

Continued

Xylose isomerase (EC 5.3.1.5.)	D-xylose = D-xylulose	0.16
Ribosephosphate isomerase (EC 5.3.1.6.)	D-ribose 5-phosphate = D-ribulose 5-phosphate	0.30
Mannose isomerase (EC 5.3.1.7.)	D-mannose = D-fructose	2.45
Mannosephosphate isomerase (EC 5.3.1.8.)	D-mannose 6-phosphate = D-fructose 6-phosphate	1.78
Glucosephosphate isomerase (EC 5.3.1.9.)	D-glucose 6-phosphate = D-fructose-6-phosphate	0.298
Glucuronate isomerase	D-glucuronate = D-fructuronate	0.82
Arabinosephosphate isomerase (EC 5.3.1.13.)	D-arabinose-5-phosphate = D-ribulose 5-phosphate	0.295
L-rhamnose isomerase (EC 5.3.1.14.)	L-rhamnose = L-rhamnulose	1.5
Phosphoglycerate phosphomutase (EC 5.4.2.1.)	2-phospho-D-glycerate = 3-phosphoglycerate	5.0
L-methylmalonyl-CoA mutase (EC 5.4.99.2.)	L-methylmalonyl-CoA = succinyl-CoA	~20
Muconate cycloisomerase (EC 5.5.1.1.)	(+)-4-carboxymethyl-4-hydroxyisocrotonolactone = cis-cis-muconate	4.03×10^{-2}
Valyl-sRNA synthetase (EC 6.1.1.9.)	ATP + L-valine + sRNA = AMP + PPi + L-valyl-sRNA	0.32
Acetyl-CoA synthetase (EC 6.2.1.1.)	ATP + acetate + CoA = AMP + PPi + acetyl-CoA	0.86
Acyl-CoA synthetase (EC 6.2.1.2.)	ATP + an acid + CoA = AMP + PPi + an acyl-CoA	~1.5
Succinyl-CoA synthetase (EC 6.2.1.5.)	ATP + Succinate + CoA = ADP + Pi + Succinyl-CoA	0.27
Glutamine synthetase (EC 6.3.1.2.)	ATP + L-glutamate + NH_3 = ADP + Pi + L-glutamine	1.2×10^{-3}
Adenylosuccinatesynthetase (EC 6.3.4.4.)	GTP + IMP + L-aspartate = GDP + P_i + adenylosuccinate	2.9 - 10
Propionyl-CoA carboxylase (EC 6.4.1.3.)	ATP + propionyl-CoA + CO_2 + H_2O= ADP + Pi + methylmalonyl-CoA	5.7

reactions are usually considered non-controlling reactions in a pathway, but they can be interesting for antagonic metabolic pathways (*i.e.* glycolysis and gluconeogenesis), as depending on the intermediate concentrations, they can be redirected to the products or the substrates.

References

[1]   Alberty, R.A., Cornish-Bowden, A., Goldberg, R.N., Hammes, G.G., Tipton, K. and Westerhoff, H.V. (2011) Recommendations for Terminology and Databases for Biochemical Thermodynamics. *Biophysical Chemistry*, **155**, 89-103. http://dx.doi.org/10.1016/j.bpc.2011.03.007

[2]   Hofmeyr, J.-H.S. and Cornish-Bowden, A. (1997) The Reversible Hill Equation: How to Incorporate Cooperative Enzymes into Metabolic Models. *CABIOS*, **13**, 377-385.

[3]   King, E.L. and Altman, C. (1956) A Schematic Method of Deriving the Rate Laws for Enzyme-Catalyzed Reactions. *The Journal of Physical Chemistry*, **60**, 1373-1378. http://biokin.com/king-altman/index.html http://dx.doi.org/10.1021/j150544a010

[4]   Barman, T.E. (1969) Enzyme Handbook. Springer-Verlag, Berlin. http://dx.doi.org/10.1007/978-3-642-86602-9

17

Graves' Disease and Down Syndrome: Case Report

Fábio Ferreira do Espírito Santo[1], Denise Rosso Tenório Wanderley Rocha[1], Alberto Krayyem Arbex[1,2]

[1]Division of Endocrinology, IPEMED Medical School, Salvador, Brazil
[2]Visiting Scientist of the Harvard T. H. Chan School of Public Health, Harvard University, Boston, USA
Email: dante_de_cerberus@hotmail.com

Abstract

Down syndrome (DS) is the most common chromosomal abnormality in humans, and the most frequent cause of mental retardation. Patients affected by this syndrome show an increased prevalence of autoimmune diseases. The most common of those is Hypothyroidism. We present a case report describing the association of Down syndrome with Hyperthyroidism. An 18-year-old patient presented with a history of recurrent throat infections and intermittent diarrhea, having developed a total *alopecia areata* within one month from the first visit to the physician. After consultations with general practitioners, he was directed to an Endocrinology Ambulatory and diagnosed with a clear case of Graves' disease associated with Down syndrome. Treatment was started with methimazole 20 mg/day, and after two months, was adjusted to 40 mg/day. The patient reached adequate clinical and laboratory balance after five months of treatment. Thus, the association between Down syndrome and Graves' Disease is relevant in medical practice, due to its specific characteristics on diagnosis, and the need of an adequate treatment regarding this disease association.

Keywords

Down Syndrome, Graves' Disease, Alopecia Areata, Methimazole, Thyroid Gland

1. Introduction

The thyroid gland is the first endocrine gland that arises in the human embryo, developing as a diverticulum of the primitive pharynx in the third week of intrauterine life. In the human embryo, the primary thyroid follicles are recognized in the eighth week. The function of the follicular cells mainly depends on the protein synthesis of thyroglobulin and thyroid peroxidase. The synthesis of thyroglobulin begins between the ninth and tenth week, and the ability to perform iodine uptake and organification, as well as to incorporate it into thyroglobulin molecule begins around the tenth and eleventh week. The final function of the follicles (colloid accumulation in the interior) is observed around the thirteenth and fourteenth week [1].

As part of the hypothalamic-pituitary-thyroid axis, the thyrotropin-releasing hormone (TRH) is synthesized by the hypothalamus and acts on the anterior pituitary controlling the synthesis and release of thyrotropin (TSH). TSH binds to thyroid receptors and stimulates the synthesis and release of thyroid hormones (TH): triiodothyronine (T3) and tyroxine (T4). In turn, the TH binds to specific nuclear receptors inhibiting the secretion of TRH in hypothalamic level and TSH in hypophyseal level ("negative feedback") [2] [3].

There are several conditions that may cause thyroid hypofunction and hyperfunction, diagnosed by TSH and free T4 lab tests. Goiter means any increase in thyroid volume, and it can be diffuse or nodular.

2. Hyperthyroidism, Thyrotoxicosis and Graves' Disease

Hyperthyroidism refers to the excessive synthesis and high secretion of thyroid hormones. Thyrotoxicosis, in turn, is a clinical syndrome that results from high circulation levels of thyroid hormones, causing a generalized acceleration of metabolism. By far the most common cause of thyrotoxicosis is Graves' disease, followed by multinodular goiter and toxic adenoma [3].

Graves' disease is an autoimmune disease in which the thyroid gland is stimulated by autoantibodies against the TSH receptor (TRAB). It was described completely in 1835 by Robert Graves and comprises 80% of the cases of hyperthyroidism. Women are affected 5 to 10 times more than men. It is uncommon before 5 years of age, increases during puberty and has its peak incidence observed between 20 and 40 years of age. It is a less common disease in blacks, but equally prevalent in Caucasians and Asians [2] [4]-[8].

Despite a strong familial predisposition, to date, no specific gene has been linked to Graves' disease. Thus, there must be also environmental factors that exert great influence on the development of the pathology. Stress, smoking, infection (viral or bacterial) and excessive intake of iodine (particularly in geographical areas poor on this element) would be some of these risk factors [2] [4] [7].

Furthermore, Graves' disease may be associated with other autoimmune endocrine disorders (type 1 *diabetes mellitus*, Addison's disease, autoimmune oophoritis, ACTH isolated deficiency, etc.) and non-endocrine (*myasthenia gravis*, systemic lupus erythematosus, rheumatoid arthritis, Sjögren's disease, pernicious anemia, chronic active hepatitis, vitiligo, Down's syndrome, etc.) [7] [9]-[11].

Graves' disease presents with three classic clinical features: hyperthyroidism with diffuse goiter, infiltrative ophthalmopathy and dermopathy ("pretibial myxedema"). The most common manifestations of hyperthyroidism include nervousness, insomnia, fatigue, hot and dry skin, excessive sweating, tachycardia, palpitation, weight loss, polyphagia, diarrhea, tremors and heat intolerance. Regarding goiter, Graves' disease it is typically diffuse (97%). It can be asymmetrical or lobular with variable volume. But there is a finding considered exclusive of the disease: the presence of "thrilling" murmur of the gland, produced by the notable increase in local blood flow. Any patient presenting with a diffuse goiter and hyperthyroidism should raise the hypothesis of Graves' disease as a diagnosis until otherwise proven [2] [6] [7]. The ophtalmopathy is present in 50% of patients with Graves' disease. It is due to the increased volume of extra ocular muscles and retro bulbar fat, generating an increase in intraorbital pressure. Consequently, protrusion of the eyeball may occur (called "exophthalmia" or "proptosis") along with decreased venous drainage resulting in per orbital edema, conjunctiva hyperemia and chemosis. Both orbits are affected, but in the beginning the manifestations may be clinically unilateral (20%). The most common ocular manifestation in Graves' disease is eyelid retraction, fixed or scared look and "*lid-lag*" signal (delayed descent of the upper eyelid when the eyeball is moved down). The periorbital edema and exophthalmiasstrongly suggest the diagnosis of Graves' disease [2] [7] [12].

Thyroid dermopathy or pretibial myxedema is exclusively found in Graves' disease. Considered a rare condition, it consists of a thickening of the skin, particularly over the lower region of the tibia, due to the accumulation of glycosaminoglycans. It affects only 5% to 10% of patients, being more common among women than in men (3.5:1) and is almost always associated with infiltrative ophthalmopathy (often severe) and high levels of TRAB. The lesions present as plaques, with very thickened skin, an aspect of orange peel and violet color. In less than 1% of the cases, it may be seen in other locations, such as hands and shoulders [6] [7].

Another common manifestation of Graves' disease is onycholysis ("Plummer's nail") which is best described as its separation from the nail layer due to faster nail growth [2] [7].

2.1. Laboratory Diagnosis

Classical laboratory findings in hyperthyroidism include TSH suppression, T3 and free T4 increase.

Occasionally, in about 5% of cases, only the T3 is high, following the suppression of TSH ("T3-toxicosis"). This situation is shown more common in the early stage of the disease or in cases of relapse. Furthermore, it is possible to find initially only low levels of TSH, with normal T4 and T3 levels (subclinical hyperthyroidism). On the other hand, in seriously ill patients a TSH suppression can be found, together with low levels of free T4 (FT4) and T3, characterizing the "Sick Euthyroid Syndrome"[2] [7].

Antithyroid antibodies such as antithyroglobulin (anti-Tg) and anti-thyroperoxidase (anti-TPO) are observed in many patients with Graves' disease, but at lower titles than those found in Hashimoto's thyroiditis. However, the presence of TRAB has a great specificity for Graves' disease, indicating disease activity [2] [7].

2.2. Treatment

As an autoimmune disease, Grave' disease has a tendency to develop relapses and remissions. There is no cure and optimal treatment, correcting the autoimmune responses, is not available. The management consists of interventions that reduce the thyroid's ability to respond to abnormal stimulation by TRAB. The three basic treatment options are antithyroid medications (thioamides), surgery and radioactive iodine [2] [4] [6] [7].

There are three antithyroid drugs: methimazole (MMI), carbimazole (used mainly in the UK and parts of the British Commonwealth) and propylthiouracil (PTU). In general, therapy with antithyroid drugs as a first treatment option is most useful in young patients with small glands and mild disease. The therapy is usually initiated with higher doses and, when the patient becomes biochemically euthyroid, one can make maintenance therapy at a lower dose. The drug is usually administered for 1 - 2 years and then it is assessed if the dose is adjusted or discontinued in order to evaluate whether the patient had remission (normal thyroid function one year after drug discontinuation) [2] [7] [13].

As for the side effects of thioamides, the frequency is added to the first 6 months of treatment. The most common reactions are allergic in nature (itching and rash) and epigastralgia, from 5% to 10% of patients. Among the serious side effects have agranulocytosis (absolute granulocyte count $< 500/mm^3$, occurring at 0.2% to 0.5% of patients and can be life threatening if the drug is not discontinued) and hepatotoxicity (PTU can cause fulminant hepatic necrosis, and potentially fatal, while the MMI can cause potentially cholestatic liver toxicity) [2] [7].

Radioiodine has been used to treat hyperthyroidism since 1941. In the United States of America, is the preferred treatment for most patients over 21 years of age. It aims to control hyperthyroidism, the gland destroying and making the hypothyroid patient. It is administered orally (in solution or capsules) and has low cost. It can be used as initial therapy or as definitive therapy of second line, when there were relapses after antithyroid drugs. Most cost-effective therapy is considered the optimal dose of radioactive iodine is still controversial: most experts prefer the use of fixed dose (10, 12 or 15 mCi), while others prefer the method in which the dose is calculated based on the size of the thyroid and its ability to capture iodine. The relative contraindications to this treatment include: Graves' eye disease, bulky goiters and refusal of the patient. However, pregnancy and lactation are absolute contraindications [2] [6] [7] [14].

Surgery (total thyroidectomy) is indicated in very bulky goiters (>150 g), in the existence of compressive symptoms in allergic patients or non-adherent to drug therapy, in patients who refuse treatment with radioactive iodine or in pregnant women with severe Graves' disease who are allergic or develop reactions to antithyroid drugs. Preoperatively, the patient should be prepared with a thyonamide (preferably 4 - 6 weeks are needed). In the 10 days before the procedure, should also be given potassium iodide in the form of saturated or Lugol solution 3 times/day mixed in water or juice. This scheme reduces the vasculature of the gland, reducing blood loss during surgery [2] [6] [7] [15].

3. Down Syndrome

Chromosomes may occasionally undergo some changes during mitosis and meiosis processes, resulting in chromosomal abnormalities. The clinically significant abnormality type is aneuploidy (abnormal number of chromosomes due to an extra chromosome or autosomal trisomy (three instead of the normal pair of one chromosome) is the most frequent aneuploidy. The most common type of viable human aneuploidy is Down syndrome or trisomy at chromosome band 21q22, corresponding to 95% of cases. John Langdon Down, the British physician, was the first to describe the syndrome characteristics that bears his name. He presented detailed description of Down syndrome in 1866 [16] [17].

Although its etiology is not yet clearly established, there are endogenous and exogenous risk factors related to it. One of the main risk factors is advanced maternal age. As for external factors, exposure to ionizing radiation, consumption of alcohol, tobacco and illicit drugs are cited as causal factors of aneuploidy. [14] [18]

3.1. Disease Profile: Down Syndrome

Individuals with Down syndrome show a variable delay in mental development, and specific phenotypic characteristics, such as brachycephalia (very small frontal-occipital diameter, palpebral fissures with upper slope, epicanthal folds, flat nasal bridge and hypoplasia of the middle region of the face). Short neck is also common; a single palmar fold may be present; the tongue is protruding and hypotonic; there is clinodactyly of the fifth chirodactyl and increased distance between the big toe and the second toe. Frequently, children with Down syndrome also have generalized muscle hypotonic [18].

3.2. Health Problems Related to Down Syndrome

Children with Down syndrome are more likely to present a health impairment due to congenital abnormalities and predispositions characteristics of the syndrome. Among the major commitments are: [11] [15] [19]:

1) Cardiac disorders: Congenital heart defects are present in 50% of cases. The most common problems are atrioventricular canal defect, ventricular septal defect, atrial septal defect and tetralogy of Fallot.

2) Lung diseases: Most children with Down syndrome have frequent colds and recurrent pneumonia. This is due to an immune predisposition and the hypotonic muscles of the respiratory tract.

3) Atlantoaxial instability: This modification consists in an increase in the intervertebral space between the first and second vertebrae of the cervical spine, caused by anatomical abnormalities (hypoplasia of the odontoid process) and muscle-ligamentous hypotonic. It reaches 10% - 20% of children and young people with Down syndrome and may lead to subluxation and spinal cord injury at the cervical level, causing neurological impairment (both sensitive and motor) or death (secondary to respiratory arrest due to injury of the medullary respiratory center).

4) Endocrinopathies: The most common hormonal dysfunction in individuals with Down syndrome is hypothyroidism, occurring in approximately 10% of children and 13% to 50% of adults. The presence of this pathology contributes to obesity in these patients, as well as harms the intellectual development of the child, if not correctly treated.

5) Visual problems: are very common in children with the syndrome. Myopia (50%), hyperopia (20%), astigmatism, strabismus, amblyopic, nystagmus and cataracts are the most common disorders.

6) Hearing problems: About 60% to 80% of children with the syndrome have uni- or bilateral hearing loss. Hearing deficits are mild or moderate in most cases and can be caused by the increase of cerumen in the ear canal, accumulation of secretions in the middle ear and frequent ear infections (due to the abnormal form of the ossicles in the middle ear). Hearing loss can also harm the overall development of the child.

7) Other associated problems: humor disorders, depression, Alzheimer's disease, autism and leukemia are associated with Down syndrome.

4. Case Report

G.J.M., 18 years old, male, melanoderm, born and raised in Feira de Santana, Northeastern region of Brazil, was admitted to an Endocrinology Ambulatory on 09 November 2014. According to his mother, he presented vomiting complaints, recurrent sore throat, fever and hair loss.

His mother also reported that 1 year before the patient began presenting repeated sore throat episodes, always accompanied by fever (not measured) and vomiting. The patient told he was always taken to the Basic Health Unit (BHU) in the neighborhood where he lives, with improvement in symptoms after the use of medications that he was not aware of. But in recent months the frequency of seizures increased and, in the last 30 days, progressive hair loss was observed.

He denied headache, dizziness, earache, runny nose, cough, dyspnea, chest pain, palpitations, abdominal pain, diarrhea, constipation, dysuria, urinary burning and insomnia, but claimed observing "him more restless, distressed" and "thickening of the legs". He denied rash or skin lesions prior or concomitant to loss of nails, but complained about the occurrence of fragile and brittle nails.

As for past medical history, the mother said that the patient is carrier of Down syndrome. It was denied that he made use of continuous medication and or would have hypertension, dyslipidaemia or diabetes *mellitus*.

Born preterm natural childbirth (approximately 32 weeks), the mother claimed that the patient had low weight and required hospitalization before hospital discharge. He described having had repetitive situations of viral infections and verminosis during childhood, not specified.

The mother denies other cases of Down syndrome in the family. She denied systemic arterial hypertension, diabetes *mellitus*, dyslipidaemia, thyroid diseases or alopecia areata. She also pointed out that the patient never attended schools or institutions specializing in care for the disabled, citing a lack of resources. Denied the use of alcohol, tobacco or illicit drugs, it has positive epidemiology for schistosomiases and negative for Chagas disease.

On physical examination, the patient has good general and nutritional status, is lucid, eupneic, flushed and anicteric. Anthropometric data: Body mass = 57.0 kg. Height = 165.0 cm. Body mass index = 20.94 kg/m^2. Radial pulse = 96 bpm. Respiratory rate = 16 ipm. Blood pressure = 120 × 80 mmHg.

HEAD: Symmetric, brachycephaly; no scalp and face injuries; absence of hair, eyebrows and eyelashes (**Figure 1**).

NECK: Symmetric; topic thyroid with normal volume, fibroelastic, mobile, painless, without palpable nodules, and no murmurs or thrills; absence of lymphadenopathy

CHEST: Symmetric; absence of skin lesions; lack of hair.

RESPIRATORY TRACT: Preserved expandability; normal thoracolumbar vocal tremor; vesicular murmur and distributed without adventitious sounds.

CARDIOVASCULAR TRACT: Quiet precordium; stroke invisible, but palpable in 5th left intercostal space in the mid-clavicular line; rhythmic sounds phonetically normal in two times, no murmurs.

ABDOMEN: Symmetric; plain; absence of hair; flaccid; painless on palpation; without masses or visceromegaly; no murmurs; normal hydro-aerial noises.

GENITALIA: Absence of pubic hair; absence of ulcers or secretions; topics testicles, painless, mobile and trophic; absence of mass in inguinal regions. Tanner: G5.

EXTREMITIES: Symmetric upper limb without skin lesions, hairless, well perfused and without edema; Symmetrical legs with discrete cutaneous thickening plates in lower third of the legs, hairless, well perfused and without edema; absence of onycholysis.

NEUROLOGICAL EXAMINATION: normal walk; tremors in hands; normal patellar reflexes.

The mother reported that the patient underwent a preliminary assessment with an otolaryngologist that would

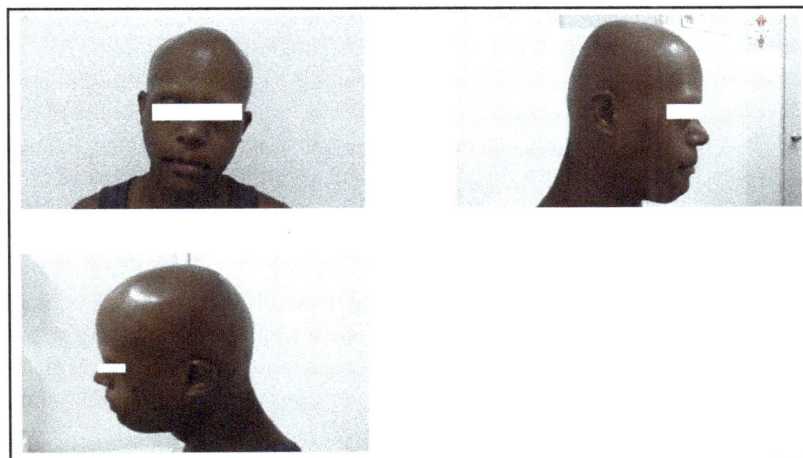

Figure 1. Characteristics of patient G.J.M. in 09/05/2014. Symmetrical and brachycephalia head; no scalp and face injuries; complete absence of hair, eyebrows and eyelashes.

have diagnosed rhinitis and requested a thyroid ultrasound. The results of this exam were, on 15/08/2014: "a topic thyroid, with regular borders and heterogeneous echogenicity. Multiple hypoechoic and echogenic areas, diffusely throughout its parenchyma; right lobe measuring 4.3 × 1.7 × 2.0 cm with volume of 8.1 cm^3; left lobe measuring 4.5 × 1.6 × 1.9 cm with volume of 7.5 cm^3; isthmus without alterations, with a volume of 0.9 cm^3; total volume of the gland 16.5 cm3 [NR - 4.8 to 12.0 cm^3]).

Based on the clinical history, the physical examination and complimentary exams, the diagnosis of DIFFUSE GOITER was defined, with its probable etiology related to Hyperthyroidism: GRAVES' DISEASE. To confirm this diagnosis and allow a proper beginning of drug therapy, complementary exams were requested. On 09/09/2014 a TSH < 0.008 mU/L (suppressed TSH) was found. FT4 = 6.79 ng/dl (increased). FT3 > 20 ng/dl, TRAB > 40.0 U/L, Anti-TPO > 600 U/ml.

In face of these lab results, the diagnosis of SECONDARY DIFFUSE GOITER DUE TO GRAVES' DISEASE was confirmed. Methimazole 10 mg was prescribed (dose: 2 tablets in the morning), and thorough instructions were made regarding the disease's characteristics and its treatment, as well as the possibility of any serious side effects of the medication (with instructions on the procedures to be adopted in case of side effects). Follow-up tests after 45 days of the start of drug treatment were required.

On 27/11/2014 the patient returned to the ambulatory. The patient's mother reported that he was in continuous use of methimazole, as prescribed. The patient kept, however, postprandial vomiting and diarrhea episodes, although with a decreased frequency. She reported that the patient was taken to the gastroenterologist who prescribed "verminosis treatment". On that consultation, he also presented new exams: (27/11/2014) TSH < 0.008 mU/L, FT4 > 30.0 µg/dl, T3 = 544.0 ng/dl.

The doctors decided to double the dosage of the medication: 40 mg of methimazole in a single dosage in the morning. Control tests were recommended to be carried out after 45 days.

On 03/02/2015, the patient and the mother returned. According to their report, the patient showed a significant improvement in symptoms of the gastrointestinal tract and did not present fever or sore throat during that period. They were glad because of a discrete hair growth in the scalp and of the eyelashes during this period. The results of required control tests on 05/01/2015 were: FT4 = 1.55 ng/dl, FT3 = 5.8 ng/dl, TRAB ≥ 40.0 U/L. Based on the important clinical recovery and on these results, an option to keep the drug therapy was made, with recommendation for further tests after 60 days.

However, the patient returned after five months in continuous use of prescribed medication, with reversal of alopecia areata (**Figure 2**) and bringing new control tests: on 06/05/2015, FT4 = 1.5 ng/dl, TRAB = > 40.0 U/L. The conduct adopted was to maintain methimazole dose.

5. Conclusions

Patients affected by Down syndrome, a condition associated with impairment of the immune system, are more likely to develop recurrent infections and autoimmune diseases. Amongst the autoimmune diseases that affect these patients, type 1 diabetes *mellitus*, autoimmune thyroiditis, alopecia, celiac disease and the early development of Alzheimer's disease are the most important medical diagnoses to be looked for.

When it comes to thyroid disorders, autoimmune thyroiditis is the most common condition in patients with Down syndrome. The most common form in children and adolescents is Hashimoto's thyroiditis. Hyperthyroidism manifests itself less frequently in patients with Down syndrome. When it does, it usually presents as Graves' disease, showing the same characteristics of this pathology in the general population, except for presenting at earlier ages (children and adolescents), showing no female predominance, low incidence of ophthalmopathy and reduced clinical remission with methimazole.

In this presented case, it is important to point out the fact that the symptoms of hyperthyroidism occurred gradually, prevailing the altered bowel habits. Because the patient had repeated throat infections and intermittent diarrhea history, this symptom inadvertently went unnoticed at first, having caused a delayed diagnosis.

Alopecia areata was also a very significant sign in this case, presenting the universal form and quick installation due to the combination of genetic factors (change in chromosome 21) and immunologic (circulating autoantibodies).

It is necessary to lead a regular treatment towards normalization of signs and symptoms as well as thyroid hormone levels. Hyperthyroidism therapy in patients with Down syndrome basically does not differ from that employed in individuals without this clinical condition. Current medical literature suggested to treat Hypothyroi-

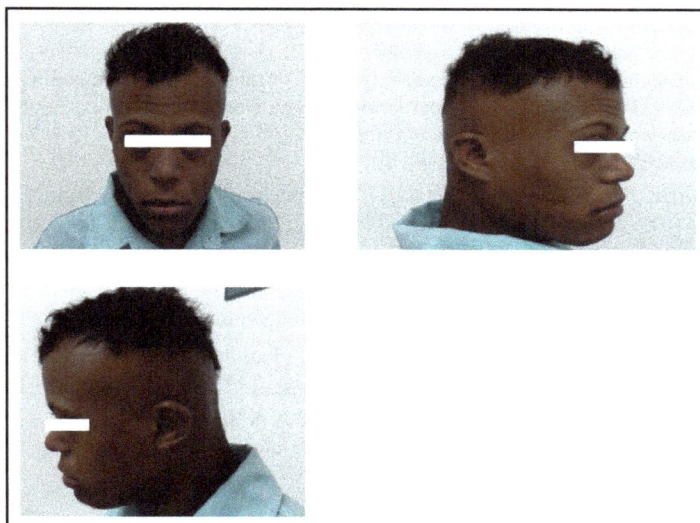

Figure 2. Patient G.J.M., characteristics on 04/09/2015, 5 months after continuous use of methimazole.

dism clinically up to 2 years after diagnosis, using thioamides (if serious side effects do not arise), and then planed the necessary definitive therapy, which would be radioiodine or surgery.

Acknowledgements

The authors would like to thank IPEMED Brazil for supporting continuing medical education.

References

[1] Kimura, E.T. and Zago, D.A. (2001) Embriologia e Histologia. In: Rosa, J.C. and Romão, L.A., Eds., *Glândula Tireoide*: *Funções e Disfunções, Diagnóstico e Tratamento*, 2nd Edition, Lemos Editorial, São Paulo, 19-25.

[2] Cooper, D.S. and Ladenson, P.W. (2013) Glândula Tireoide. In: Gardner, D.G. and Shoback, D., Eds., *Endocrinologia básica e clínica de Greenspan*. 9th Edition, AMGH, Porto Alegre, 163-226.

[3] Gadelha, P.S., Azevedo, M.F. and Montenegro, R.M. (2013) Interpretação dos Testes de Função Tireoidiana. In: Vilar, L., Ed., *Endocrinologia Clínica*, 5th Edition, Guanabara Koogan, Rio de Janeiro, 249-259.

[4] Weetman, A.P. (2000) Graves' Disease. *The New England Journal of Medicine*, **343**, 1236-1248. http://dx.doi.org/10.1056/NEJM200010263431707

[5] Sandrini, R., França, S.N., de Lacerda, L., *et al.* (2001) Tratamento do Hipertireoidismo na Infância e Adolescência. *Arquivos Brasileiros de Endocrinologia & Metabologia*, **45**, 32-36. http://dx.doi.org/10.1590/S0004-27302001000100006

[6] Neves, C., *et al.* (2008) Doença de Graves. *Arquivos de Medicina*, **22**, 137-146.

[7] Freitas, M.C., Mota, V.C. and Vilar, L. (2013) Diagnóstico e Tratamento da Doença de Graves. In: Vilar, L., Ed., *Endocrinologia Clínica*, 5th Edition, Guanabara Koogan, Rio de Janeiro, 310-327.

[8] Wasniewska, M., *et al.* (2014) Epidemiological, Pathophysiological and Clinical Peculiarities of Graves' Disease in Children with Down and Turner Syndrome: A Literature Review. *Health*, **6**, 1447-1452. http://dx.doi.org/10.4236/health.2014.612178

[9] Karlsson, B., *et al.* (1998) Thyroid Dysfunction in Down's Syndrome: Relation to Age and Thyroid Autoimmunity. *Archives of Disease in Childhood*, **79**, 242-245.

[10] Goday-Arno, A., Cerda-Esteva, M., Flores-Le-Roux, J.A., *et al.* (2009) Hyperthyroidism in a Population with Down Syndrome (DS). *Clinical Endocrinology*, **71**, 110-114. http://dx.doi.org/10.1111/j.1365-2265.2008.03419.x

[11] Iughetti, L., *et al.* (2015) Thyroid Function in Down syndrome. *Expert Review of Endocrinology & Metabolism*, **10**, 1-8. http://dx.doi.org/10.1586/17446651.2015.960846

[12] Bloise, W. (2001) Oftalmopatia da Moléstia de Graves. In: Rosa, J.C. and Romão, L.A., Eds., *Glândula Tireoide*: *Funções e Disfunções, Diagnóstico e Tratamento*, 2nd Edition, Lemos Editorial, São Paulo, 249-254.

[13] Young, E.T., *et al.* (1988) Prediction of Remission after Antithyroid Drug Treatment in Graves' Disease. *Quarterly Journal of Medicine*, **66**, 175-189.

[14] Cruz Júnior, A.F., Takahashi, M.H. and Albino, C.C. (2006) Tratamento Clínico com Drogas Antitireoidianas ou Dose Terapêutica de Iodo-131 no Controle do Hipertireoidismo na Doença de Graves: Avaliação dos Custos e Benefícios. *Arquivos Brasileiros de Endocrinologia e Metabologia*, **50**, 1096-1101. http://dx.doi.org/10.1590/S0004-27302006000600017

[15] Andrade, V.A., Gross, J.L. and Maia, A.L. (2001) Tratamento do Hipertireoidismo da Doença de Graves. *Arquivos Brasileiros de Endocrinologia e Metabologia*, **45**, 609-618. http://dx.doi.org/10.1590/S0004-27302001000600014

[16] Nakadonari, E.K. and Soares, A.A. (2006) Síndrome de Down: Considerações Gerais sobre a Influência da Idade Materna Avançada. *Arquivos doMudi*, **10**, 5-9.

[17] Matos, S.B., *et al.* (2007) Síndrome de Down: Avanços e perspectivas. *Revista Saúde.com*, **3**, 77-86.

[18] Silva, N.L.P. and Dessen, M.A. (2001) Deficiência Mental e Família: Implicações para o Desenvolvimento da Criança. *Psicologia: Teoria e Pesquisa*, **17**, 133-141. http://dx.doi.org/10.1590/s0102-37722001000200005

[19] Moreira, L.M.A., El-Hani, C.N. and Gusmão, F.A.F. (2000) A Síndrome de Down e sua Patogênese: Considerações sobre o Determinismo Genético. *Revista Brasileira de Psiquiatria*, **22**, 96-99. http://dx.doi.org/10.1590/s1516-44462000000200011

18

Effect of Soy Bean Isoflavon on Lipid Accumulation in 3T3-L1 Adipocytes

Teruhiko Matsushima, Noriko Yoshimura, Yuumi Koseki

Department of Human Life Science, Jissen Women's University, Tokyo, Japan
Email: matshima@nifty.com

Abstract

Several nutrition and food ingredients are supposed to have beneficial effects, but precise cell biological mechanism has not been elucidated. Among food ingredients, polyphenols such as soy bean isoflavon genistein and wine resveratrol have been reported to have effects on lipid metabolism and cardiovacular diseases (1). In order to elucidate the effect of genistein on obesity, we cultured adipocyte and observed of genisten to lipid accumulation in cells. Triglyceride accumulation was suppressed by genistein when it was added at the time of differentiation but not when added after differentiation. Genistein is considered to suppress lipid accumulation by suppressing the differtiation of adipocytes.

Keywords

Obesity, Adipocyte, Genistein, Resveratrol

1. Introduction

Obesity is one of world-wide problem leading to disseases including atherosclerosis. Several nutrition and food ingredients are considered to have beneficial effects [1], but precise cell biological mechanism has not been elucidated. Among food ingredients, polyphenols such as soy bean isoflavon genistein and green tea epigallo-cathecin gallate have been reported effects on lipid metabolism and cardiovacular diseases [2]. In this paper we studied the effects of genistein and EGCG on differentiation to adipocyte and lipid accumulation in 3T3L1 preadipocytes.

2. Methods

2.1. Cell Culture

3T3L1 preadipocytes derived from mice skin fibroblast were obtained from American Tissue Culture Collection. Cells were cultured in Dulbecco's modified essential medium (DMEM) including 10% fetal calf serum (FCS) in atmosphere of 5% CO_2 at 37°C. Two days after confluency, ells were differenciated to adipocyte by standard procedure [3], by adding differentiation mix at final concentration of 5 μg/ml insulin, 1.0 μM dexamethazone and 400 μM isobutyl methyl xanthine. Afer 2 days, the medium was changed to DMEM ontaining 0.1 mg/ml insulin and 10% FCS and the culture was continued.

2.2. Experiments

Genistein, epigallocatech ingallate (EGCG) and β-estradiol was purchased from Sigma. Genisteinn and β-estradiol was dissolved in dimethylsulfoxide and EGCG was dissolved in water. In experiment A, testing materials were added to the cells simultaneously at the time of differentiation and lipid accumulated in cells was extracted and triglyceride was quantified at 3, 5, 7 and 10 days. In experiment B, testing materials were added seven days after differentiation and triglyceride was quantified at 5, 10, 15 and 21 days.

2.3. Lipid Staining

Cells on culture dishes were washed twice with phosphate buffered saline (PBS), fixed with 10% formalin for 10min, soaked in 60% isopropanol for one minute and staind with fleshly prepared 1.8% Oil-Red O stain solution in 60% isopropanol for one hour. Cells were washed with 60% isopropanol and then tap water, and stained with hematoxylin solution for 10 min. After washing the cells with tap water, the cells were observed by microscope.

2.4. Lipid Extraction and Quantification

Cells on dishes were washed twice by PBS, scraped off in 25 mM Tris-HCl 1mM Ethylenediaminetetraacetic acid pH7.4 and disrupted by sonication in ice-water for 10 min. Lipid was extracted from cell lysate by equal volume of 1:1 chloroform-methanol. After adding 20 ml of Triton X100-methanol (1:1) the organic solvent was browed out by nitrogen gas flow and the solution was diluted by 220 μl water. Triglyceride concentration was quantified by enzymatic method using Triglyceride E-test (Wako).

3. Results

After differentiation, cells gradually accumulated lipid and lipid droplets became visible around the third or the forth days. In experiment A (**Figure 1**), where the reagents were added to cells at the timing of differentiation, cellular triglyceride accumulation was suppressed to 26.3% of control by genistein and to 78.8% by EGCG and 43.2% by β-estradiol respectively. At the 10th days, further accumulation of lipid was observed but it was also suppressed to 17.8% by genistein and to 54.8% by EGCG and 41.0% by β-estradiol. On the other hand, in experiment B (**Figure 2**), where the reagents were added 7 days after differentiation, no difference was observed in triglriceride accumulation at any point of time course.

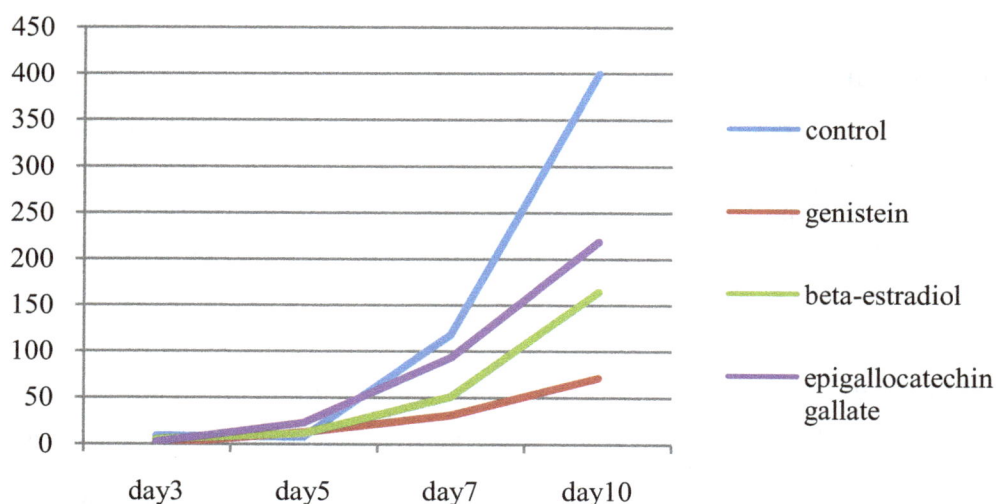

Figure 1. Time course of triglyceride content in 3T3L1 cells. Reagents were added at the timing of cell differentiation.

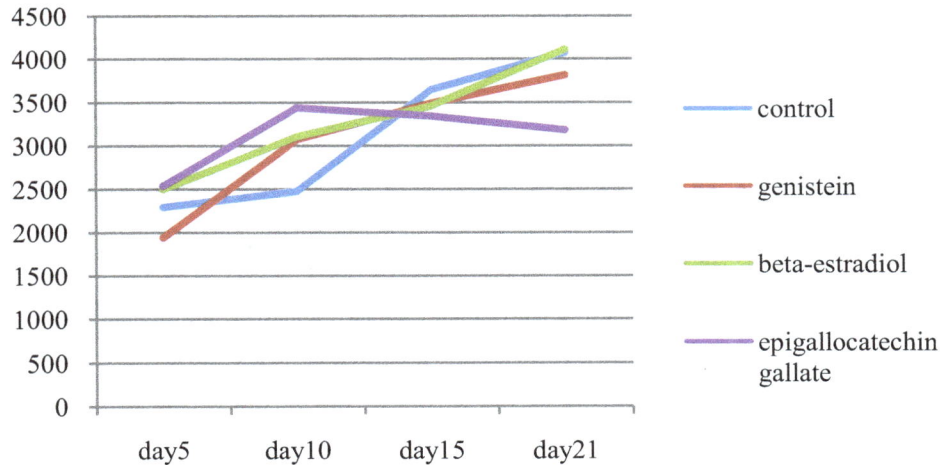

Figure 2. Time course of triglyceride content in 3T3L1 cells. Reagents were added 7days after differentiation.

4. Discussion

Soy isoflavon was reported to increase lypolysis and oxidation in 3T3L1 when adminstered together with L-carnitine [3]. It was also confirmed in mice that isoflavone increase energy expenditure and decrease adiposity [4]. In this study, we found that genistein, soy bean isoflavone, suppresses triglyceride accumulation in 3T3L1 cells when it was added at the time of differenciation but not when added later. It suggests that after differentiation, genistein has no effect on lipid accumulation, suggesting that genistein may have influence on adipocyte differentiation. Further studies on differentiation, such as about transcriptional factor PPAR-g or CEBP are necessary.

Acknowledgements

This study was supported by Grant-for-Aide No. 24650503 from the Ministry of Education and Science, Japan.

References

[1]   Moriguchi, E.H., Moriguchi, Y. and Yamori, Y. (2004) Impact of Diet on the Cardiovascular Risk Profile of Japanese Immigrants Living in Brazil: Contributions of World Health Organization CARDIAC and MONALISA Studies. *Clinical and Experimental Pharmacology and Physiology*, **31**, S5-S7. http://dx.doi.org/10.1111/j.1440-1681.2004.04119.x

[2]   Anderson, J.W., Smith, B.M. and Washnock, C.S. (1999) Cardiovascular and Renal Benefits of Dry Bean and Soybean Intake. *The American Journal of Clinical Nutrition*, **70**, 464S-474S.

[3]   Murosaki, S., Lee, T.R., Muroyama, K., Shin, E.S., Cho, S.Y., Yamamoto, Y. and Lee, S.J. (2007) A Combination of Caffeine, Soy Isoflavones, and L-Carnitine Enhances both Lipolysis and Fatty Acid Oxidation in 3T3-L1 and HepG2 Cells *in Vitro* and in KK Mice *in Vivo*. *Journal of Nutrition*, **137**, 2252-2257.

[4]   Cederroth, C.R., Vinciguerra, M., Kühne, F., Madani, R., Doerge, D.R., Visser, T.J., Foti, M., Rohner-Jeanrenaud, F., Vassalli, J.D. and Nef, S. (2007) A Phytoestrogen-Rich Diet Increases Energy Expenditure and Decreases Adiposity in Mice. *Environmental Health Perspectives*, **115**, 1467-1473. http://dx.doi.org/10.1289/ehp.10413

19

Mathematical Modeling of a Metabolic Network to Study the Impact of Food Contaminants on Genomic Methylation and DNA Instability

Etienne Z. Gnimpieba[1]*, Souad Bousserouel[2], Abalo Chango[1]

[1]Department of Nutritional Sciences and Health, EGEAL UPSP: 2007.05.137-Institut Polytechnique Lasalle Beauvais, Beauvais, France
[2]Laboratoire de Prévention Nutritionnelle du Cancer, Inserm U682-IRCAD, Strasbourg, France
Email: souadbousserouel@gmail.com

Abstract

Environmental contamination of food is a worldwide public health problem. Folate mediated one-carbon metabolism plays an important role in epigenetic regulation of gene expression and mutagenesis. Many contaminants in food cause cancer through epigenetic mechanisms and/or DNA instability *i.e.* default methylation of uracil to thymine, subsequent to the decrease of 5-methyltetrahydrofolate (5 mTHF) pool in the one-carbon metabolism network. Evaluating consequences of an exposure to food contaminants based on systems biology approaches is a promising alternative field of investigation. This report presents a dynamic mathematical modeling for the study of the alteration in the one-carbon metabolism network by environmental factors. It provides a model for predicting "the impact of arbitrary contaminants that can induce the 5 mTHF deficiency. The model allows for a given experimental condition, the analysis of DNA methylation activity and dumping methylation in the *de novo* pathway of DNA synthesis.

Keywords

DNA-Methylation, DNA Instability, Mathematical Modeling, Logic Programming, Metabolic Network, Food Contaminant

1. Introduction

An inadequate methyl group donor enhances the risk of cancer because the one-carbon unit (CH_3) has critical functions in biological methylation reactions such as DNA-cytosine methylation, and in DNA synthesis or repair [1]-[3]. The methylation of DNA is a fundamental mechanism for epigenetic control of gene expression and the maintenance of genomic integrity, as well as uracil methylation into thymidine for the maintenance of DNA sta-

---

*Current address: Computer Science Department, University of South Dakota, USA.

bility to ensure chromosomal integrity during replication process [4]. Low 5-methytetrahydrofolate (5 mTHF) (**Figure 1**) reduces DNA methylation, and thymidylate synthase-mediated methylation of deoxyuridylate (dU) to thymidylate (dT). This results in a higher dU/dT ratio, increase in uracil misincorporation into DNA, inefficient DNA repair, and chromosomal breakage [5]-[7].

The role of dietary factors in DNA methylation processes diseases following folate repletion, and the consequences of genetic defect has been underlined in 2001 during the Trans-HHS Workshop in the USA [8]. Abnormal DNA methylation has been reported in disease prevention such as cancer, hepatotoxicity, pancreatic toxicity, diabetes, atherosclerosis, birth defects, and neurological disturbances. Poirier *et al.*, [9] have suggested three major causes of diseases related to methyl group insufficiency: dietary deficiency, genetic polymorphism, and a third prospective cause, chemicals. Evidence now suggest that some environmental contaminants, including exogenous chemicals such as polyhalogenated compounds, metals, some mycotoxins, and others, can produce abnormal methylation processes or abnormal folate uptake [10] linked to the etiology of diseases. Recently, Lawley *et al.* (2011) [11] demonstrates the application of a mathematical model to arsenic methylation in human studies in Bangladesh. However, in their model, various biochemical aspect of arsenic metabolism have been greatly simplified.

DNA hypomethylation and uracil misincorporation/repair are not exclusive mechanisms and both could be important in diagnostics. Since both aspects of DNA modification are strongly associated with 5 mTHF metabolism and carcinogenesis, development of methods for analyzing DNA-cytosine methylation and DNA-uracil in the aetiology of diseases is of great interest.

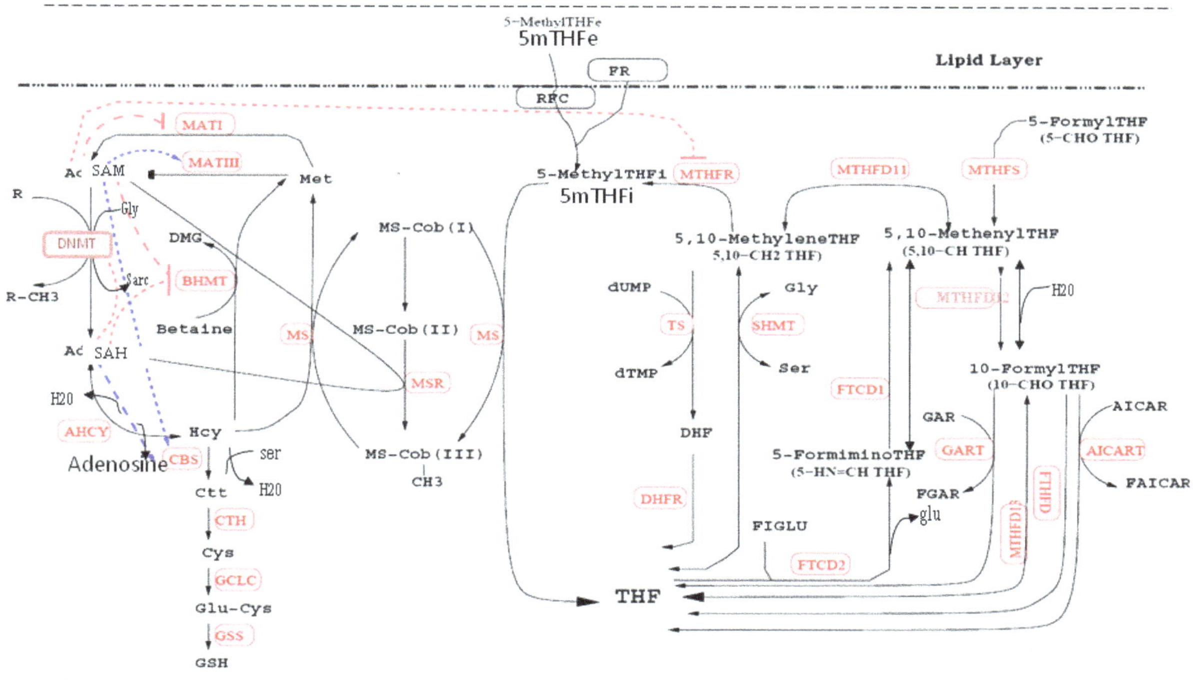

Figure 1. The Folate-mediated one carbon metabolism network [12]. Légende: Black arrow: normal reaction; Red arrow: inhibition (negative regulation); Blue arrow: activation (positive regulation). Red box: Enzyme catalyzes reaction; Black no box text: metabolites. Abbreviation: AHCY: S-adenosylhomocysteine hydrolase. AICART: Aminoimidazole carboxamide ribonucléotide (AICAR) formyltransférase; BHMT: betaine homocysteine methyltransferase. CBS: cystathionine beta-synthase; CTH: cystathionine gamma-lyase; DHFR: dihydrofolate reductase. FR: folate receptor; DNA MéthylTransférase; FTCD: formiminotransferase cyclodeaminase. GART: Phosporibosylglycinamide formyltransferas, phosphoribosylglycinamide synthase, phosphoribosylaminoimidazole synthase; GLCL: gammaglutamylcysteine synthase; GSS: glutathion synthase. (MATI/MATIII): adénosylmethionine transferase gene I/III. MS: methionine synthase. MSR: methionine synthase reductase; MTs: Methyltransferase MTHFD: methylenetetrahydrofolate dehydrogenase, methenyltetrahydrofolate cyclohydrolase, formyltetrahydrofolate synthase. MTHFR: 5,10-methylenetetrahydrofolate reductase. MTHFS: 5,10-methylenetetrahydrofolate synthase 5-formyltetrahydrofolate cycloligase. RFC: reduced folate; AdoMet: S-adénosylmethionine; AdoHcy: S-adénosylhomocystéine; SHMT: serine hydroxymethyltransferase; TS: tymidylate synthase. 5mTHF: 5-methyltetrahydrofolate.

2. Motivation

One of the major difficulties when working at the cellular level is describing the dynamic regulation of metabolites accurately to explain how subcellular processes such as DNA methylation or uracil methylation, are driven by environmental conditions such as 5 mTHF deficiency. Besides featuring complex networks in a living cell, with interconnecting pathways that consist of hundreds of reactions, there is need to take into account that the metabolism is subject to control and regulatory mechanisms. During the last ten years, there were many attempts to develop mathematical models for the study of cellular functions or cellular processes. We recently, built a mathematical model that integrates experimental conditions using logic programming for the study of the folate-mediated one-carbon metabolism regulation (FOCM) [12]. Here, we present the model, simulating the impact of environmental conditions such as the presence of a specific food contaminant on the network.

3. Contaminant Agents and the Alteration of Methylation Processes

Among mechanisms by which environmental agents can induce tumor formation are DNA hypomethylation associated with gene expression modification and uracil misincorporation into DNA leading to chromosomal breaks, micronucleus formation. Studies have showed that several classes of environmental chemicals that modify epigenetic marks, including metals (cadmium, arsenic, nickel, chromium, methylmercury), peroxisome proliferators (trichloroethylene, dichloroacetic acid, trichloroacetic acid), air pollutants (particulate matter, black carbon, benzene), and endocrine-disrupting/reproductive toxicants (diethylstilbestrol, bisphenol A, persistent organic pollutants, dioxin). Most studies conducted so far have been centered on DNA methylation [9] [13]. There is a need to explore the causes of many other environmental effects on methylation processes. Several paths of interaction of these contaminants on the methylation process: alteration of 5 mTHF uptake, of methyltranferase activity, or other key enzyme of the network. In this report we are interested to the interaction impinging on the availability of 5 mTHF in the cell. This is the case for instance of arsenic which may alter the expression of folate carrier and reducing the 5 mTHF uptake by cells [14].

4. Principle and Interest of Mathematical Modeling

Models describing biological systems such as the one-carbon metabolism network are too complex to be analyzed manually and therefore typically are solved numerically, using computers to solve the mathematical equations. With appropriated mathematical tools and the availability of computer-based techniques for solving equations, it is possible to predict and analyze the responses of a biological system to different conditions. In many cases the computer simulations called "dry experiments" require much lower investment and much less time compared with the typically more time-consuming and expensive biological experiments ("wet experiments"). Among benefits offer by mathematical models there are the fact that discrepancies between systems behaviors predicted by a mathematical model and actual behaviors measured in experiments can point to components that still are missing from the mathematical model, thereby assisting in developing a more comprehensive picture of a biological process. Even if it is not clear which components are missing from the system under investigation, the results obtained with the mathematical model may help to guide the design of additional experiments to clarify the issue (Systems: http://pubs.niaaa.nih.gov/publications/arh311/49-59.htm). The rationale of modeling is that it assists investigators in the analysis of the system in various possible experimental conditions. Predictions (or modeling results) are then compared to experimental measurements.

5. The One-Carbon Metabolism Network

Folate-mediated one-carbon metabolism is fundamental for cell growth and differentiation. In cells, folate uptake in the 5 mTHF form is converted to THF by transfer of the methyl group to homocysteine forming methionine and THF (**Figure 1**) [15]. Methionine can then be converted to S-adenosyl-methionine (AdoMet). AdoMet is involved in more than 100 reactions, and at least 80 AdoMet-dependent enzymes have been identified [16]. S-Adenosyl-homocysteine (AdoHcy), the by-product of methyl transfer reactions, is hydrolyzed, thus regenerating homocysteine, which then becomes available to start a new cycle of methyl-group transfer. In most tissues, homocysteine is re-methylated back to methionine through two pathways: the methionine synthase/methionine synthase reductase (MS/MSR) pathway. In the folate cycle, the THF reacts with serine synthetizing $N_{5,10}$-methyleneTHF (5,10-CH$_2$-THF) in a reaction catalyzed by serine hydroxymethyltransferase (SHMT). The 5,10-CH$_2$-THF is reduced into 5-CH$_3$-THF by the enzyme methylenetetrahydrofolate reductase (MTHFR), or oxidized into

5,10-methenylTHF by a reversible reaction catalyzed by methylenetetrahydrofolate dehydrogenase (MTHFD). 5,10-methenyl-THF can be converted to 10-formyl-THF by 5,10-methenyl-THF cyclohydrolase. Folate serves for DNA methylation in the transmethylation pathways [17], for synthesis of purines and a pyrimidine nucleoside (thymidine). It provides carbon units for *de novo* purine and thymidylate biosynthesis. Purine biosynthesis requires 10-formyl-THF for the C2 and C8 carbons of the purine ring catalyzed by glycinamide ribonucleotide transformylase (GART). Thymidylate biosynthesis requires CH_2-THF for the reductive methylation of deoxyuridylate catalyzed by the enzyme thymidylate synthase (TS).

The OCM system, presented in the **Figure 1**, considers an extracellular 5 mTHF uptake and a set of enzyme reactions. We considered a "generic" mammalian cell OCM including 26 enzymes reactions (*i.e.* 30 variables and 27 reactions involved). The model emphasises three functional units: one for the folate uptake and internalisation, one for the folate cycle, and one for methionine/homocysteine cycle. Each unit consists of a pool of interconnected metabolites by enzymatic reactions. The set of these reactions produces a system that we simulate using a mathematical framework. Mathematical model and reaction kinetic laws involved in the OCM model were reported in our previous study [12]. We modeled the kinetics of reactions of the OCM system using Ordinary Differentials Equations (ODE). Metabolites represent the system variables and variations of their concentration indicate the difference between their synthesis and catabolism levels.

6. Experimental Conditions and Logic Programming

We have proposed the use of the logic programming that represents an automatic way to study the possible impact of exogenous contaminant on the OCM network [12]. It consists of an automatic generation of a model based on data and knowledge available. This approach, developed in the laboratory takes into account several experimental conditions, which are considered as a set of constraints, in addition to the kinetic descriptions and as an original contribution to the standard mathematical modeling.

In the logic programming we encoded the set of data as a set of rules or facts. Each rule is encoded in the form "*IF* condition *THEN* conclusion". The first approach allows to study the structure of the biological system of interest, whereas the second proposes an analysis of the qualitative properties. As a complementary approach, we propose herein to apply such a theoretical framework for estimating the values of parameters in accuracy with the available experimental knowledge. The kinetic rates and known parameters (P') were inferred by using the logic programming inference as follow. All existing data (including experiments and literature based knowledge) are gather in a knowledge base (KB). We proceed to an inference by a back-tracking technique using the logic programming tool. In the KB, data are spread into a fact base (FB), that represents encoded biological knowledge (extracted from the literature) of our model; and the rule base (RB) that sums up the biological conditions monitoring the system behaviours. Formally, a given biological knowledge BK_i consists of sets of facts $F_i = \{F_{ij}\}$ and rules $R_i = \{R_{ij}\}$, where F_{ij} and R_{ij} are respectively atomics fact and rules obtained from BK_i. At first, the KB is empty and noted KB = { } (null). For each biological knowledge BK_i, KB is updated using a simple unification principle when a novel biological knowledge is added. The Fact Based (FB) is then completed by the new Fact set F_i and the Rules Base (RB) by the R_i ones.

The constraints are either the biological referential in which the OCM is observed (*i.e.* tissue, cell, etc...), the clinical conditions (*i.e.* healthy or pathological), and if needed, experimental parameters (*i.e.* temperature and pH of *in vitro* enzyme reactions). Each constraint represents a condition in which the model must behave accurately with given known experimental conditions. Logic programming is a well-investigated domain of machines learning artificial intelligence. Logical constraints are used to verify biological model behaviors during environmental perturbations via model-checking methods. The set of data is encoded as a set of rules or facts which gives rise of the opportunity to automatically learn novel rules by induction or deduction. Each rule is encoded in the form "*IF* condition *THEN* conclusion". The first approach allows studying the structure of the biological system of interest, whereas the second proposes an analysis of the qualitative properties. As a complementary approach, we propose herein to apply such a theoretical framework for estimating the values of parameters accurately with the available experimental knowledge. The parameters identification, inference of known parameters and the model validation are reported elsewhere [12].

7. Simulating the Impact of Contaminants by Reducing 5 mTHF Level in the Network

Food contaminants such as arsenic, fumonisin B1 and other, decreases intracellular 5 mTHF pool by reducing the activity of 5 mTHF transporter [10] [14]. In a previous in vitro study using HepG2 cell line grown either in experimental complete medium or in folate-depleted medium, we shown global hypomethylation of genomic DNA induced by the absence of folic acid in folate-depleted medium and significant increase of uracil residues in the same DNA sample [15].

We simulate the impact of arbitrary contaminants that can induce the 5 mTHF deficiency. 5 mTHF was computed by testing 50% and 25% of extra cellular 5 mTHF (5 mTHFe) input compared to 100% (10 nM[1]) (**Figure 2**). With 25% of 5 mTHFe major metabolites were quite insensitive while other metabolites show differential behavior. About AdoHcy, the methyl group donor, we observe an inverse tendency. For 50% and 100%, there was decreasing from 22.87 Units to 5.21 Units at 0.27 h and rapid increase to 25.12 Units at 1h of running, then a second level of rapid increasing to 88.97 Units at 1.5h was observed. With 25%, AdoHcy shows a different behavior from 2.5 Units increasing slowly to reach 18.94 Units at 2.6 h to remain constant. Finally, the curve of AdoMet/AdoHcy ratio increased at the beginning of running, reaching the highest level at 0.42 h with a ratio of

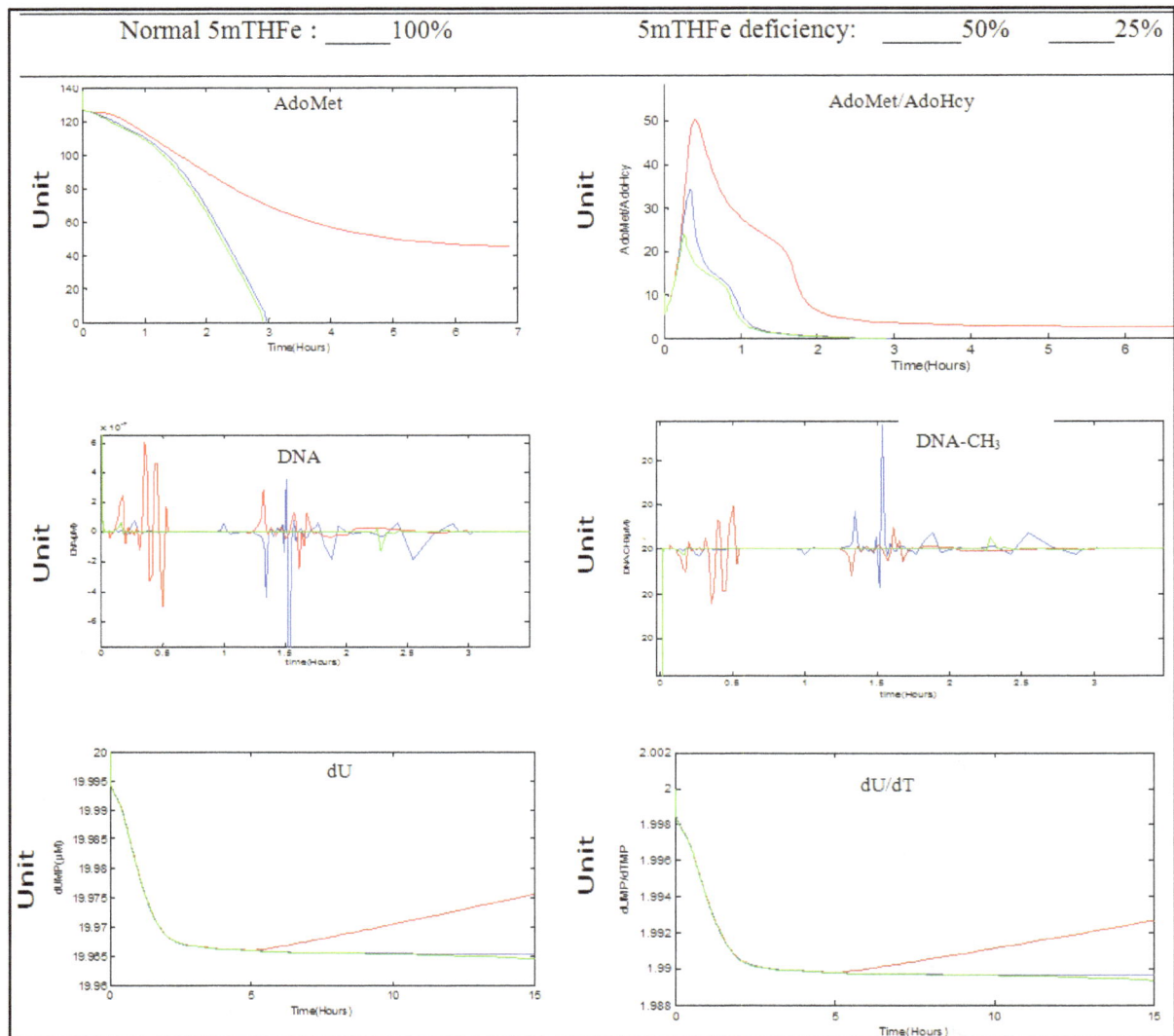

Figure 2. Result of simulating 5-methyltetrahydrofolate (5mTHF) deficiency [12]. Figure shows the variations relate to the transmethylation pathway, and the uracil methylation pathway. Disruptions of these subsystems are represented here by the behavior of state variables (metabolite concentrations over time). Thus, we observe an overall weak disturbance between the state without deficit (100% green) and the state with 50% deficit (blue). But the disruption is greater with 25% (red). Abbreviation AdoMet: S-adenosylmethionine; AdoHcy: S-adénosylhomocystéine: dU: deoxyuridylate, dT: thymidylate.

---

[1]This value represents also the simulation units (Units) that was at the nanomolar scale for 5mTH and other folate derived metabolites.

22; 34 and 50 respectively for 100%; 50% and 25% of 5 mTHFe condition respectively. In regard of the trans methylation reaction, results of time course DNA methylation process did not show characteristic differential behaviours with the three 5 mTHFe conditions. However, at steady state there are two oscillations of variable amplitude. These oscillations show lower amplitudes on methylated DNA (DNA-CH$_3$). The observed oscillations are not clear. However it is interesting to note that physiologically folate deficiency produce both global genomic DNA hypomethylation and gene specific hyper methylation. For dU, after a rapid decreasing with the three 5 mTHFe conditions, we observed a progressive increasing with 25% condition from 19.96 Units at 5h of running to 19.97 Units at 15 h of running. Finally with 100% of 5 mTHFe, dU/dT ratio reaches the steady-state 1.95 after 2.5 h compared to 1.99 after 2 h with 25% of 5 mTHF.

Finally, the model demonstrates that dependent of the impact of a contaminant on the decrease of 5 mTHF pool, there are different profiles of the dynamical behavior of the network. The questions emerging from such a study is how the stability of the critical reaction in the cycle is maintained when large localized changes occur either within the system or the input, and what is the significant of observed oscillations for DNA and DNA-CH$_3$ curves for cell. Otherwise a recent study from Nijhout *et al.* [18] have shown the inhibition of *GNMT* by 5 mTHF and consequently the existing long-range interactions stabilize DNA methylation. This report didn't include this particular finding that will need to include in the future.

8. Conclusion

The model allowed successfully the simulation of many key regulatory processes in one-carbon metabolism network. However it may be refined and used as tool in predictive nutritional toxicology to provide novel hypotheses for pathogenesis. It can be a predictive tool and could, therefore, be substituted in the future to experimental techniques in some cases.

Acknowledgements

This study has been supported by the Comité de l'Oise de la Ligue Contre le Cancer.

References

[1] Duthie, S.J., Narayanan, S., Brand, G.M. and Grant, G. (2000) DNA Stability and Genomic Methylation Status in Colonocytes Isolated from Methyl-Donor-Deficient Rats. *European Journal of Nutrition*, **39**, 106-111. http://dx.doi.org/10.1007/s003940070026

[2] Friso, S. and Choi, S.W. (2002) Gene-Nutrient Interactions and DNA Methylation. *Journal of Nutrition*, **132**, 2382S-2387S.

[3] Gabriel, H.E., Crott, J.W., Ghandour, H., Dallal, G.E., Choi, S.W., Keyes, M.K., Jang, H., Liu, Z., Nadeau, M., Johnston, A., Mager, D. and Mason, J.B. (2006) Chronic Cigarette Smoking Is Associated with Diminished Folate Status, Altered Folate Form Distribution, and Increased Genetic Damage in the Buccal Mucosa of Healthy Adults. *The American Journal of Clinical Nutrition*, **83**, 835-841.

[4] Toyota, M. and Suzuki, H. (2010) Epigenetic Drivers of Genetic Alterations. *Advances in Genetics*, **70**, 309-323. http://dx.doi.org/10.1016/B978-0-12-380866-0.60011-3

[5] Blount, B.C., Mack, M.M., Wehr, C.M., MacGregor, J.T., Hiatt, R.A., Wang, G., Wickramasinghe, S.N., Everson, R.B. and Ames, B.N. (1997) Folate Deficiency Causes Uracil Misincorporation into Human DNA and Chromosome Breakage: Implications for Cancer and Neuronal Damage. *Proceedings of the National Academy of Sciences of the USA*, **94**, 3290-3295. http://dx.doi.org/10.1073/pnas.94.7.3290

[6] Chango, A., Abdel Nour, A.M., Niquet, C. and Tessier, F.J. (2009) Simultaneous Determination of Genomic DNA Methylation and Uracil Misincorporation. *Medical Principles and Practice*, **18**, 81-84. http://dx.doi.org/10.1159/000189803

[7] James, S.J., Pogribny, I.P., Pogribna, M., Miller, B.J., Jernigan, S. and Melnyk, S. (2003) Mechanisms of DNA Damage, DNA Hypomethylation, and Tumor Progression in the Folate/Methyl-Deficient Rat Model of Hepatocarcinogenesis. *Journal of Nutrition*, **133**, 3740S-3747S.

[8] Ross, S.A. and Poirier, L. (2002) Proceedings of the Trans-HHS Workshop: Diet, DNA Methylation Processes and Health. *Journal of Nutrition*, **132**, 2329S-2332S.

[9] Poirier, L.A. (2002) The Effects of Diet, Genetics and Chemicals on Toxicity and Aberrant DNA Methylation: An Introduction. *Journal of Nutrition*, **132**, 2336S-2339S.

[10] Abdel Nour, A.M., Ringot, D., Gueant, J.L. and Chango, A. (2007) Folate Receptor and Human Reduced Folate Car-

rier Expression in HepG2 Cell Line Exposed to Fumonisin B1 and Folate Deficiency. *Carcinogenesis*, **28**, 2291-2297. http://dx.doi.org/10.1093/carcin/bgm149

[11] Lawley, S.D., Cinderella, M., Hall, M.N., Gamble, M.V., Nijhout, H.F. and Reed, M.C. (2011) Mathematical Model Insights into Arsenic Detoxification. *Theoretical Biology and Medical Modelling*, **8**, 31. http://dx.doi.org/10.1186/1742-4682-8-31

[12] Gnimpieba, E.Z., Eveillard, D., Gueant, J.L. and Chango, A. (2011) Using Logic Programming for Modeling the One-Carbon Metabolism Network to Study the Impact of Folate Deficiency on Methylation Processes. *Molecular BioSystems*, **7**, 2508-2521. http://dx.doi.org/10.1039/c1mb05102d

[13] Baccarelli, A. and Bollati, V. (2009) Epigenetics and Environmental Chemicals. *Current Opinion in Pediatrics*, **21**, 243-251. http://dx.doi.org/10.1097/MOP.0b013e32832925cc

[14] Chango, A., Bousserouel, S., Ge, Z., Abdel Nour, A.N.N. and Abdennebi-Najar, L. (2011) Effects of Arsenic Exposure and Folate Deficiency on Methyl Metabolism in Human Fibroblast Cell Lines. *The FASEB Journal*, **25**, 592-598.

[15] Chango, A., Nour, A.A., Bousserouel, S., Eveillard, D., Anton, P.M. and Gueant, J.L. (2009) Time Course Gene Expression in the One-Carbon Metabolism Network Using HepG2 Cell Line Grown in Folate-Deficient Medium. *The Journal of Nutritional Biochemistry*, **20**, 312-320. http://dx.doi.org/10.1016/j.jnutbio.2008.04.004

[16] Kagan, K.O., Avgidou, K., Molina, F.S., Gajewska, K. and Nicolaides, K.H. (2006) Relation between Increased Fetal Nuchal Translucency Thickness and Chromosomal Defects. *Obstetrics Gynecology*, **107**, 6-10. http://dx.doi.org/10.1097/01.AOG.0000191301.63871.c6

[17] Mihai, D., Niculescu, M.D. and Zeisel, S.H. (2002) Diet, Methyl Donors and DNA Methylation: Interactions between Dietary Folate, Methionine and Choline. *Journal of Nutrition*, **132**, 2333S-2335S.

[18] Nijhout, H.F., Reed, M.C., Anderson, D.F., Mattingly, J.C., James, S.J. and Ulrich, C.M. (2006) Long-Range Allosteric Interactions between the Folate and Methionine Cycles Stabilize DNA Methylation Reaction Rate. *Epigenetics*, **1**, 81-87. http://dx.doi.org/10.4161/epi.1.2.2677

20

"*Withered Tree*" *Concept Host,* Achieved by Global Contraception and Abortion, Secondary to Fragmented Germ Cells, Agonizingly Reduced Endogenous Estrogen/Androgen, Defaulted Genomic Repertoire, Deranged Cell Metabolism, Metabolic Syndrome, *Result in Failure of Pharmacological Therapeutics with Advanced Technologies*

Elizabeth Jeya Vardhini Samuel[1], Nagarajan Natarajan[2], Sri Kumar[3]

[1]Department of General Medicine, MM Hospital, Tanjore, India
[2]Department of General Medicine, Pondicherry Institute of Medical Sciences, Pondicherry, India
[3]Dhonavur Fellowship Hospital, Dhonavur, India
Email: elizabethjsamuel@gmail.com

Abstract

Background: In spite of advanced technologies and drug discoveries, morbidity and mortality were undoubtedly increasing in the era of contraception and abortion. Aims: Altruistic correlation of increasing morbidity, mortality, with contraception, abortion was planned for. Methods: In 2012, a retrospective analysis of prevalence of mortality in 350 patients of 20 - 35 years, 35 - 50 years and >50 years from data collected between 2003 and 2012 by convenient, stratified random sampling, from community, hospital, and its association with contraception and abortion status was undertaken; simultaneously, serum estrogen levels obtained from 105 patients were analyzed. In 2014, randomly chosen 8 males, of the 3 age groups, from a different community, whose life partners had undergone sterilization, were assessed for their serum testosterone levels. Results: Contraception users exhibited 3 - 4 fold increased mortality [p < 0.0005] amongst 20 - 50 years and 6 fold increased mortality among >50 years [p < 0.0005]. Endogenous estrogen was reduced in 75% [p < 0.0005] of contraceptive users. Plasma testosterone was reduced in males observing contraception, to less than 50% of normal, e.g. 1.3 ng/ml; 66.6% contraception users aged 20 - 35 years had reduced [p < 0.0005] testosterone; 100% of male contraception users aged 36 - 70 years showed reduced testosterone [p < 0.0005]. Conclusion: The "withered tree akin host" concept is contraception, abortion, with smashed fragmentation of germ cells. Reduced endogenous estrogen, androgen [dried up, destroyed life factors] result in deranged cell metabolism, cell cycle, and defaulted genomic repertoire, leading to failure of all established pharmacological therapeutics, including advanced technologies which yield gratifying results in non contracepted people today and in every one, before the era of contraception; subsets of people, host with contraception, with destroyed life factors, behave helplessly, concerning therapeutic applications, compared with subsets of people, host without contraception, with intact genomic repertoire, God ordained Life factors, make a remarkable recovery. Contraception reversal replants the germ cells [germ cells destruction stops], hormones rejuvenate to 79.9% of age normal, and diseases abate with recovery.

Keywords

Withered Tree Concept Host, Deranged Cell Metabolism, Defaulted Genomic Repertoire, Deranged Mitochondrial Pathways, Contraception Reversal, Metabolic Syndrome Reverts

1. Introduction

After the implementation of contraception, abortion, specially permanent sterilization-tubectomy, and vasectomy in our country, with a presumption of no associated side effects, *i.e.* there was no study done prior to assessing the presumed safety or therapeutic indication of sterilization procedures, contracepted couple experienced illnesses like obesity, diabetes mellitus, and acute coronary syndrome, including early demise at the young age; as the implementation of global contraception/abortion stealthily increased, global incidence, prevalence of diseases, and mortality had increased glaringly and undoubtedly and could not be explained as to its cause, otherwise.

Molecules which were performing remarkably, as per pharmacological therapeutics, before the era of contraception, were failing to achieve their therapeutic goals with a set back; in order to explain the failure of therapeutics [after the era of contraception-presumed to have no side effects-vacuum in information towards cause and effect phenomenon], help was sought by calculating odds ratios, hazard ratio, confidence interval, and number to treat and to give power to medicines, which had already been established with detailed pharmacological profile, but was of no avail.

Metabolic defect of reduced formation of high density lipo protein from low density lipo protein was observed, suggesting defaulted cell membrane synthesis and steroid hormone synthesis; metabolic syndrome was recognized globally, with achievement of global contraception; acquired mitochondrial pathologies were identified; basically, cell metabolism, which was under the surveillance of endogenous estrogen and androgen, got deranged consequent to wantonly acquired germ cells destruction, and secondary to contraception abortion, to result in possible mutations, degenerative diseases, and neoplasms. Concept of host resembling "withered tree" stems as etiology, to explain globally increased prevalence of morbidity, mortality.

Hence, an altruistic analysis for association of morbidity and mortality, with status of contraception and abortion in the host, was planned.

2. Methods

Data collected was divided into 3 age groups, namely, 20 - 35 years, 36 - 50 years, and >50 years; though people from the community are visiting the hospital, analysis of hospital patients alone can create a bias, hence data from the community, hospital, health screening camps, of different geographical locations were included; data from each person depicted, prevalent diseases, status of contraception, hysterectomy, type of oil ingested, life style, level of nutrition, presence of anemia; the data was tabulated as prevalent morbidity, mortality, matched against the variables in each age group; retrospective bio-informatics analysis was done, by plotting histograms for the 3 age groups and cumulative graphs for each disease and mortality in 2012; an example of tabulation of the data is provided in the supplementary file.

In 2003 house to house survey [1] in the community, spread over 3 weeks, was conducted by the corresponding Author, to collect data of prevalent diseases of 100 people; the people who were present during the survey were included at random, by convenient sampling into the 3 age groups, namely, 20 - 35 years, 35 - 50 years, and >50 years, to include a minimum of 30 people in each age group; serum estrogen estimation was done for 12 people as per their request; the reduced estrogen levels [5 - 8 pg] found in young contraceptive users, was the eye opener, leading to further data analysis.

In 2004 data of 93 hospital patients was collected over a period of 6 months, including prevalent diseases, mortality, Status of contraception, life style, nutrition, type of oil ingested, level of hemoglobin and were assigned to the 3 age groups, by stratified random sampling with a minimum of 30 patients in each age group; serum estrogen estimation was done for all 93 patients; the data was tabulated matching diseases, mortality against status of contraception and other variables; one patient was a foreign national.

In 2011, 96 people [43 couples] working in different states of our nation had attended a health screening camp conducted in the community, spread over 3 days and their data was analyzed after assigning into the 3 age groups at random, for association of diseases , mortality with status of contraception, hysterectomy and other variables; effect of contraception in both partners also could be analyzed; none had sedentary life style, low nutrition or anemia or had worn tight attires around the pelvis.

In 2012, data of 61 hospital patients including a foreign resident, from another geographical location, was collected over a span of 6 months, assigned to the 3 age groups at random and was pooled to the other data from 2003, 2004, 2011 and retrospective bio informatics analysis was undertaken for the 350 patients in 2012, by Histogram, for the 3 age groups and cumulative graphs for each disease and mortality.

Every participant was informed about their data being included for study purpose and the concerned hospital Authorities were also informed; an engineering college student did the bio informatics analysis as his project.

In 2014, randomly chosen 8 males, [2] of the 3 age groups, from a different community, whose life partners had undergone sterilization, were assessed for their serum testosterone levels.

3. Results

Variables like nutrition, lifestyle, presence of anemia, tight attires around pelvis were nullified, since none of them were malnourished, or anemic, or wore tight attires around the pelvis. Contraception users **Figure 1** exhibited 3 - 4 fold increased mortality [$p < 0.0005$] among 20 - 50 years and 6 fold increased mortality among >50 years [$p < 0.0005$]. Contraception users depicted 275% increase in diseases **Figure 2** among 20 - 35 years, 35 - 50 years age group [$p < 0.0005$]; >50 years people without contraception also develop degenerative diseases, since the endogenous estrogen, androgen decrease after 37 years of age, naturally to 15 pg, <2.6 ng respectively. Absence of diseases was seen by the analysis of heath screening camps, 80% - 90% [$p < 0.0005$] **Figure 3** in the people without contraception only in 20 - 35 years age, 35 - 50 years age group. Contraception correlates absolutely with increased morbidity, mortality, in young age < 50 years; absence of contraception correlates absolutely with absence of diseases, in young age < 50 years. Endogenous estrogen [3] was reduced in 75% [$p < 0.0005$] of contraceptive users.

Plasma testosterone was reduced in males observing contraception, to less than 50% of age normal, e.g. 1.3 ng/ml; 66.6% contraception users aged 20 - 35 years had reduced [$p < 0.0005$] testosterone; 100% male contraception users, aged 36 - 70 years showed reduced testosterone [$p < 0.0005$].

4. Discussion

Population aging is transforming the world in dramatic and fundamental ways, age distribution of populations have changed and will continue to change radically, due to long term declines in [4] fertility rates; its predicted in another 30 years, younger age group of < 5 years will become 5% [alas unchecked, disappearing human race].

Global contraception, abortion with resultant smashed destruction of [5] germ cells, associated reduction in endogenous estrogen, androgen, on whose surveillance the cell cycle, cell metabolism is dependent upon, leads to deranged cell metabolism, metabolic syndrome, [6] [7] defaulted genomic repertoire, with consequent in-

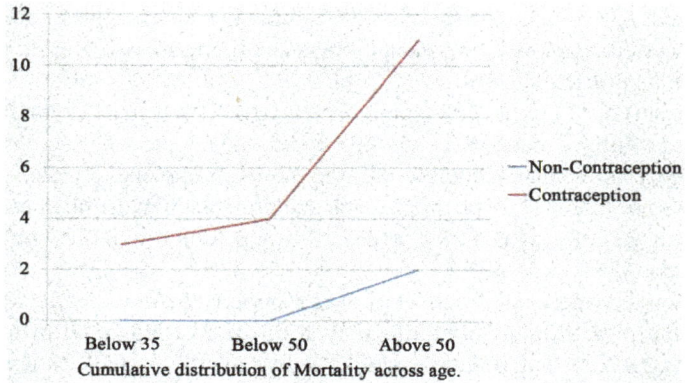

Figure 1. Prevalence of mortality, contraception.

Disease Prevalence and age group.

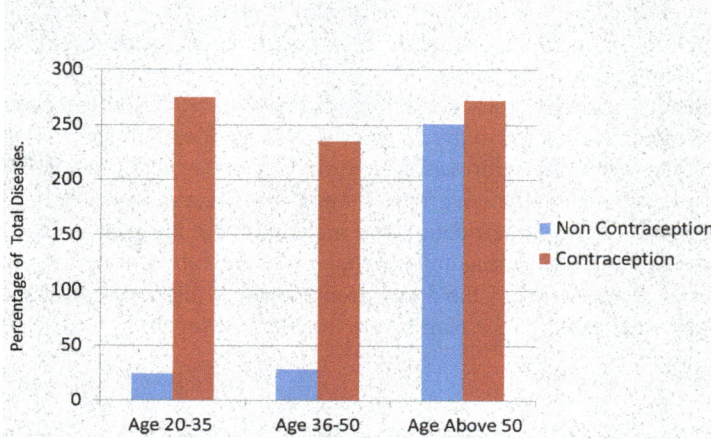

Figure 2. Prevalence of diseases, contraception.

Absence of disease- nil contraception

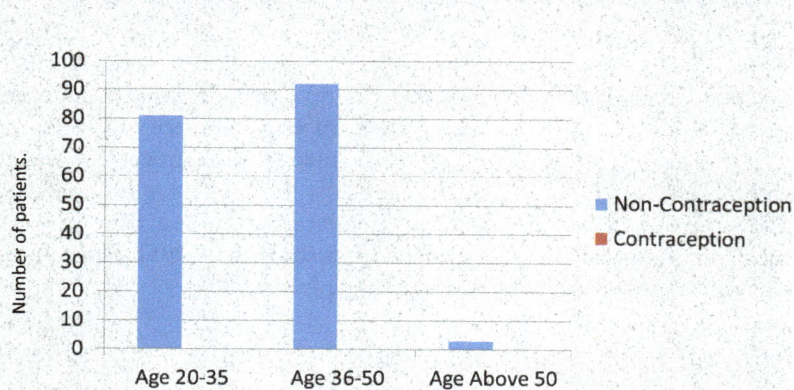

What a Bliss to have no disease with nil contraception!!
With contraception no disease is not seen i.e., no escape as per human physiology
from degenerative diseases – painful tragedy-prevalent-true, but not recognized
by doctors/govt./people

Figure 3. Prevalence of absence of disease, non-contraception.

crease in degenerative diseases—"withered tree concept host"—e.g. T2 diabetes mellitus, hypertension, rising by 15 - 50 fold [8] amongst 20 - 50 years of people using contraception.

The fragmented germ cells, *i.e.* ring chromosomes, acentric fragments, chromatid breaks are identified as foreign and autoimmune antibodies are detected to the above fragmented chromatids resulting in entire spectrum of auto [9] immune diseases increasing by 15 - 40 fold amongst 20 - 50 years of contraception users.

The concept is when the endogenous estrogen, androgen decrease with contraception, abortion, [withered tree concept Host] cell cycle of differentiation followed by controlled multiplication, defaults leading to increase in [10] neoplasms, cancers, mutations of, e.g. glucokinase, hepatocyte nuclear transcription factors leading to MODY, including mitochondrial pathologies; 10 - 20 fold increase in breast cancer, 20 - 30 fold increase in prostate cancer, 20 - 40 fold increase in cancer cervix is seen amongst contraception users of 20 - 50 years of age.

Secondary to aborted blood pollution, contraceptive menstrual blood pollution, evidenced by rising environmental estrogen, α feto protein, β human chorionic gonadotropins, infectious [11] [12] diseases' prevalence have increased for e.g. tuberculosis which had earlier been documented as curable in the era before contraception, has increased by 15 - 30 fold amongst contraception users, progressing to destroyed lungs; the concept is, the host with contraception, abortion is akin to "withered tree" damaged {eaten up} easily by soaring virulent infections promoted by environmental aborted blood pollution [Alas! Young parents with contraception, abortion, die like flies by infectious diseases including severe sepsis, less virulent fungal infections, tuberculosis, rickettsial infections, in spite of newer antimicrobials, protocols, policies, because their physique is akin to "withered tree", achieved unaware, by wantonly acquired, globally permitted, without evidence based practice-contraception, abortion].

Mitochondrial pathologies are transmitted [13] by matrilineal fashion, non-coding region of mitochondrial chromosome, referred to as D loop, is highly polymorphic, alterations in the mitochondrial DNA affect enzymes required for oxidative phosphorylation, leading to reduction of ATP supply, generation of free radicals, induction of apoptosis; contraception can culminate in mitochondrial pathologies by deranged cell metabolism, defaulted genomic repertoire, mutations achieved by reduced endogenous androgen, estrogen surveillance as a result of smashed fragmentation of germ cells.

The concept is [as portrayed above] with contraception, abortion the germ cells destruction and their associated hormonal reduction, leads to withered tree akin host, resulting in 3 - 6 fold increase in mortality amongst contraception users of 20 - >50 years in spite of advanced technologies, drug discoveries, therapeutic protocols, and policies.

Our therapies capitalize on the cells healing capacity, which defaults in the "withered tree" concept host, by acquired contraception, abortion, secondary to destruction of germ cells and associated decrease in endogenous estrogen, androgen, on whose surveillance the cell cycle, cell differentiation, controlled multiplication, genomic repertoire, cell metabolism is dependent upon.

Contraception reversal, specially including tubal [14] recanalisation, for permanent sterilization, replants the germ cells, *i.e.* stops destruction of the germ cells, associated with 79.9% restored synthesis of endogenous estrogen, androgen, correcting the defaulted genomic repertoire, deranged cell metabolism, thereby reversing metabolic syndrome [figures-supplementary files [14]. Since after hysterectomy the endogenous estrogen decreases to 0.4 pg/ml, there's associated 500% increase in morbidity in this subset of people.

When a molecule is analyzed for, e.g. Olmesartan, [15] enalapril maleate, why they are not effective as they ought to be in nephropathy, cardiac failure, or some unusual side effects which is not detailed in the product monograph or pharmacology therapeutics text, by using odds ratio, number to treat, power to medicines, the studies cannot find the answer; molecule will perform as portrayed in the pharmacological text, in normal live human body, unaltered by acquired contraception, abortion, with intact germ cells, endogenous estrogen, androgen, robust cell cycle, metabolism, genomic repertoire; whereas in people with acquired contraception, abortion, the host is akin to "withered tree" with ongoing, perennial germ cells` destruction, [specially in permanent sterilization] reduced endogenous estrogen, androgen, defaulted genomic repertoire, metabolic syndrome secondary to deranged cell metabolism, cell cycle, cell differentiation, similar to, no possible effect of the therapeutic molecules in dead body, can they have any effect?; how can the molecule perform the same way, in physique with acquired contraception, abortion, with defaulted genomic repertoiret; we have to reconcile with facts of "withered tree" concept host in subset of people using contraception, with acquired 275% increase in neoplastic, degenerative, infectious, auto immune diseases, mortality and offer rectification as cause and effect phenomenon, to reverse permanent modes of contraception, halt, eradicate contraception, abortion from the face of the earth.

5. Conclusions

Global contraception and abortion, results in smashed destruction of germ cells, consequent gross reduction in endogenous estrogen, and androgen, leading to deranged cell metabolism, defaulted cell cycle of differentiation, controlled multiplication, metabolic syndrome, and mutations including mt DNA similar to "withered tree", *i.e.* human live body, deprived of life factors by unaware, wantonly acquired contraception, and abortion, form the basis of failure of therapies, technologies, and molecules which otherwise will have been a success in subsets of people without contraception and abortion, but are blessed with uncurbed child birth, unlike people practising small family norms and one child policy.

This has resulted in 3 - 6 fold increase in mortality in contraception users, aged 20 - >50 years, consequent to rise in infectious diseases, neoplastic diseases, and degenerative and auto immune diseases, in spite of advanced technologies and therapeutics.

Another significant finding is that "withered tree" springs forth by 79.9%, *i.e.* on contraception reversal including tubal recanalization, the germ cells destruction stops, replant of germ cells with regain in synthesis of endogenous estrogen, androgen by 79.9% of corresponding normal for age, results in decline in degenerative, neoplastic, autoimmune, infectious diseases; cell's healing capacity-genomic repertoire, cell metabolism is restored; metabolic syndrome regresses marvelously, e.g. new nail beds, hair follicles, angiogenesis, collaterals spring forth; embryo like healing capacity in the cells-genomic repertoire is restored 79.9% on reversing contraception and abortion.

Let the medical fraternity and the medical curriculum pave way for this awareness of, wantonly acquired early demise in young parents, by global contraception and abortion similar to "withered tree", and plan global protocols, policies and strategies, to revert and eradicate global contraception and abortion, destroying young lives in disguise.

6. Key Points

- Contraception, abortion achieves "withered tree" concept host, by destruction of germ cells leading to agonizingly reduced endogenous estrogen, androgen;
- Smashed destruction of germ cells, agonizingly reduced endogenous estrogen, androgen result in deranged cell metabolism, defaulted genomic repertoire, leading to 3 - 6 fold increase in mortality and unwanted early demise in young parents;
- Advanced technologies, therapeutics fail to reduce mortality in contraception users aged 20 - 50 years;
- 3 - 6 fold increase in mortality amongst contraception users aged 20 - >50 years, since the host component has become like withered tree [deprived of life factors];
- Contraception reversal restores cell function, metabolism by 79.9%, since the germ cells destruction stops, endogenous estrogen, androgen's synthesis rises again by 79.9% of age normal, equal to flourishing back of "withered tree" concept host, materializing cause and effect phenomenon.

References

[1]   Samuel, E.J.V., *et al.* (2014) Increasing Prevalence of Osteoporosis, Hypothyroidism and Endogenous Estrogen with Germ Cells. *Open Journal of Rheumatology and Autoimmune Diseases*, **4**, 131-137. http://dx.doi.org/10.4236/ojra.2014.43019

[2]   Elizabeth, J.S. (2014) Survival in Severe Sepsis and Non Fragmented Germ Cells. Virulent Infections in Children and Aborted Blood, Contraceptive Menstrual Blood Environmental Pollution. *Global Journal of Medical Research: F Diseases*, **14**, 1-9.

[3]   Samuel, E.J. (2012) Increased Prevalence of Neuroleptic Malignant Syndrome, Dementia and Fragmented Germ Cells with Reduced Endogenous Estrogen. *International Journal of Science and Research (IJSR)*, **3**, 1694-1700.

[4]   Suzman, R. and Haaga, J.G. (2012) World Demography of Aging Harrisons Principles of Internal Medicine. 18th Edition, Vol. 1, McGraw Hill Medical, New York, 556.

[5]   Gilliland, B.G. (1987) Systemic Sclerosis, Harrisons Principles of Internal Medicine. 11th Edition, Vol. 2, McGraw Hill Book Company, New York, 1429.

[6]   Mendelsohn, J. (1987) Cancer Biology; Harrisons Principles of Internal Medicine. 11th Edition, Vol. 1, McGraw Hill Book Company, New York, 422.

[7]   Elizabeth, J.S. (2014) Increased Prevalence of Renal Diseases-Metabolic Syndrome and Fragmented Germ Cells with

Reduced Endogenous Estrogen, Androgen. *International Journal of Innovative Research and Studies (IJIRS)*, **3**, 80-83.

[8]   Samuel, E.J.V., Natarajan, N., George, S., Gkulirankal, K. and Eapen, G. (2014) Increased Incidence of Diabetes Mellitus, Systemic Hypertension and Germ Cells with Endogenous Estrogen. *Open Journal of Preventive Medicine*, **4**, 481-488. http://dx.doi.org/10.4236/ojpm.2014.46056

[9]   Elizabeth, J.S. (2014) Autoimmunity and Fragmented Germ Cells. *IOSR Journal of Dental and Medical Sciences (IOSR-JDMS)*, **13**, 99-105.

[10] Elizabeth, J.S. (2014) Cancer and Germ Cells. *Open Journal of Preventive Medicine*, **4**, 606-615.

[11] Elizabeth, J.S. (2014) Increased Prevalence of Solar Keratoses, Infectious Diseases and Rising Environmental Estrogen Equating with Aborted Blood Pollution with Consequent Ozone Depletion. *IOSR Journal of Environmental Science, toxicology and Food Technology (IOSR-JESTFT)*, **8**, 74-80.

[12] Samuel, E.J. (2014) Increasing Prevalence of Chronic Obstructive Pulmonary Disease, Tuberculosis, Lung Cancer and Rising Environmental Estrogen. *International Journal of Science and Research (IJSR)*, **3**, 1591-1598

[13] Larry Jameson, J. and Kopp, P. (2012) Genes the Environment and Disease, Mitochondrial Disorders; Harrisons Principles of Internal Medicine. 18th Edition, Vol. 1, McGraw Hill Medical, New York, 501.

[14] Samuel, E.J. (2014) Abortion, Contraception Reversal-Medical Miracle-Autologous Germ Cells Replant-Decline in Global Degenerative, Autoimmune, Neoplastic, Infectious Diseases, Decline in Rising Environmental Estrogen, Equating with Aborted Blood Pollution and Decline in Depletion of Ozone. *IOSR Journal of Dental and Medical Sciences (IOSR-JDMS)*, **13**, 93-102.

[15] Haller, H., Ito, S., Izzo Jr., J.L., Januszewicz, A., katayama, S., Menne, J., Mimran, A., Rabelink, T.J., Ritz, E., Ruilope, L.M., Rump, L. and Viberti, G. (2011) Olmesartan for the Delay or Prevention of Microalbuminuria in Type 2 Diabetes. *The New England Journal of Medicine*, **364**, 907-917. http://dx.doi.org/10.1056/NEJMoa1007994

Supplementary Files: Figures in Reference 7

Endogenous estrogen, androgen surveillance
Cell cycle/metabolism

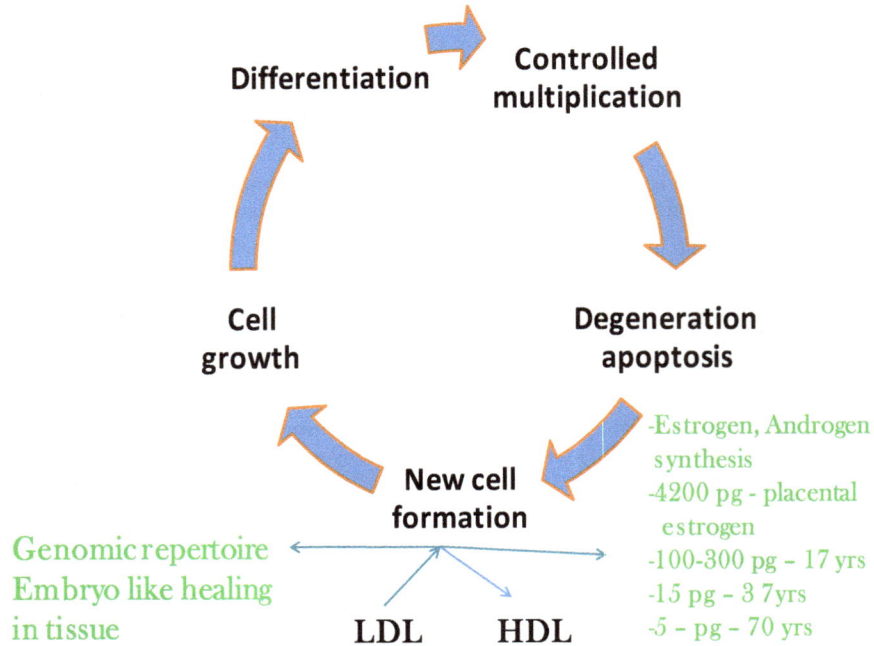

Differentiation → **Controlled multiplication**

Cell growth

Degeneration apoptosis

New cell formation

-Estrogen, Androgen synthesis
-4200 pg - placental estrogen
-100-300 pg – 17 yrs
-15 pg – 3 7yrs
-5 – pg – 70 yrs

Genomic repertoire
Embryo like healing
in tissue

LDL   HDL

Reduced Endogenous estrogen, androgen
Contraception, Abortion - Deranged Cell cycle/metabolism

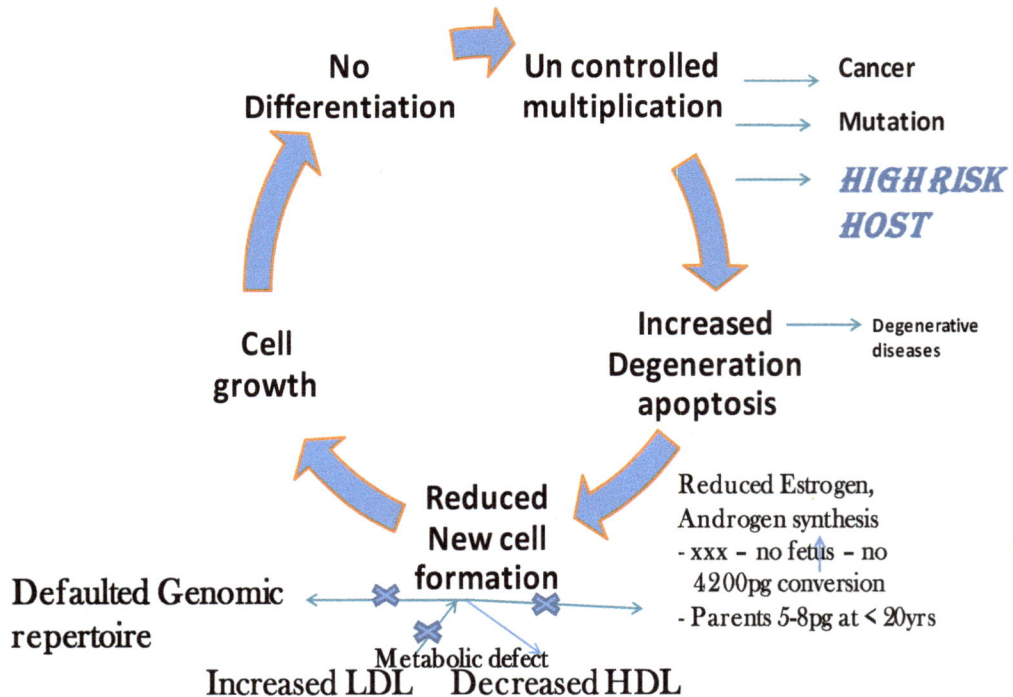

No Differentiation → **Un controlled multiplication** → Cancer

→ Mutation

→ *HIGH RISK HOST*

Increased Degeneration apoptosis → Degenerative diseases

Cell growth

Reduced New cell formation

Reduced Estrogen, Androgen synthesis
- xxx – no fetus – no 4200pg conversion
- Parents 5-8pg at < 20yrs

Defaulted Genomic repertoire

Metabolic defect
Increased LDL   Decreased HDL

Supplementary Files: Figures in Reference 13

Degenerative Diseases with. Contraception at young age.

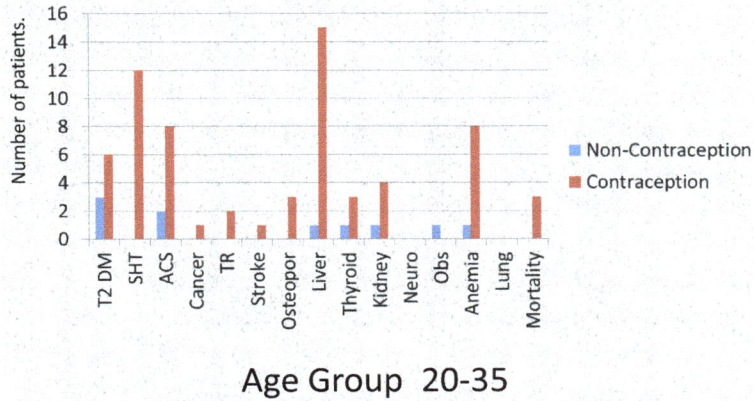

Age Group 20-35

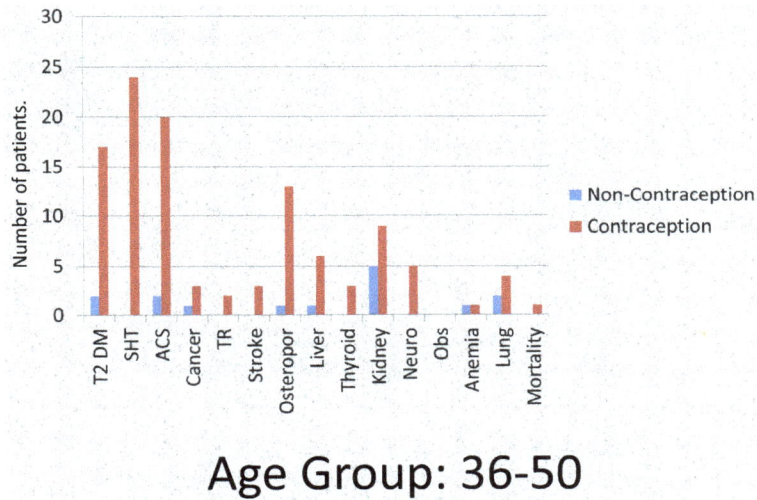

Age Group: 36-50

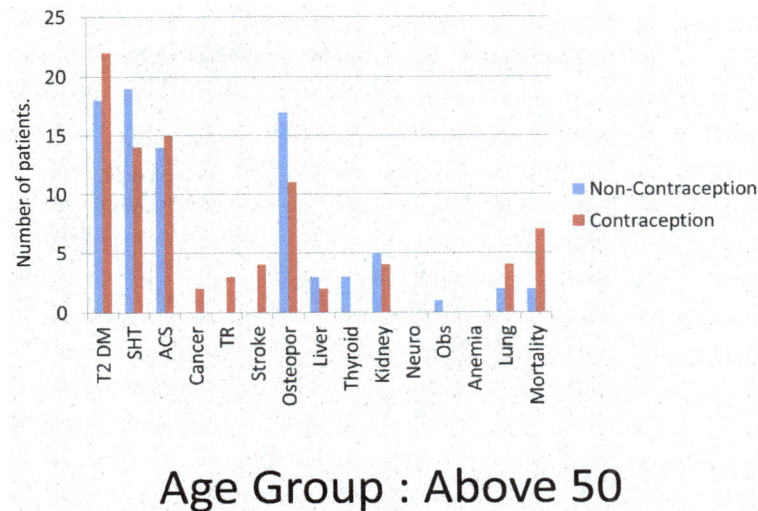

Age Group : Above 50

- **Diseases in both partners** (Husband and wife) (in **young age-20-50 years**)In**Contraception only**

In **non contraceptive users both husband and wife exhibit** **no disease** **in 20 – 35 and 35-50 age groups**. Hysterectomy there was no patient in 20-35 age group

Diseases/morbidity-contraception/hysterectomy.

Tubal Recanalization – mandatory/essential - will return life factors – result in decreased diseases. Hysterectomy should be reserved only for PPH/Uterine Cancers. Hysterectomy to be replaced by tubal-recanalization, myomectomy, Pelvic Floor Repair.

Contraception Reversal-Decline in Diseases (Medical Miracle)

21

Effects of Ranolazine on Carbohydrate Metabolism in the Isolated Perfused Rat Liver

Márcio Shigueaki Mito, Cristiane Vizioli de Castro, Rosane Marina Peralta, Adelar Bracht*

Laboratory of Liver Metabolism, Department of Biochemistry, University of Maringá, Maringá, Brazil
Email: *adebracht@uol.com.br

Abstract

The action mechanism of ranolazine, an antiangina drug, could be at least partly metabolic, including inhibition of fatty acid oxidation and stimulation of glucose utilization in the heart. The purpose of the present work was to investigate if ranolazine affects hepatic carbohydrate metabolism. For this purpose, the hemoglobin-free isolated perfused rat liver was used as the experimental system. Ranolazine increased glycolysis and glycogenolysis and decreased gluconeogenesis. These effects were accompanied by an inhibition of oxygen consumption. The drug also changed the redox state of the NAD^+-NADH couple. For the cytosol, increased $NADH/NAD^+$ ratios were observed both under glycolytic conditions as well as under gluconeogenic conditions. For the mitochondria, increased $NADH/NAD^+$ ratios were found in the present work in the absence of exogenous fatty acids in contrast with the previous observation of a decreasing effect when the liver was actively oxidizing exogenous oleate. It seems likely that ranolazine inhibits gluconeogenesis and increases glycolysis in consequence of its inhibitory actions on energy metabolism and fatty acid oxidation and by deviating reducing equivalents in favour of its own biotransformation. This is in line with the earlier postulates that ranolazine diminishes fatty acid oxidation, shifting the energy source from fatty acids to glucose.

Keywords

Glycogenolysis, Glycolysis, NAD^+-NADH Redox Potentials, Gluconeogenesis, Ketogenesis

1. Introduction

Ranolazine is an agent for angina medication, commercialized under the trade name of Ranexa™. Its action mechanism is not clear and there are at least two different hypotheses. The first one postulates that ranolazine

---

*Corresponding author.

diminishes fatty acid oxidation, shifting the energy source from fatty acids to glucose [1]-[5]. An alternative interpretation with increasing experimental support postulates that ranolazine could exert its effects by improving the deficient functioning of sodium channels [6]-[8].

Irrespective of its clinical importance, alterations in fatty acid metabolism by ranolazine were in fact observed. A concomitant reduction in fatty acid oxidation and increase in glucose oxidation, for example, were found in experiments with the perfused rat heart [4]. These effects were accompanied by a reduction in the levels of acetyl-CoA in the heart tissue [4]. In the liver, which is the site of ranolazine biotransformation [9], it has been shown that ranolazine inhibits oleate net uptake (40% at 200 μM ranolazine) by diminishing the transfer of this fatty acid from the extracellular albumin site to the intracellular space [10]. No effect on the coefficient for intracellular sequestration of oleate was found. Inhibition of net uptake is thus not the consequence of an acyl-CoA synthetase inhibition. Consistently, ranolazine also inhibits the extra oxygen consumption caused by oleate, as well as the extra ketogenesis induced by this substrate. It seems thus that in the liver ranolazine acts on fatty acid metabolism by at least two mechanisms: inhibition of cell membrane permeation and inhibition of the mitochondrial electron transfer via pyridine nucleotides [10]. The latter involves possibly the NADH dehydrogenase, but a direct effect on specific enzymes, especially β-hydroxybutyrate dehydrogenase, cannot be excluded.

Fatty acid and carbohydrate metabolism are always interconnected in mammalian cells. It is well known, for example, that fatty acid oxidation increases gluconeogenesis [11] [12], that the availability of carbohydrates enhances fatty acid synthesis and also that ketogenesis, even from endogenous sources, is strongly influenced by the presence of gluconeogenic substrates such as lactate [13] [14]. These interrelationships are caused by many factors which include activation/deactivation of key enzymes, alterations in the redox status of the cytosolic and mitochondrial NAD^+-NADH systems and alterations in energy metabolism. Considering, thus, the action of ranolazine on fatty acid metabolism, it seems also worth to investigate its possible actions on carbohydrate metabolism. In the present work the actions of ranolazine on both glycolysis from endogenous sources and gluconeogenesis driven by exogenous substrates were measured in addition to the adenine nucleotide levels, in the hope of expanding knowledge about the actions of this drug in the liver.

2. Materials and Methods

2.1. Materials and Animals

First, the liver perfusion apparatus was built in the workshops of the University of Maringá. Enzymes and coenzymes used in the assay procedures and fatty acid-free bovine serum albumin were purchased from Sigma Chemical Co. (St. Louis, USA). All other chemicals were of at least 98% - 99% purity.

Male albino rats (Wistar strain; 220 - 250 g) were used. They received a standard laboratory diet and water ad libitum prior to the surgical removal of the liver. Animal handling and experiments were done in accordance with the world-wide accepted ethical guidelines for animal experimentation.

2.2. Liver Perfusion

For the surgical procedure the rats were anesthetized by intraperitoneal injection of sodium pentobarbital (50 mg/kg). The criterion of anesthesia was the lack of body or limb movement in response to a standardized tail clamping stimulus. Hemoglobin-free, non-recirculating perfusion was done according to the technique described elsewhere [15] [16]. After cannulation of the portal and cava veins the liver was positioned in a plexiglass chamber. The hepatic artery was closed (monovascular perfusion) and the bile duct was left open. The flow was maintained constant by a peristaltic pump (Minipuls 3, Gilson, France) and was adjusted to between 30 and 35 mL·min^{-1}, depending on the liver weight. The perfusion fluid was Krebs/Henseleit-bicarbonate buffer (pH 7.4), saturated with a mixture of oxygen and carbon dioxide (95:5) by means of a membrane oxygenator with simultaneous temperature adjustment at 37°C. The composition of the Krebs/Henseleit-bicarbonate buffer is [15] [16]: 115 mM NaCl, 25 mM NaHCO$_3$, 5.8 mM KCl, 1.2 mM Na$_2$SO$_4$, 1.18 mM MgCl$_2$, 1.2 mM NaH$_2$PO$_4$ and 2.5 mM CaCl$_2$. Substrates and ranolazine were dissolved in the perfusion fluid according to necessity. Samples of the effluent perfusion fluid were collected at 4-minute intervals and analyzed for their metabolite content.

2.3. Analytics

The following compounds in the outflowing perfusate were assayed by means of standard enzymatic procedures

[17]: lactate, pyruvate, glucose, β-hydroxybutyrate and acetoacetate. The oxygen concentration in the outflowing perfusate was monitored polarographically employing a teflon-shielded platinum electrode adequately positioned in a plexiglass chamber at the exit of the perfusate [16] [18].

2.4. Determination of the Hepatic Contents of Adenine Mononucleotides

The perfused liver was rapidly frozen in liquid nitrogen and a portion weighing between 2 and 4 g triturated and used for extraction. The adenine mononucleotides (AMP, ADP, ATP) were extracted with a 0.6 M perchloric acid solution. After mixing the liver powder with 6 to 12 mL of the perchloric acid solution the suspension was homogenized in a van-Potter homogenizer. The homogenate was centrifuged at 2°C (10 minutes at 3000 g) and the supernatant was neutralized with potassium carbonate. The neutralized extract was kept in ice bath until HPLC analysis.

The adenine mononucleotides in the samples were separated and quantified by HPLC. The apparatus (Shimadzu, Japan) consisted in a system controller SCL-10AVP, two pumps model LC10ADVP, a column oven model CTO-10AVP, and a UV-VIS detector model SPD-10AVP. A reversed-phase column C18 HRC-ODS (5 lm; 150 × 6 mm I.D.; Shimadzu, Japan), protected with a pre-column GHRC-ODS (5 μm; 10 × 4 mm I.D.; Shimadzu, Japan), was used with a gradient from reversed-phase 0.044 M phosphate buffer solution pH 6.0 to 0.044 M phosphate buffer solution plus methanol (1.1) pH 7.0 at 0.8 mL·min^{-1}. The gradient was (in % of methanol): 0 min, 0%; 2.5 min, 0.5%; 5 min, 3%; 7 min, 5%; 8 min, 12%; 10 min, 15%; 12 min, 20%; 20 min, 30%. Temperature was kept at 35°C and the injection volume was always 20 μL. The UV-absorbance detector was auto-zeroed at the start of each chromatogram and the absorbance was measured at 254 nm.

The identification of the peaks of the investigated compounds was carried out by comparison of their retention times with those obtained injecting standards in the same conditions, as well as by spiking liver samples with stock standard solutions. The concentrations of the identified compounds in the extract samples were calculated by means of the regression parameters obtained from calibration curves. The calibration curves were constructed by separating chromatographically standard solutions of the compounds. Linear relationships were obtained between the concentrations and the areas under the absorbance curves.

2.5. Statitical Analysis

The error parameters presented in the text and tables are standard errors of the means. Differençes between pairs of means were analyzed by means of Student's t test or Student's paired t-test according to the context. The 5% level (p < 0.05) was adopted as a criterion of significance.

3. Results

3.1. Glycogen Catabolism and Glycolysis

In order to investigate the action of ranolazine on glycogen catabolism and glycolysis, livers from fed rats were perfused with substrate-free perfusion fluid, in an open system. Under these conditions, the livers release glucose, lactate and pyruvate as a result of glycogen degradation [15] [19]. Lactate plus pyruvate production are a good estimate for the glycolytic activity because, under these conditions, the processing of pyruvate by the pyruvate dehydrogenase complex and pyruvate carboxylase proceeds at very low rates [20] [21]. **Figure 1** shows the time course of the experiments in which 100 μM ranolazine was infused. Oxygen uptake was diminished (p < 0.05, paired t-test) and remained so during the entire ranolazine infusion period. Lactate and glucose productions were both increased shortly after initiation of ranolazine infusion (p < 0.05). Both variables also remained elevated during the ranolazine infusion. Pyruvate production was not affected. Due to the elevated lactate production, the lactate to pyruvate ratio was increased, meaning also an elevated cytosolic NADH/NAD$^+$ ratio, due to the lactate dehydrogenase equilibrium [13] [22]. Upon cessation of the infusion all variables tended to return to values close to those before initiation of ranolazine infusion (basal rates).

3.2. Lactate Gluconeogenesis and Ketogenesis from Endogenous Sources

For investigating the action of ranolazine on glucose synthesis livers from 24 hours fasted rats were used in order to minimize the interference by glycogen catabolism [13]. The liver cells under these conditions can survive

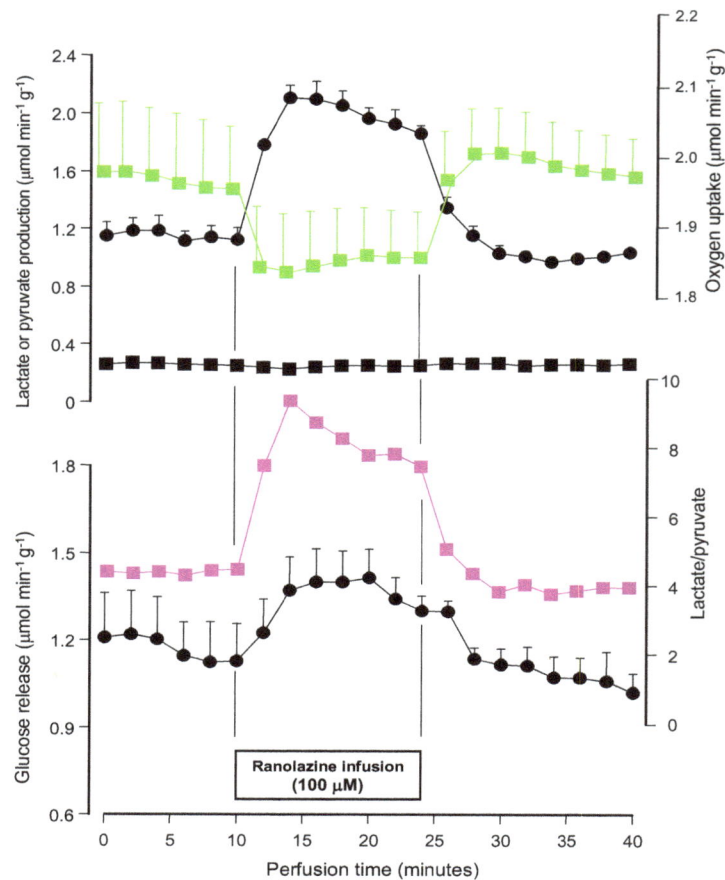

Figure 1. Time course of the effects of 100 μM ranolazine on metabolic fluxes derived from glycogen catabolism and on oxygen uptake in livers from fed rats. Livers were perfused with Krebs/Henseleit-bicarbonate buffer (pH 7.4) as described in the Materials and Methods section. Samples of the effluent perfusate were collected for glucose, lactate and pyruvate assay. Oxygen in the outflowing perfusate was monitored polarographically. The data represent the means (±SEM) of three liver perfusion experiments.

mainly at the expense of the oxidation of endogenous fatty acids and amino acids. The intense β-oxidation increases the acetyl-CoA levels, which in turn leads to a significant ketogenesis (β-hdyroxybutyrate + acetoacetate production), as revealed by panels A and B of **Figure 2**. The introduction of ranolazine under these conditions produced a rapid decrease in ketogenesis and oxygen uptake ($p < 0.05$; **Figure 2(A)**). The β-hydroxybutyrate to acetoacetate ratio, on the other hand, was increased by ranolazine. This effect differs from that observed when ketogenesis was mainly due to exogenous oleate oxidation, where the introduction of ranolazine decreased the β-hydroxybutyrate/acetoacetate ratio [10]. The introduction of 5 mM lactate further decreased ketogenesis and increased the β-hdyroxybutyrate/acetoacetate ratio. It also produced increments in oxygen uptake and glucose production. The latter effect, however, was much less pronounced than that found when lactate was infused in the absence of ranolazine, as shown in **Figure 2(B)**. This means that ranolazine inhibited gluconeogenesis, with an inhibition degree of 85% ($p < 0.05$). It should be remarked that lactate alone also decreased ketogenesis ($p < 0.05$; **Figure 2(B)**) to the same low levels as those found when ranolazine and lactate were both present (**Figure 2(A)**). Lactate also increased the β-hydroxybutyrate/acetoacetate ratio, either alone (**Figure 2(B)**) or when ranolazine was also present (**Figure 2(A)**). This observation, in addition to the increment in oxygen uptake caused by lactate in the presence of ranolazine, indicates that the reducing equivalents derived from lactate oxidation were transferred to the mitochondria. It should be noted that the β-hydroxybutyrate to acetoacetate ratio reflects the mitochondrial NADH to NAD$^+$ ratio [13] [22].

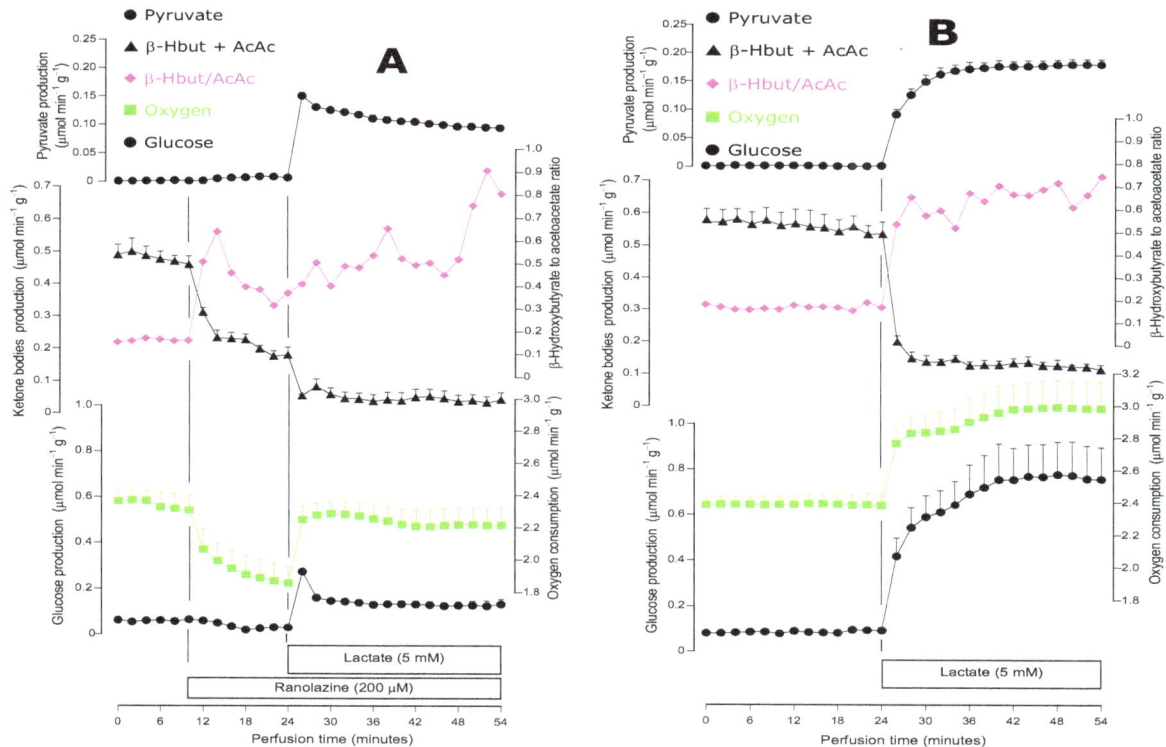

Figure 2. Effects of ranolazine on lactate gluconeogenesis and ketogenesis from endogenous sources. Livers from 24 hours fasted rats were perfused with substrate-free medium initially and with 5 mM lactate containing medium at the times indicated in the bars near to the time scale. In the experiments of panel A 200 μM ranolazine was infused as indicated. Perfusate samples were collected for metabolite measurements by means of enzymatic procedures. Oxygen uptake was measured polarographically. Data are means plus mean standard errors of 4 (panel A) and 5 (panel) liver perfusion experiments. Legends: β-Hbut, β-hydroxybutyrate; AcAc, acetoacetate.

3.3. Pyruvate Gluconeogenesis and Ketogenesis from Endogenous Sources

The same kind of experiments that were done with 5 mM lactate as gluconeogenic substrate were also done with 5 mM pyruvate. The infusion of lactate induces a highly reducing state in the cell whereas the infusion of pyruvate induces the opposite, *i.e.*, a highly oxidizing condition [22]. Concerning ketogenesis, the actions of pyruvate were similar to those of lactate: an additional inhibition in the presence of ranolazine (p < 0.05; **Figure 3(A)**) and a strong inhibition in the absence of the drug (p < 0.05; **Figure 3(B)**). The β-hydroxybutyrate/acetoacetate ratio was considerably increased by pyruvate in the presence of ranolazine, even though strong fluctuations were apparent (**Figure 3(A)**). In the absence of ranolazine, unlike to what happened with lactate, the increase in the β-hydroxybutyrate/acetoacetate ratio caused by pyruvate was relatively modest (**Figure 3(B)**), an expected phenomenon if one considers that the transformation of pyruvate generates much less reducing equivalents than that of lactate. The response of gluconeogenesis to pyruvate in the presence of ranolazine differed from that of lactate: it was slower (**Figure 3(A)**) when compared to the control condition (**Figure 3(B)**) with a progressive increase so that at the end of the experiment the inhibition of gluconeogenesis was relatively small, only 17% (p < 0.05). Lactate production from pyruvate, finally, was 25% higher in the presence of ranolazine (p < 0.05).

3.4. Adenine Mononucleotide Levels

Table 1 lists the hepatic contents of AMP, ADP and ATP in livers from fed rats perfused with substrate-free medium in the absence (control) and presence of ranolazine. The levels of AMP, ADP and ATP are very close to those found under exactly the same conditions (substrate-free perfused rat liver of fed rats) using enzymatic assays [23]-[25]. As revealed by **Table 1**, 200 μM ranolazine did not produce significant changes in the cellular

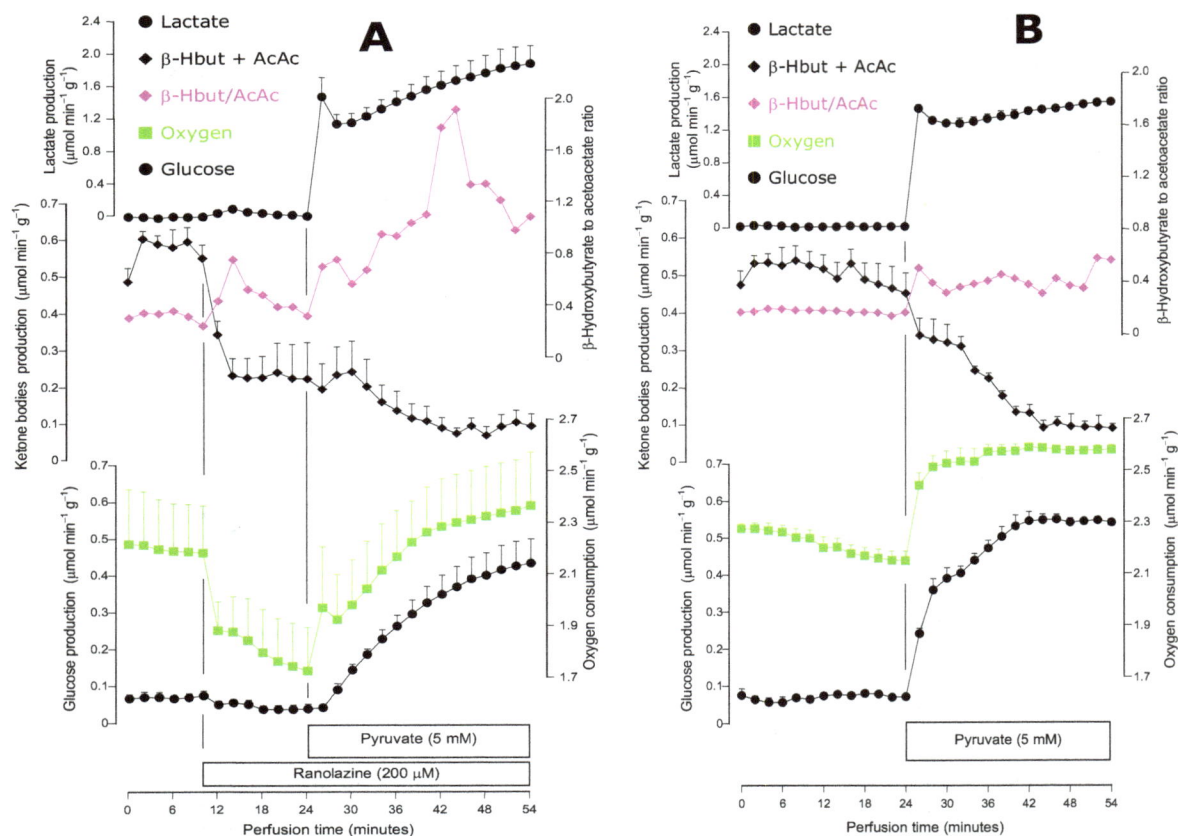

Figure 3. Effects of ranolazine on pyruvate gluconeogenesis and ketogenesis from endogenous sources. Livers from 24-hours fasted rats were perfused with substrate-free medium initially and with 5 mM pyruvate containing medium at the times indicated in the bars near to the time scale. In the experiments of panel A 200 μM ranolazine was infused as indicated. Perfusate samples were collected for metabolite measurements by means of enzymatic procedures. Oxygen uptake was measured polarographically. Data are means plus mean standard errors of 4 (panel A) and 5 (panel) liver perfusion experiments. Legends: β-Hbut, β-hydroxybutyrate; AcAc, acetoacetate.

Table 1. Contents of adenine mononucleotides of livers from fed rats in the presence and absence of 200 μM ranolazine. The extraction and assay procedures are described in the Materials and Methods section. Error parameters are mean standard errors. The p values refer to student's t test.

	Control	Ranolazine (200 μM)	p
	μmol (gram liver wet weight)$^{-1}$		
ATP	2.08 ± 0.16 (n = 6)	2.20 ± 0.25 (n = 3)	>0.05
ADP	0.88 ± 0.07 (n = 6)	0.76 ± 0.07 (n = 3)	>0.05
AMP	0.36 ± 0.07 (n = 6)	0.12 ± 0.01 (n = 3)	<0.05

ATP and ADP contents, although a tendency toward diminished ADP levels is apparent. The AMP levels, however, were significantly diminished. This means also increased ATP/AMP ratios in the presence of ranolazine.

Table 2 shows the hepatic contents of AMP, ADP and ATP in livers from 24-hours fasted rats perfused with lactate as the gluconeogenic substrate. Under these conditions the ATP content was diminished by 200 μM ranolazine (−21%). The AMP and ADP contents, under these conditions, were not affected by ranolazine.

4. Discussion

The results obtained in the present work confirm the general hypothesis stated in the Introduction, namely, that

Table 2. Contents of adenine mononucleotides of livers from fasted rats in the presence of 5 mM lactate and 5 mM lactate + 200 μM ranolazine. The extraction and assay procedures are described in the materials and methods section. Error parameters are mean standard errors. The p values refer to Student's t test.

	5 mM lactate	5 mM lactate + 200 μM ranolazine	p
	μmol (gram liver wet weight)$^{-1}$		
ATP	1.986 ± 0.083 (n = 5)	1.566 ± 0.031 (n = 3)	<0.05
ADP	0.999 ± 0.111 (n = 5)	1.091 ± 0.063 (n = 3)	>0.05
AMP	0.313 ± 0.018 (n=5)	0.354 ± 0.060 (n = 3)	>0.05

ranolazine could be active on carbohydrate metabolism in the liver. In principle one is authorized to say that the drug increases glycolysis and decreases gluconeogenesis. Additionally it tends to increase the NADH/NAD$^+$ ratio in both the cytosolic and in the mitochondrial compartment, as indicated by the lactate/pyruvate and β-hydroxybutyrate/acetoacetate ratios [12] [13]. For the cytosolic NADH/NAD$^+$ ratio, increases were observed both under glycolytic conditions as well as under gluconeogenic conditions when pyruvate was the substrate (increased lactate production). For the mitochondrial NADH/NAD$^+$ ratio, increases were observed in the present work in the absence of exogenous fatty acids, but it should be remarked that the opposite was found when the liver was actively oxidizing an exogenous fatty acid [10].

An important cause for the increased glycolysis and diminished gluconeogenesis is probably the inhibition of oxygen uptake caused by ranolazine and the consequently diminished rate of oxidative phosphorylation. It is well established by studies with other inhibitors that such an action usually causes stimulation of glycolysis and inhibition of gluconeogenesis [13] [26]. Inhibition of mitochondrial oxygen uptake, in turn, may have two causes. The first one is a direct inhibition of electron transfer at complex I [27]; the second cause is a direct inhibition of fatty acid oxidation, as suggested by experiments in which the oxidation of palmitoyl-CoA and oleoyl-CoA by isolated mitochondria was measured [10]. The fact that ranolazine inhibited the ketone body production from endogenous sources strongly corroborates the view of a direct inhibition of fatty acid oxidation. The latter may be even more important than complex I inhibition as suggested by the observation that the infusion of lactate or pyruvate in the presence of ranolazine still increased oxygen uptake to levels close to those found before the infusion of ranolazine suggesting that the reducing equivalents generated by the oxidation of lactate or pyruvate were still partly able to reach the cytochrome c oxidase system, a phenomenon that requires the participation of complex I. Even so, it is likely that complex I is inhibited to a certain extent, because the increased β-hydroxybutyrate to acetoacetate ratios in the presence of ranolazine indicate a diminished capacity of oxidizing the mitochondrial NADH [22].

Since ranolazine inhibits oxygen uptake, it seems reasonable to assume that this also represents diminished mitochondrial ATP production. Corroborating this, a diminution of the ATP content was found in the perfused liver of fasted rats and under gluconeogenic conditions. However, no such diminution was found in the liver of fed rats under glycogenolytic and glycolytic conditions. The fact that the ATP content was not affected by ranolazine in the fed state is most probably an event caused by the compensatory ATP production in the glycolytic pathway, which is stimulated by ranolazine (**Figure 1**). Actually, in the case of the experiments shown in **Figure 1**, in which 100 μM ranolazine was infused, the excess lactate production was approximately equal to 0.7 μmol min$^{-1} \cdot$g^{-1}. On stoichiometric grounds, this corresponds also to a net ATP production rate of 0.7 μmol·min$^{-1} \cdot$g^{-1}. The diminution of oxygen uptake, on the other hand, was around 0.1 μmol O$_2$ min$^{-1} \cdot$g^{-1} (or 0.2 μg-atom oxygen min$^{-1} \cdot$g^{-1}), which corresponds to a decrease of 0.5 μmol·min$^{-1} \cdot$g^{-1} in mitochondrial ATP production if one assumes a P/O ratio of 2.5 [21]. The diminished phosphorylation is, thus, fully compensated, or even exceeded, by the increased glycolysis, what explains the absence of effects of ranolazine on the cellular ATP contents.

Another phenomenon that can be contributing for gluconeogenesis inhibition is the deviation of reducing equivalents and intermediates of the gluconeogenic pathway because of the extra NADPH consumption in the microsomal electron transport chain due to ranolazine transformation [9]. The strong influence of this phenomenon on gluconeogenesis has been unequivocally demonstrated by experiments with aminopyirine [28]. That this may be occurring with ranolazine is corroborated by the previous observations that the drug was able to increase hepatic oxygen consumption in the presence of 2 mM cyanide, a condition where changes in oxygen consumption no longer reflect the mitochondrial respiratory chain [10]. This increase was equal to 0.14 ± 0.02

$\mu\text{mol·min}^{-1}\text{·g}^{-1}$ with 200 μM ranolazine and it requires a constant supply of NADPH which must come from the reactions catalyzed by the NADPH-supplying dehydrogenases [28]. Two of them, the malic enzyme and the glucose 6-phosphate dehydrogenase interfere with gluconeogenesis because their action drains away or recycles intermediates of the gluconeogenic pathway [28] [29].

5. Conclusion

In conclusion, it seems likely that ranolazine inhibits gluconeogenesis and increases glycolysis in consequence of its inhibitory actions on energy metabolism and fatty acid oxidation and by deviating reducing equivalents in favour of its own biotransformation. Lactate gluconeogenesis, which is more strongly inhibited, is particularly important because of the predominance of high lactate to pyruvate ratios under *in vivo* conditions. All these observations are in line with the earlier postulates that ranolazine diminishes fatty acid oxidation, shifting the energy source from fatty acids to glucose [1]-[5]. Nevertheless, there were also indications that the action of ranolazine on metabolism may not be restricted to the sites of action that were already identified in the present and previous work [10] [27]. The unusual response of pyruvate gluconeogenesis in the presence of ranolazine, for example, suggests a more complex mechanism of action. Identification of other sites of action depends no doubt on additional experimental work.

Acknowledgements

This work was supported by grants from the Conselho Nacional de Desenvolvimento Científico e Tecnológico (CNPq) and from the Programa Nacional de Núcleos de Excelência (PRONEX, Fundação Araucária-CNPq).

References

[1]   Anderson, J.R. and Nawarskas, J.J. (2005) Ranolazine, a Metabolic Modulator for the Treatment of Chronic Stable Angina. *Cardiology in Review*, **13**, 202-210. http://dx.doi.org/10.1097/01.crd.0000161979.62749.e7

[2]   Clarke, B., Spedding, M., Patmore, L. and McCormack, J.G. (1993) Protective Effects of Ranolazine in Guinea-Pig Hearts during Low-Flow Ischaemia and Their Association with Increases in Active Dehydrogenase. *British Journal of Pharmacology*, **109**, 748-750. http://dx.doi.org/10.1111/j.1476-5381.1993.tb13637.x

[3]   Clarke, B., Wyatt, K.M. and McCormack, J.G. (1996) Ranolazine Increases Active Pyruvate Dehydrogenase in Perfused Normoxic Rat Hearts: Evidence for an Indirect Mechanism. *Journal of Molecular and Cellular Cardiology*, **28**, 341-350. http://dx.doi.org/10.1006/jmcc.1996.0032

[4]   McCormack, J.G., Barr, R.L., Wolff, A.A. and Lopaschuk, G.D. (1996) Ranolazine Stimulates Glucose Oxidation in Normoxic, Ischemic and Reperfused Ischemic Rat Hearts. *Circulation*, **93**, 135-142. http://dx.doi.org/10.1161/01.CIR.93.1.135

[5]   Fragasso, G. (2007) Inhibition of Free Fatty Acids Metabolism as a Therapeutic Target in Patients with Heart Failure. *International Journal of Clinical Practice*, **61**, 603-610. http://dx.doi.org/10.1111/j.1742-1241.2006.01280.x

[6]   Marx, S. and Sweeney, M. (2006) Mechanism of Action of Ranolazine. *Archives of Internal Medicine*, **166**, 1325-1326. http://dx.doi.org/10.1001/archinte.166.12.1325-b

[7]   Verrier, R.L., Kumar, K., Nieminen, T. and Belardinelli, L. (2013) Mechanisms of Ranolazine's Dual Protection against Atrial and Ventricular Fibrillation. *Eurospace*, **15**, 317-324. http://dx.doi.org/10.1093/europace/eus380

[8]   Kahlig, K.M., Hirakawa, R., Liu, L., George Jr., A.L., Belardinelli, L. and Rajamani, S. (2014) Ranolazine Reduces Neuronal Excitability by Interacting with Inactivated States of Brain Sodium Channels. *Molecular Pharmacology*, **85**, 162-174. http://dx.doi.org/10.1124/mol.113.088492

[9]   Jerling, M., Huan, B.L., Leung, K., Chu, N., Abdallah, H. and Hussein, Z. (2005) Diltiazem, or Simvastatin during Combined Administration in Healthy Subjects. Studies to Investigate the Pharmacokinetic Interactions between Ranolazine and Keto-Conazole. *Journal of Clinical Pharmacology*, **45**, 422-433. http://dx.doi.org/10.1177/0091270004273992

[10] Mito, M.S., Constantin, J., Castro, C.V., Ono, M.K.C. and Bracht, A. (2010) Effects of Ranolazine on Fatty Acid Transformation in the Isolated Perfused Rat Liver. *Molecular and Cellular Biochemistry*, **345**, 35-44. http://dx.doi.org/10.1007/s11010-010-0557-8

[11] Williamson, J.R., Browning, E.T. and Scholz, R. (1969) Control Mechanisms of Gluconeogenesis and Ketogenesis. I. Effects of Oleate on Gluconeogenesis in Perfused Rat Liver. *Journal of Biological Chemistry*, **244**, 4607-4616.

[12] Veiga, R.P., Silva, M.H.R.A., Teodoro, G.R., Yamamoto, N.S., Constantin, J. and Bracht, A. (2008) Metabolic Fluxes

in the Liver of Rats Bearing the Walker-256 Tumour: Influence of the Circulating Levels of Substrates and Fatty Acids. *Cell Biochemistry and Function*, **26**, 51-63. http://dx.doi.org/10.1002/cbf.1398

[13] Soboll, S., Scholz, R. and Heldt, H.W. (1978) Subcellular Metabolite Concentrations. Dependence of Mitochondrial and Cytosolic ATP Systems on the Metabolic State of Perfused Rat Liver. *European Journal of Biochemistry*, **87**, 377-390. http://dx.doi.org/10.1111/j.1432-1033.1978.tb12387.x

[14] Sugden, M.C., Ball, A.J., Ilk, V. and Williamson, D.H. (1980) Stimulation of [1-^{14}C]oleate Oxidation to ^{14}CO$_2$ in Isolated Rat Hepatocytes by Vasopressin: Effects of Ca^{2+}. *FEBS Letters*, **116**, 37-40. http://dx.doi.org/10.1016/0014-5793(80)80523-0

[15] Scholz, R. and Bücher, T. (1965) Hemoglobin-Free Perfusion of Rat Liver. In: Chance, B., Estabrook, R.W. and Williamson, J.R., Eds., *Control of Energy Metabolism*, Academic Press, New York, 393-414. http://dx.doi.org/10.1016/B978-1-4832-3161-7.50048-3

[16] Bracht, A., Ishii-Iwamoto, E.L. and Kelmer-Bracht, A.M. (2003) O estudo do metabolismo no fígado em perfusão. In: Bracht, A. and Ishii-Iwamoto, E.L., Eds., *Métodos de Laboratório em Bioquímica*, Editora Manole, São Paulo, 275-289.

[17] Bergmeyer, H.U. (1974) Methods of Enzymatic Analysis. Verlag Chemie-Academic Press, Weinheim-London.

[18] Clark, L.C. (1956) Monitoring and Control of Blood O$_2$ Tension. *Transactions of the American Society of Artificial Internal Organs*, **2**, 41-49.

[19] Bazotte, R.B., Constantin, J., Hell, N.S. and Bracht, A. (1990) Hepatic Metabolism of Meal-Fed Rats: Studies *in Vivo* and in the Isolated Perfused Liver. *Physiology & Behavior*, **48**, 247-253. http://dx.doi.org/10.1016/0031-9384(90)90308-Q

[20] Thurman, R.G. and Scholz, R. (1977) Interaction of Glycolysis and Respiration in Perfused Liver. Changes in Oxygen Uptake Following the Addition of Ethanol. *European Journal of Biochemistry*, **75**, 13-21. http://dx.doi.org/10.1111/j.1432-1033.1977.tb11499.x

[21] Kimmig, R., Mauch, T.J. and Scholz, R. (1983) Actions of Glucagon on Flux Rates in Perfused Rat Liver. 2. Relationship between Inhibition of Glycolysis and Stimulation of Respiration by Glucagon. *European Journal of Biochemistry*, **136**, 617-620. http://dx.doi.org/10.1111/j.1432-1033.1983.tb07785.x

[22] Sies, H. (1982) Nicotinamide Nucleotide Compartmentation. In: Sies, H., Ed., *Metabolic Compartmentation*, Academic Press, New York, 205-231.

[23] Gasparin, F.R.S., Salgueiro-Pagadigorria, C.L., Bracht, L., Ishii-Iwamoto, E.L., Bracht, A. and Constantin, J. (2003) Action of Quercetin on Glycogen Catabolism in the Rat Liver. *Xenobiotica*, **33**, 587-602. http://dx.doi.org/10.1080/0049825031000089100

[24] Pereira, S.R.C., Darronqui, E., Constantin, J., Silva, M.H.R.A., Yamamoto, N.S. and Bracht, A. (2004) The Urea Cycle and Related Pathways in the Liver of Walker-256 Tumor-Bearing Rats. *Biochimica et Biophysica Acta*, **1688**, 187-196. http://dx.doi.org/10.1016/j.bbadis.2003.12.001

[25] Pivato, L.S., Constantin, R.P., Ishii-Iwamoto, E.L., Kelmer-Bracht, A.M., Yamamoto, N.S., Constantin, J. and Bracht, A. (2006) Metabolic Effects of Carbenoxolone in the Rat Liver. *Journal of Biochemical and Molecular Toxicology*, **20**, 230-240. http://dx.doi.org/10.1002/jbt.20139

[26] Acco, A., Comar, J.F. and Bracht, A. (2004) Metabolic Effects of Propofol in the Isolated Perfused Rat Liver. *Basic & Clinical Pharmacology & Toxicology*, **95**, 166-174. http://dx.doi.org/10.1111/j.1742-7843.2004.pto950404.x

[27] Wyatt, K.M., Skene, C., Veitch, K., Hue, L. and McCormack, J.G. (1995) The Antianginal Ranolazine Is a Weak Inhibitor of the Respiratory Complex I, but with Greater Potency in Broken or Uncoupled than in Coupled Mitochondria. *Biochemical Pharmacology*, **50**, 1599-1606. http://dx.doi.org/10.1016/0006-2952(95)02042-X

[28] Scholz, A., Hansen, W. and Thurman, R.G. (1973) Interaction of Mixed-Function Oxidation with Biosynthetic Processes. 1. Inhibition of Gluconeogenesis by Aminopyrine in Perfused Rat Liver. *European Journal of Biochemistry*, **38**, 64-72. http://dx.doi.org/10.1111/j.1432-1033.1973.tb03034.x

[29] Orrenius, S. and Sies, H. (1982) Compartmentation of Detoxification Reactions. In: Sies, H., Ed., *Metabolic Compartmentation*, Academic Press, New York, 485-520.

22

The Effects of Adiponectin on Bone Metabolism

Yuan Yu Lin[1], Ching Yi Chen[1], Chih Chien Chen[1], Han Jen Lin[1], Harry John Mersmann[1], Shinn Chih Wu[1], Shih Torng Ding[1,2]*

[1]Department of Animal Science and Technology, National Taiwan University, Taiwan
[2]Institute of Biotechnology, National Taiwan University, Taiwan
Email: *sding@ntu.edu.tw

Abstract

Osteoporosis and its related bone fractures are growing medical problems, especially in industrial countries, and thus the knowledge of regulation of bone metabolism is critical to develop therapeutic approaches. Bone adipocytes share common mesenchymal precursors with osteoblasts and chondrocytes and their numbers in bone marrow are altered in various pathophysiological conditions. Several findings suggest that accelerated adipogenesis in bone marrow, known as fatty marrow, is associated with the progression of osteoporosis. Apart from its demonstrated anti-atherosclerogenic and insulin-sensitizing actions, the adipokine adiponectin and its receptors have been shown to be expressed in bone tissues and participate in bone metabolism. Here we review recent findings regarding the regulation of bone metabolism by adiponectin and its receptors and the underlying mechanisms. We also provide future perspectives for research.

Keywords

Adiponectin, Mesenchymal Stem Cells, Bone and Osteoporosis

1. Introduction

The relationship between bone and fat formation within the bone marrow microenvironment is complex and remains an area of active investigation. Clinical and experimental findings suggest that acceleration of adipogenesis in bone marrow, known as fatty marrow, is associated with the progression of osteoporosis and aging [1] [2]. It is now clear that adipose tissue is a complex, essential and highly active metabolic and endocrine organ [3] [4]. Adipocytes express and secrete various endocrine hormones such as leptin, adiponectin (ApN), TNF-α and

---

*Corresponding author.

IL-6 [4]. Among these hormones, leptin is the first adipokine found to have function in both energy and bone metabolism [5] [6]. These observations suggest that energy metabolism and bone mass are regulated by the same hormones. Over the past decades, ApN and its receptors (AdipoR1 and AdipoR2) have been found to regulate energy homeostasis and have protective functions for metabolic and cardiovascular diseases [7]. In addition, accumulating evidences indicate that ApN measurement may serve as a useful screening tool for predicting osteoporosis [8]. ApN and its receptors are expressed in cells of osteoblastic and osteoclastic lineages, suggesting that they play roles in regulating bone metabolism [9] [10]. Here, we summarize the effects of ApN on bone metabolism and propose future research directions.

2. ApN and Its Receptors

ApN was originally identified by four independent groups and was named Acrp30 [11] and AdipoQ [12] in mice, and apM1 [13] or GBP28 [14] in humans. It belongs to the complement 1q family [15] and forms multimer complexes through the collagen-like domain in the circulatory system. Multi-mer complexes include trimers, hexamers and high-molecular-weight (HMW) forms [16]. ApN-deficient mice exhibit features of insulin resistance, dyslipidemia and hypertension [17]. ApN exerts its insulin-sensitizing effect by regulating glucose utilization and fatty acid metabolism [7]. Administration of ApN to mice decreases the plasma concentration of glucose, free fatty acids and triglycerides, increases muscular fatty acid oxidation, induces weight loss [18] and reverses obesity-associated insulin resistance [19].

Yamauchi *et al.* first cloned the cDNA encoding adiponectin receptors 1 (AdipoR1) and 2 (AdipoR2) from humans and mice [20]. Our group, then cloned the porcine counterparts [21]. AdipoR1 and AdipoR2 contain seven transmembrane domains with structure, topology and function distinct from those of the G-protein-coupled receptors [20]. AdipoR1 and AdipoR2 serve as the major AdipoRs *in vivo*, with the former activating the AMP kinase (AMPK) pathway and the latter activating the peroxisome proliferator-activated receptor alpha (PPARα) pathway in liver to enhance insulin sensitivity and decrease inflammation [7]. Disruption of both AdipoR1 and R2 exterminate ApN binding and downstream actions including abolishment of ApN-induced AMPK activation and decreased activity of the PPAR-α signaling pathway; The result of disruption is to increase tissue triglyceride content, inflammation, oxidative stress, insulin resistance and glucose intolerance [22]. Recent research indicates ApN has anti-proliferative effects on cancer cells and a cardio-protective role increasing longevity [23]. **Figure 1** represents the effects of adiponectin on peripheral tissues and hypoadiponectinemia related diseases.

3. Bone Remodeling

Bone remodeling is a continuous process throughout adult life consisting of the resorption of senescent bone

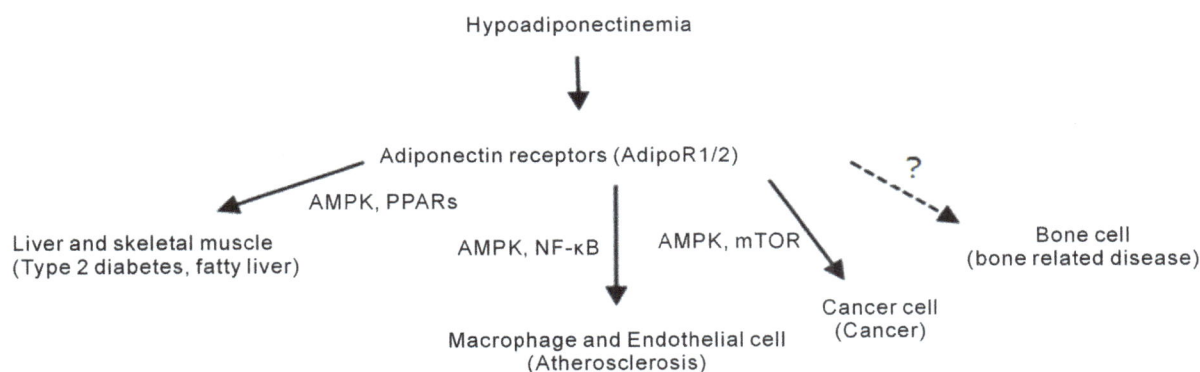

Figure 1. Current targets and mediators of adiponectin and its receptors. Adiponectin and its receptors (AdipoR1/R2) play critical roles in the regulation of peripheral tissue functions and development of obesity-related disease, such as type 2 diabetes, fatty liver, atherosclerosis, bone related disease or cancer. AdipoR1/2 serve as receptors for adiponectin actions, which are mediated by AMPK, PPARs, NF-κB and mTOR. The related diseases are indicated in parentheses. (AMPK, 5' adenosine monophosphate-activated protein kinase; PPARs, peroxisome proliferative activated receptors; NF-κB, nuclear transcription factor κB; mTOR, mammalian target of rapamycin; modified from [23]).

by osteoclasts (Oc) and the formation of new bone from osteoblasts (Ob). Differentiated Oc are derived from hematopoietic stem cells [24], whereas Ob are derived from mesenchymal stem cells [25]. In the process of bone remodeling, Oc adhere to bone to remove the exterior rigid structure by acidification and proteolytic digestion. Once the resorption site is created, Ob intrude and begin new bone formation along with the secretion of osteoid, a mineralizing factor. The process is completed by coverage of the bone surface by lining cells, a type of terminally differentiated Ob [26]. Bone disease is caused by an imbalance in bone remodeling. At the physiological level, mechanisms of bone remodeling are regulated locally by cytokines and systemically by hormones [27]. PTH and 1,5-dihydroxy vitamin D have anabolic actions, which are opposed by calcitonin [27]-[29]. Several systemic regulators, such as, insulin-like growth factor (also acting through local regulators) [30], glucocorticoids [31], thyroid hormone [32] and estrogen [33] contribute to bone formation and bone resorption. In addition, local factors derived from bone cells, like TGF-β, have inhibitory functions on osteoclastogenesis [34] regulate cell growth and differentiation and induce anabolic activity in Ob [35]. IL-1 and TNF-α serve to quiesce Oc and participate in bone resorption pathophysiology [36]. The receptor activator of NF-κB ligand (RANKL), RANK and osteoprotegrin (OPG) are essential for Oc differentiation. RANKL is expressed by Ob as a soluble factor that binds with RANK on Oc with recruitment of tumor necrosis factor receptor-associated factor 6 (TRAF6) and activation of the transcription factor, nuclear factor of activated T-cells cytoplasmic 1 (NFATc1) to induce of Ob differentiation related genes via the NF-κB pathway [37] [38]. OPG is a decoy receptor for RANKL which plays an inhibitory role in osteoclastogenesis [39]. OPG-deficient mice exhibit a decrease in total bone density and develope osteoporosis [40]. The regulation of bone remodeling not only involves osteoblastic and osteoclastic cell lineages but also other marrow cells. Adipocytes are derived from the same progenitor cells as Ob, and the equilibrium between the two cell types is important in bone remodeling [41] [42]. Several regulatory pathways of adipocyte differentiation from bone marrow mesenchymal stem cells interact with osteoblast differentiation pathway [43]. The major adipogenic transcriptional factors, C/EBPα and PPARγ, are regulated by extracellular signaling involved in osteoblastgenesis [43]. Mesenchymal stem cell differentiation into Ob requires Wnt signaling activation, which stimulates osteoblastogenesis and suppresses adipogenesis by blocking PPARγ and C/EBPα [44] [45]. Cell lineage allocation in the bone marrow microenvironment is shown in **Figure 2**.

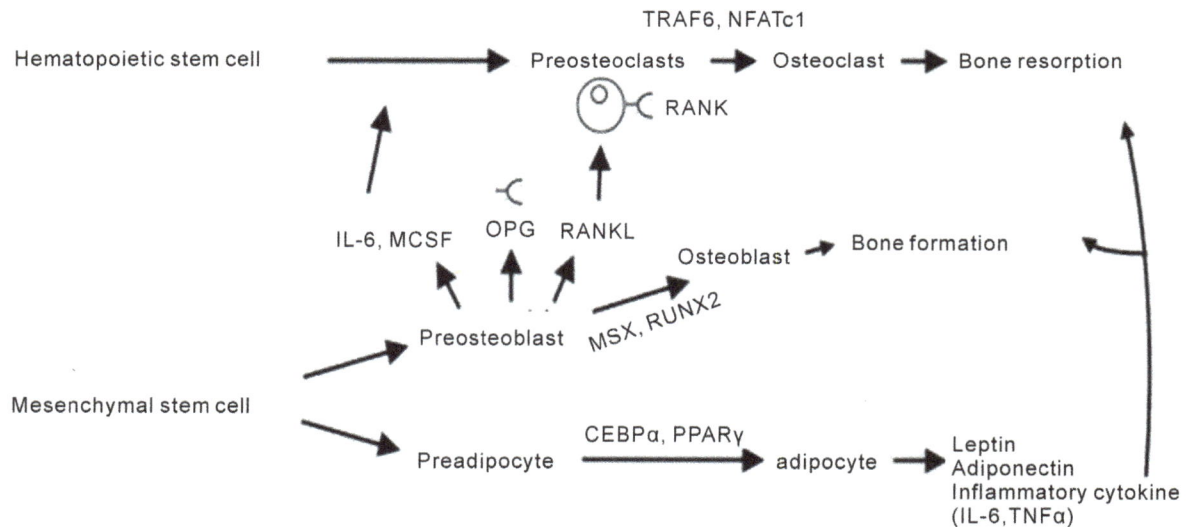

Figure 2. Cell lineage allocation and regulation in the bone marrow microenvironment (modified from [30]). Osteoblasts and adipocytes are derived from the same progenitors, the mesenchymal stem cells. To achieve full differentiated status, multiple critical transcription factors must be activated. RANKL is expressed by osteoblasts as a soluble factor, which binds to RANK on osteoclasts. Further recruitment of TRAF6 and activation of NFATc1 induce osteoclast differentiation. Cytokines released from the adipocytes participate in the bone remodeling process. (CEBPα, CAAT/enhancer binding protein α; PPARγ, peroxisome proliferative activated receptor γ; RANK, receptor activator of nuclear transcription factor κB; RANKL, receptor activator of nuclear transcription factor κB ligand; OPG, osteoprotegerin; IL, interleukin; MCSF, macrophage colony stimulating factor; MSX, MSH homeobox homolog; RUNX, runt-related transcription factor; TRAF6, tumor necrosis factor receptor-associated factor 6; NFATc1, nuclear factor of activated T-cells cytoplasmic 1).

4. The Actions of Adiponectin on Bone Metabolism

4.1. Effects of ApN on Bone Metabolism and on Osteoblast and Osteoclast Differentiation

ApN stimulates osteoblastogenesis and chondrocytogenesis, but suppresses osteoclastogenesis and therefore promotes bone formation [9] [46]. There are three distinct ApN actions in bone formation: 1) a direct positive endocrine action through circulating ApN; 2) an autocrine/paracrine action; 3) indirect endocrine effects by interacting with other signaling pathways such as insulin and bone morphogenetic protein 2 (BMP2).

Several studies confirm the positive endocrine role of ApN in bone formation. Challa *et al*. suggest that ApN increases chondrocyte proliferation, proteoglycan synthesis and matrix mineralization by upregulating the expression of type II collagen and Runx2 and increasing the activities of alkaline phosphatase [46]. Similarly, Oshima *et al*. (2005) demonstrated that ApN-treated C57BL/6J mice have increased trabecular bone mass and enhanced mineralization of Ob, accompanied by a decreased number of Oc and bone resorption activity [47]. Potential mechanisms for circulating ApN to modulate Oc differentiation are that ApN augmentes gene expression of several osteogenic markers and increases Ob differentiation in mesenchymal progenitor cells [48]. Moreover, ApN activates p38 mitogen-activated protein kinase via AdipoR1, which results in c-Jun activation and upregulation of the target gene, cyclooxygenase-2 (COX-2). ApN also stimulates BMP2 expression in a COX2-dependent manner and therefore increases Ob differentiation [48]. An alternative action of ApN, discovered by Huang *et al*. is that ApN stimulates osteoblast differentiation by increasing BMP-2 expression with involvement of AMPK, p38 and NF-κB [49].

ApN regulates bone formation in an autocrine/paracrine manner. ApN and its receptors are expressed in osteoblastic and osteoclastic cells, indicating participation in bone metabolism not only through an endocrine pathway, but also locally in the bone [9]. The authors analyzed cultures of bone marrow cells from ApN-knockout (Ad−/−) and WT mice and find a significant decrease of osteogenesis in Ad−/− marrow cell culture, compared to WT. Collectively, these results suggest a positive autocrine/paracrine action of ApN on bone formation.

ApN also has indirect effects on bone, possibly through modulating growth factor action or insulin sensitivity. In the presence of insulin and BMP2 (but not IGF-1), ApN stimulates Ob differentiation in bone marrow cells [9]. Co-culture of Ob with the secretory products of adipocytes produces an inhibitory effect on Ob differentiation, which can be reversed by knockdown of adipoR1 [50].

4.2. Involvement of Insulin Signaling, Long Term Adaption and Compensation in ApN-Modulated Bone Metabolism

Most studies indicate that the effects of ApN and its receptors have a positive role on bone metabolism, but some opposite aspects are also described [51]. One confounding factor is insulin signaling. Shinoda *et al*. (2006) treated a bone marrow cell culture with insulin or recombinant mouse ApN and found that insulin impairs the effect of ApN treatment on osteogenesis and restores the number of colonies. In addition, long term adaption and compensation in transgenic or knockout mice may modify ApN-modulated bone metabolism. Analyses of bone characteristics by radiological and histological examination of the femur, tibia and vertebrae in male WT and Ad−/− littermates indicates no difference between WT and Ad−/− mice [9]. Williams *et al*. (2009) also observed the same results in WT and Ad−/− 22 wk old mice [51]. In this circumstance, long term adaption and compensation produced no change in bone development *in vivo* in ApN knockout mice. Tu *et al*. (2011) isolated the bone cells from genetically double-labeled mBSP9.0Luc/β-ACT-EGFP transgenic mice and transplanted them into ApN−/− or wild type mice to investigate the effect of temporary exposure to ApN on bone growth and metabolism; growth of bone explants in ApN−/− mice is significantly retarded. Moreover, micro-CT analysis and tartrate-resistant acid phosphatase staining revealed decreased bone volume, cortical bone and increased Ob number in bone explants in ApN−/− mice [52]. ApN inhibits RANKL-induced osteoclastogenesis from RAW264.7 cells, down-regulates RANKL-enhanced osteoclastogenic regulators, and increases Oc apoptosis [52]. The effects of ApN on bone metabolism including the *in vivo* mouse model are shown in **Table 1**.

5. Involvement of AMPK in ApN-Modulated Bone Metabolism

Bone remodeling is an energy intensive process and bones need to balance energy constantly in response to nutrient availability during growth and bone turnover. During the last decade adenosine 5'-monophosphate-activated protein kinase (AMPK) emerged as a key in the regulation of energy homeostasis and as the mediator of

Table 1. Effects of ApN on bone metabolism.

Main idea	Animal model	Cell model	Approach	Ref.
In vivo: ↑ trabecular bone mass ↓ decreased osteoclast number and serum NTx *In vitro*: ↓ osteoclast differentiation ↑ expression of alkaline phosphatase and mineralization in MC3T3-E1 cells	C57BL/6J mice treated with adenovirus expressing lacZ or adiponectin	Treat MC3T3-E1, CD14+ cells, bone marrow macrophage with adiponectin	Micro-CT, EIA (NTx), Histological examination (TRAP+), real-time (ALP), Alizarin Red S staining	[47]
In vivo: No difference between overexpressing adiponectin and WT *In vitro*: 1. ↓ osteogenesis in Ad−/− mice bone marrow cell 2. Treat adiponectin recombinant protein inhibit osteogenesis	Ad−/− mice, Ad-Tg mice	Bone marrow cell (from adult mouse long bones, neonatal calvarial osteoblasts, osteoclast precursor M-CSF-dependent bone marrow macrophage, ST2 cells	Histtological analysis, osteoclast formation assay, immunoprecipitation and immunoblotting	[9]
In vivo: ↑ Trabecular bone volume and trabecular number in 14 week Ad KO mice. *In vitro*: ↓ osteoclastogenesis in rat and human osteoclast	AdKO mice (C57BL/6J)	Rat and human primary osteoblast, osteoclast	Micro-CT, primary osteoblast culture	[51]
In vivo: ↓ osteoclastogenesis and bone resorption via APPL1-mediated suppression of AKT1 *In vitro*: ↓ osteoclast differentiation by RANKL in RAW264.7 and decreased expression of osteoclastogenic regulator (NFAT2, TRAF6)	ADN-KO mice	RAW264.7	Histological examination, micro CT	[52]

central and peripheral effects of numerous hormones [53]. In addition, AMPK signaling activates ApN receptor signaling pathways in liver, muscle and adipose tissues [54]-[57]. *In vitro* studies demonstrate that AMPK modulates bone cell differentiation and function. AMPK is expressed in mouse tibia and ROS 17/2.8 osteoblastic cells [58]. Murine Ob and human mesenchymal stem cells treated with AMPK activators (AICAR or metformin) stimulate Thr-172 phosphorylation of AMPK in a dose/time-dependent manner. In contrast, treatment with the AMPK inhibitor (compound C) or knockdown of AMPK by shRNA-lentivirus infection inhibits AMPK phosphorylation and induces osteogenesis [58] [59]. Shah *et al.* (2010) analyzed the bone phenotype of 4 month-old male WT and AMPKα1−/−knockout mice by micro-CT. The AMPKα1−/−KO mice have less trabecular bone [58]. Furthermore, AMPK acts as a negative regulator in differentiation of Oc [60]. Treatment of pre-Oc with compound C (AMPK inhibitor) potentiates bone resorption and formation of TRAP-positive multinucleated cells in a dose-dependent manner [60]. Treatment with the globular form of ApN inhibits TNF-α/RANKL-induced Oc formation from a RAW264 clone via AMPK signaling [61]. The elucidation of the importance of AMPK signaling in bone is still in early stage, but already reveals that AMPK activation affects bone formation and bone mass; therefore, AMPK signaling might act as a significant pathway in skeletal physiology.

6. Conclusions and Future Perspectives

ApN and its receptors are expressed in bone and bone stromal cells which suggest that they play critical roles in bone metabolism. The present review summarizes effects of ApN on bone metabolism, both in physiological states and in Ob or Oc culture *in vitro*. There are still several controversial results on the correlation of ApN and bone mineral density or other bone parameters. The critical role of ApN in the bone remodeling process and bone metabolism is an indisputable fact. Herein, we propose some possible future research directions.

1) In the circulatory system, ApN exists multi-mer complexes, such as trimers, hexamers and HMW forms [16]. Several researches suggest that different forms of ApN may give rise to different activities and have different roles in insulin sensitivity [62] [63]. In both mice and human diabetic patients, an increased ratio of HMW ApN to total ApN in the plasma correlates with improvement in insulin sensitivity during treatment with an insulin-sensitizing drug, TZD; there is no corelation with total amount of ApN [63]. Only one research group indicates that HMW ApN affects bone metabolism in both male and female hemodialysis patients [64]. We speculate that different multi-mer forms of ApN cause different influences on bone formation, but more molecular

level observations are needed to confirm this speculation.

2) Energy equilibrium in mammals is controlled by the actions of circulatory hormones that coordinate fuel production and utilization in metabolically active tissues. Bone remodeling can be affected by metabolic related hormones, implying that bones are involved in the control of energy homeostasis [65] [66]. Osteocalcin, the most abundant non-collagenous protein of the bone extracellular matrix regulates β-cell proliferation, insulin secretion and glucose homeostasis [66] [67]. Furthermore, there are several consistent results showing the insulin-osteocalcin endocrine loop in humans [68] [69] were decreased in adipocyte and pancreatic islets respectively co-culture with osteocalcin knockout osteoblasts [65]. Whether osteocalcin has any interaction with ApN in bone metabolism or as a feed-back loop via ApN needs further investigation.

3) Mao *et al.* [70] used the cytoplasmic domain of AdipoR1 as bait to screen a yeast two-hybrid cDNA library derived from human brain. They found that APPL1 (adaptor protein containing pleckstrin homology domain, phosphotryosine binding domain (PTB) and leucine zipper motif) interacted with ApN receptors in mammalian cells and the interaction was stimulated by ApN. It has been suggested that APPL1 mediates the effect of ApN on inhibition of osteoclastogenesis and bone resorption [52]. Although this observation is an indirect evidence, we speculate that APPL1 may have functions to mediate ApN effects on bone development. APPL1 not only has an AdipoR1 binding domain in the PTB domain, but also has a FSH receptor binding domain [71]. The existence of FSH receptor domain in APPL1 increases the possibility of APPL1 mediating the regulation of ApN on bone metabolism [71] [72]. In order to investigate this possible regulator, we have to further investigate the role of APPL1 by culture system or loss-of-function and gain-of-function model.

4) Epigenic regulation—MicroRNAs (miRNAs) are small endogenous RNA fragments (19 - 25 nt) that regulate gene expression by targeting mRNA in post-transcriptional stage [73]. Controling the differentiation of the mesenchymal stem cells into osteogenic or adipogenic lineage is important for maintaining healthy bone and is necessary for prevention of bone related disease. Recently, there are some evidences showing that the differentiation between Ob and adipocytes is tightly controlled by miRNAs [74] [75]. We speculate that miRNA may have the effects on regulating expression of ApN and therefore affect bone formation or bone resorption.

5) AdipoR2 is expressed in bone-forming cells [10]. So far, there is no evidence showing the effect of ApN through AdipoR2 in bone formation or bone resorption. The role of AdipoR2 in bone metabolism must be investigated.

6) Bone marrow microenvironment and its endocrine or paracrine regulatory systems are actively studied. Osteoporosis models such as ovariectomy and senescence have been used extensively in rodents or other mammals [76] [77]. Ovariectomy mimics postmenopausal women whose bone loss is caused from acute ovary hormonal deficiency. Ovariectomy destroys the overall hormonal balance, but is a difficult model to investigate changes in bone microenvironments. More appropriate models are needed to investigate regulatory mechanisms.

Acknowledgements

The study was supported by grants from the National Science Counsel in Taiwan.

References

[1] Meunier, P., Aaron, J., Edouard, C. and Vignon, G. (1971) Osteoporosis and the Replacement of Cell Populations of the Marrow by Adipose Tissue. A Quantitative Study of 84 Iliac Bone Biopsies. *Clinical Orthopaedics and Related Research*, **80**, 147-154. http://dx.doi.org/10.1097/00003086-197110000-00021

[2] Gimble, J.M., Zvonic, S., Floyd, Z.E., Kassem, M. and Nuttall, M.E. (2006) Playing with Bone and Fat. *Journal of Cellular Biochemistry*, **98**, 251-266. http://dx.doi.org/10.1002/jcb.20777

[3] Ahima, R.S. and Flier, J.S. (2000) Adipose Tissue as an Endocrine Organ. *Trends in Endocrinology and Metabolism*, **11**, 327-332. http://dx.doi.org/10.1016/S1043-2760(00)00301-5

[4] Kershaw, E.E. and Flier, J.S. (2004) Adipose Tissue as an Endocrine Organ. *The Journal of Clinical Endocrinology and Metabolism*, **89**, 2548-2556. http://dx.doi.org/10.1210/jc.2004-0395

[5] Ducy, P., Amling, M., Takeda, S., Priemel, M., Schilling, A.F., Beil, F.T., *et al.* (2000) Leptin Inhibits Bone Formation through a Hypothalamic Relay: A Central Control of Bone Mass. *Cell*, **100**, 197-207. http://dx.doi.org/10.1016/S0092-8674(00)81558-5

[6] Karsenty, G. (2006) Convergence between Bone and Energy Homeostases: Leptin Regulation of Bone Mass. *Cell Metabolism*, **4**, 341-348. http://dx.doi.org/10.1016/j.cmet.2006.10.008

[7] Yamauchi, T. and Kadowaki, T. (2008) Physiological and Pathophysiological Roles of Adiponectin and Adiponectin Receptors in the Integrated Regulation of Metabolic and Cardiovascular Diseases. *International Journal of Obesity*, **32**, S13-18. http://dx.doi.org/10.1038/ijo.2008.233

[8] Kelesidis, I., Kelesidis, T. and Mantzoros, C.S. (2006) Adiponectin and Cancer: A Systematic Review. *British Journal of Cancer*, **94**, 1221-1225. http://dx.doi.org/10.1038/sj.bjc.6603051

[9] Shinoda, Y., Yamaguchi, M., Ogata, N., Akune, T., Kubota, N., Yamauchi, T., *et al.* (2006) Regulation of Bone Formation by Adiponectin through Autocrine/Paracrine and Endocrine Pathways. *Journal of Cellular Biochemistry*, **99**, 196-208. http://dx.doi.org/10.1002/jcb.20890

[10] Berner, H.S., Lyngstadaas, S.P., Spahr, A., Monjo, M., Thommesen, L., Drevon, C.A., *et al.* (2004) Adiponectin and Its Receptors Are Expressed in Bone-Forming Cells. *Bone*, **35**, 842-849. http://dx.doi.org/10.1016/j.bone.2004.06.008

[11] Scherer, P.E., Williams, S., Fogliano, M., Baldini, G. and Lodish, H.F. (1995) A Novel Serum Protein Similar to C1q, Produced Exclusively in Adipocytes. *The Journal of Biological Chemistry*, **270**, 26746-26749. http://dx.doi.org/10.1074/jbc.270.45.26746

[12] Hu, E., Liang, P. and Spiegelman, B.M. (1996) AdipoQ is a Novel Adipose-Specific Gene Dysregulated in Obesity. *The Journal of Biological Chemistry*, **271**, 10697-10703. http://dx.doi.org/10.1074/jbc.271.18.10697

[13] Maeda, K., Okubo, K., Shimomura, I., Funahashi, T., Matsuzawa, Y. and Matsubara, K. (1996) cDNA Cloning and Expression of a Novel Adipose Specific Collagen-Like Factor, apM1 (AdiPose Most abundant Gene Transcript 1). *Biochemical and Biophysical Research Communications*, **221**, 286-289. http://dx.doi.org/10.1006/bbrc.1996.0587

[14] Nakano, Y., Tobe, T., Choi-Miura, N., Mazda, T. and Tomita, M. (1996) Isolation and Characterization of GBP28, a Novel Gelatin-Binding Protein Purified from Human Plasma. *Journal of Biochemistry*, **120**, 803-812. http://dx.doi.org/10.1093/oxfordjournals.jbchem.a021483

[15] Wong, G.W., Wang, J., Hug, C., Tsao, T.S. and Lodish, H.F. (2004) A Family of Acrp30/Adiponectin Structural and Functional Paralogs. *Proceedings of the National Academy of Sciences of the United States of America*, **101**, 10302-10307. http://dx.doi.org/10.1073/pnas.0403760101

[16] Okamoto, Y., Kihara, S., Funahashi, T., Matsuzawa, Y. and Libby, P. (2006) Adiponectin: A Key Adipocytokine in Metabolic Syndrome. *Clinical Science*, **110**, 267-278. http://dx.doi.org/10.1042/CS20050182

[17] Kubota, N., Terauchi, Y., Yamauchi, T., Kubota, T., Moroi, M., Matsui, J., *et al.* (2002) Disruption of Adiponectin Causes Insulin Resistance and Neointimal Formation. *The Journal of Biological Chemistry*, **277**, 25863-25866. http://dx.doi.org/10.1074/jbc.C200251200

[18] Fruebis, J., Tsao, T.S., Javorschi, S., Ebbets-Reed, D., Erickson, M.R., Yen, F.T., *et al.* (2001) Proteolytic Cleavage Product of 30-kDa Adipocyte Complement-Related Protein Increases Fatty Acid Oxidation in Muscle and Causes Weight Loss in Mice. *Proceedings of the National Academy of Sciences of the United States of America*, **98**, 2005-2010. http://dx.doi.org/10.1073/pnas.98.4.2005

[19] Yamauchi, T., Kamon, J., Waki, H., Terauchi, Y., Kubota, N., Hara, K., *et al.* (2001) The Fat-Derived Hormone Adiponectin Reverses Insulin Resistance Associated with both Lipoatrophy and Obesity. *Nature Medicine*, **7**, 941-946. http://dx.doi.org/10.1038/90984

[20] Yamauchi, T., Kamon, J., Ito, Y., Tsuchida, A., Yokomizo, T., Kita, S., *et al.* (2003) Cloning of Adiponectin Receptors That Mediate Antidiabetic Metabolic Effects. *Nature*, **423**, 762-769. http://dx.doi.org/10.1038/nature01705

[21] Ding, S.T., Liu, B.H. and Ko, Y.H. (2004) Cloning and Expression of Porcine Adiponectin and Adiponectin Receptor 1 and 2 Genes in Pigs. *Journal of Animal Science*, **82**, 3162-3174.

[22] Yamauchi, T., Nio, Y., Maki, T., Kobayashi, M., Takazawa, T., Iwabu, M., *et al.* (2007) Targeted Disruption of AdipoR1 and AdipoR2 Causes Abrogation of Adiponectin Binding and Metabolic Actions. *Nature Medicine*, **13**, 332-339. http://dx.doi.org/10.1038/nm1557

[23] Yamauchi, T. and Kadowaki, T. (2013) Adiponectin Receptor as a Key Player in Healthy Longevity and Obesity-Related Diseases. *Cell Metabolism*, **17**, 185-196. http://dx.doi.org/10.1016/j.cmet.2013.01.001

[24] Teitelbaum, S.L. (2000) Bone Resorption by Osteoclasts. *Science*, **289**, 1504-1508. http://dx.doi.org/10.1126/science.289.5484.1504

[25] Owen, M. (1988) Marrow Stromal Stem Cells. *Journal of Cell Science*, 63-76. http://dx.doi.org/10.1242/jcs.1988.Supplement_10.5

[26] Manolagas, S.C. and Jilka, R.L. (1995) Bone Marrow, Cytokines, and Bone Remodeling—Emerging Insights into the Pathophysiology of Osteoporosis. *The New England Journal of Medicine*, **332**, 305-311. http://dx.doi.org/10.1056/NEJM199502023320506

[27] Raisz, L.G. (1999) Physiology and Pathophysiology of Bone Remodeling. *Clinical Chemistry*, **45**, 1353-1358.

[28] Dempster, D.W., Cosman, F., Parisien, M., Shen, V. and Lindsay, R. (1993) Anabolic Actions of Parathyroid Hormone

on bone. *Endocrine Reviews*, **14**, 690-709.

[29] Li, Y.C., Amling, M., Pirro, A.E., Priemel, M., Meuse, J., Baron, R., *et al.* (1998) Normalization of Mineral Ion Homeostasis by Dietary Means Prevents Hyperparathyroidism, Rickets, and Osteomalacia, But Not Alopecia in Vitamin D Receptor-Ablated Mice. *Endocrinology*, **139**, 4391-4396.

[30] Rosen, C.J. and Donahue, L.R. (1998) Insulin-Like Growth Factors and Bone: The Osteoporosis Connection Revisited. *Experimental Biology and Medicine*, **219**, 1-7. http://dx.doi.org/10.3181/00379727-219-44310

[31] Advani, S., LaFrancis, D., Bogdanovic, E., Taxel, P., Raisz, L.G. and Kream, B.E. (1997) Dexamethasone Suppresses *in Vivo* Levels of Bone Collagen Synthesis in Neonatal Mice. *Bone*, **20**, 41-46. http://dx.doi.org/10.1016/S8756-3282(96)00314-6

[32] Kawaguchi, H., Pilbeam, C.C. and Raisz, L.G. (1994) Anabolic Effects of 3,3',5-Triiodothyronine and Triiodothyroacetic Acid in Cultured Neonatal Mouse Parietal Bones. *Endocrinology*, **135**, 971-976.

[33] Pacifici, R. (1998) Cytokines, Estrogen, and Postmenopausal Osteoporosis—The Second Decade. *Endocrinology*, **139**, 2659-2661.

[34] Takai, H., Kanematsu, M., Yano, K., Tsuda, E., Higashio, K., Ikeda, K., *et al.* (1998) Transforming Growth Factor-Beta Stimulates the Production of Osteoprotegerin/Osteoclastogenesis Inhibitory Factor by Bone Marrow Stromal Cells. *The Journal of Biological Chemistry*, **273**, 27091-27096. http://dx.doi.org/10.1074/jbc.273.42.27091

[35] Ramirez-Yanez, G.O., Hamlet, S., Jonarta, A., Seymour, G.J. and Symons, A.L. (2006) Prostaglandin E_2 Enhances Transforming Growth Factor-Beta 1 and TGF-Beta Receptors Synthesis: An *in Vivo* and *in Vitro* Study. *Prostaglandins, Leukotrienes and Essential Fatty Acids*, **74**, 183-192. http://dx.doi.org/10.1016/j.plefa.2006.01.003

[36] Steeve, K.T., Marc, P., Sandrine, T., Dominique, H. and Yannick, F. (2004) IL-6, RANKL, TNF-Alpha/IL-1: Interrelations in Bone Resorption Pathophysiology. *Cytokine and Growth Factor Reviews*, **15**, 49-60. http://dx.doi.org/10.1016/j.cytogfr.2003.10.005

[37] Takayanagi, H., Kim, S., Koga, T., Nishina, H., Isshiki, M., Yoshida, H., *et al.* (2002) Induction and Activation of the Transcription Factor NFATc1 (NFAT2) Integrate RANKL Signaling in Terminal Differentiation of Osteoclasts. *Developmental Cell*, **3**, 889-901. http://dx.doi.org/10.1016/S1534-5807(02)00369-6

[38] Nakashima, T., Hayashi, M. and Takayanagi, H. (2012) New Insights into Osteoclastogenic Signaling Mechanisms. *Trends in Endocrinology and Metabolism*, **23**, 582-590. http://dx.doi.org/10.1016/j.tem.2012.05.005

[39] Lacey, D.L., Timms, E., Tan, H.L., Kelley, M.J., Dunstan, C.R., Burgess, T., *et al.* (1998) Osteoprotegerin Ligand Is a Cytokine That Regulates Osteoclast Differentiation and Activation. *Cell*, **93**, 165-176. http://dx.doi.org/10.1016/S0092-8674(00)81569-X

[40] Bucay, N., Sarosi, I., Dunstan, C.R., Morony, S., Tarpley, J., Capparelli, C., *et al.* (1998) *Osteoprotegerin*-Deficient Mice Develop Early Onset Osteoporosis and Arterial Calcification. *Genes and Development*, **12**, 1260-1268. http://dx.doi.org/10.1101/gad.12.9.1260

[41] Chamberlain, G., Fox, J., Ashton, B. and Middleton, J. (2007) Concise Review: Mesenchymal Stem Cells: Their Phenotype, Differentiation Capacity, Immunological Features, and Potential for Homing. *Stem Cells*, **25**, 2739-2749. http://dx.doi.org/10.1634/stemcells.2007-0197

[42] Duque, G. (2008) Bone and Fat Connection in Aging Bone. *Current Opinion in Rheumatology*, **20**, 429-434. http://dx.doi.org/10.1097/BOR.0b013e3283025e9c

[43] Muruganandan, S., Roman, A.A. and Sinal, C.J. (2009) Adipocyte Differentiation of Bone Marrow-Derived Mesenchymal Stem Cells: Cross Talk with the Osteoblastogenic Program. *Cellular and Molecular Life Sciences*, **66**, 236-253. http://dx.doi.org/10.1007/s00018-008-8429-z

[44] Ross, S.E., Hemati, N., Longo, K.A., Bennett, C.N., Lucas, P.C., Erickson, R.L., *et al.* (2000) Inhibition of Adipogenesis by Wnt Signaling. *Science*, **289**, 950-953. http://dx.doi.org/10.1126/science.289.5481.950

[45] Krishnan, V., Bryant, H.U. and Macdougald, O.A. (2006) Regulation of Bone Mass by Wnt Signaling. *Journal of Clinical Investigation*, **116**, 1202-1209. http://dx.doi.org/10.1172/JCI28551

[46] Challa, T.D., Rais, Y. and Ornan, E.M. (2010) Effect of Adiponectin on ATDC5 Proliferation, Differentiation and Signaling Pathways. *Molecular and Cellular Endocrinology*, **323**, 282-291. http://dx.doi.org/10.1016/j.mce.2010.03.025

[47] Oshima, K., Nampei, A., Matsuda, M., Iwaki, M., Fukuhara, A., Hashimoto, J., *et al.* (2005) Adiponectin Increases Bone Mass by Suppressing Osteoclast and Activating Osteoblast. *Biochemical and Biophysical Research Communications*, **331**, 520-526. http://dx.doi.org/10.1016/j.bbrc.2005.03.210

[48] Lee, H.W., Kim, S.Y., Kim, A.Y., Lee, E.J., Choi, J.Y. and Kim, J.B. (2009) Adiponectin Stimulates Osteoblast Differentiation through Induction of COX2 in Mesenchymal Progenitor Cells. *Stem Cells*, **27**, 2254-2262. http://dx.doi.org/10.1002/stem.144

[49] Huang, C.Y., Lee, C.Y., Chen, M.Y., Tsai, H.C., Hsu, H.C. and Tang, C.H. (2010) Adiponectin Increases BMP-2 Ex-

pression in Osteoblasts via AdipoR Receptor Signaling Pathway. *Journal of Cellular Physiology*, **224**, 475-483. http://dx.doi.org/10.1002/jcp.22145

[50] Liu, L.F., Shen, W.J., Zhang, Z.H., Wang, L.J. and Kraemer, F.B. (2010) Adipocytes Decrease Runx2 Expression in Osteoblastic Cells: Roles of PPARgamma and Adiponectin. *Journal of Cellular Physiology*, **225**, 837-845. http://dx.doi.org/10.1002/jcp.22291

[51] Williams, G.A., Wang, Y., Callon, K.E., Watson, M., Lin, J.M., Lam, J.B., *et al.* (2009) *In Vitro* and *in Vivo* Effects of Adiponectin on Bone. *Endocrinology*, **150**, 3603-3610. http://dx.doi.org/10.1210/en.2008-1639

[52] Tu, Q., Zhang, J., Dong, L.Q., Saunders, E., Luo, E., Tang, J., *et al.* (2011) Adiponectin Inhibits Osteoclastogenesis and Bone Resorption via APPL1-Mediated Suppression of Akt1. *The Journal of Biological Chemistry*, **286**, 12542-12553. http://dx.doi.org/10.1074/jbc.M110.152405

[53] Jeyabalan, J., Shah, M., Viollet, B. and Chenu, C. (2012) AMP-Activated Protein Kinase Pathway and Bone Metabolism. *Journal of Endocrinology*, **212**, 277-290. http://dx.doi.org/10.1530/JOE-11-0306

[54] Kadowaki, T., Yamauchi, T., Kubota, N., Hara, K., Ueki, K. and Tobe, K. (2006) Adiponectin and Adiponectin Receptors in Insulin Resistance, Diabetes, and the Metabolic Syndrome. *The Journal of Clinical Investigation*, **116**, 1784-1792. http://dx.doi.org/10.1172/JCI29126

[55] Yamauchi, T., Kamon, J., Minokoshi, Y., Ito, Y., Waki, H., Uchida, S., *et al.* (2002) Adiponectin Stimulates Glucose Utilization and Fatty-Acid Oxidation by Activating AMP-Activated Protein Kinase. *Nature Medicine*, **8**, 1288-1295. http://dx.doi.org/10.1038/nm788

[56] Tomas, E., Tsao, T.S., Saha, A.K., Murrey, H.E., Zhang, C.C., Itani, S.I., *et al.* (2002) Enhanced Muscle Fat Oxidation and Glucose Transport by ACRP30 Globular Domain: Acetyl-CoA Carboxylase Inhibition and AMP-Activated Protein Kinase Activation. *Proceedings of the National Academy of Sciences of the United States of America*, **99**, 16309-16313. http://dx.doi.org/10.1073/pnas.222657499

[57] Berg, A.H., Combs, T.P., Du, X., Brownlee, M. and Scherer, P.E. (2001) The Adipocyte-Secreted Protein Acrp30 Enhances Hepatic Insulin Action. *Nature Medicine*, **7**, 947-953. http://dx.doi.org/10.1038/90992

[58] Shah, M., Kola, B., Bataveljic, A., Arnett, T.R., Viollet, B., Saxon, L., *et al.* (2010) AMP-Activated Protein Kinase (AMPK) Activation Regulates *in Vitro* Bone Formation and Bone Mass. *Bone*, **47**, 309-319. http://dx.doi.org/10.1016/j.bone.2010.04.596

[59] Kim, E.K., Lim, S., Park, J.M., Seo, J.K., Kim, J.H., Kim, K.T., *et al.* (2012) Human Mesenchymal Stem Cell Differentiation to the Osteogenic or Adipogenic Lineage Is Regulated by AMP-Activated Protein Kinase. *Journal of Cellular Physiology*, **227**, 1680-1687. http://dx.doi.org/10.1002/jcp.22892

[60] Lee, Y.S., Kim, Y.S., Lee, S.Y., Kim, G.H., Kim, B.J., Lee, S.H., *et al.* (2010) AMP Kinase Acts as a Negative Regulator of RANKL in the Differentiation of Osteoclasts. *Bone*, **47**, 926-937. http://dx.doi.org/10.1016/j.bone.2010.08.001

[61] Yamaguchi, N., Kukita, T., Li, Y.J., Kamio, N., Fukumoto, S., Nonaka, K., *et al.* (2008) Adiponectin Inhibits Induction of TNF-Alpha/RANKL-Stimulated NFATc1 via the AMPK Signaling. *FEBS Letters*, **582**, 451-456. http://dx.doi.org/10.1016/j.febslet.2007.12.037

[62] Waki, H., Yamauchi, T., Kamon, J., Ito, Y., Uchida, S., Kita, S., *et al.* (2003) Impaired Multimerization of Human Adiponectin Mutants Associated with Diabetes. Molecular Structure and Multimer Formation of Adiponectin. *The Journal of Biological Chemistry*, **278**, 40352-40363. http://dx.doi.org/10.1074/jbc.M300365200

[63] Pajvani, U.B., Hawkins, M., Combs, T.P., Rajala, M.W., Doebber, T., Berger, J.P., *et al.* (2004) Complex Distribution, Not Absolute Amount of Adiponectin, Correlates with Thiazolidinedione-Mediated Improvement in Insulin Sensitivity. *The Journal of Biological Chemistry*, **279**, 12152-12162. http://dx.doi.org/10.1074/jbc.M311113200

[64] Amemiya, N., Otsubo, S., Iwasa, Y., Onuki, T. and Nitta, K. (2012) Association between High-Molecular-Weight Adiponectin and Bone Mineral Density in Hemodialysis Patients. *Clinical and Experimental Nephrology*, **17**, 411-415. http://dx.doi.org/10.1007/s10157-012-0723-2

[65] Lee, N.K., Sowa, H., Hinoi, E., Ferron, M., Ahn, J.D., Confavreux, C., *et al.* (2007) Endocrine Regulation of Energy Metabolism by the Skeleton. *Cell*, **130**, 456-469. http://dx.doi.org/10.1016/j.cell.2007.05.047

[66] Fulzele, K., Riddle, R.C., DiGirolamo, D.J., Cao, X., Wan, C. and Chen, D. (2010) Insulin Receptor Signaling in Osteoblasts Regulates Postnatal Bone Acquisition and Body Composition. *Cell*, **142**, 309-319. http://dx.doi.org/10.1016/j.cell.2010.06.002

[67] Ferron, M., Wei, J., Yoshizawa, T., Del Fattore, A., DePinho, R.A., Teti, A., *et al.* (2010) Insulin Signaling in Osteoblasts Integrates Bone Remodeling and Energy Metabolism. *Cell*, **142**, 296-308. http://dx.doi.org/10.1016/j.cell.2010.06.003

[68] Hwang, Y.C., Jeong, I.K., Ahn, K.J. and Chung, H.Y. (2012) Circulating Osteocalcin Level Is Associated with Improved Glucose Tolerance, Insulin Secretion and Sensitivity Independent of the Plasma Adiponectin Level. *Osteoporosis International*, **23**, 1337-1342. http://dx.doi.org/10.1007/s00198-011-1679-x

[69] Hwang, Y.C., Jeong, I.K., Ahn, K.J. and Chung, H.Y. (2009) The Uncarboxylated Form of Osteocalcin Is Associated with Improved Glucose Tolerance and Enhanced Beta-Cell Function in Middle-Aged Male Subjects. *Diabetes/Metabolism Research and Reviews*, **25**, 768-772.

[70] Mao, X., Kikani, C.K., Riojas, R.A., Langlais, P., Wang, L., Ramos, F.J., *et al.* (2006) APPL1 Binds to Adiponectin Receptors and Mediates Adiponectin Signalling and Function. *Nature Cell Biology*, **8**, 516-523. http://dx.doi.org/10.1038/ncb1404

[71] Deepa, S.S. and Dong, L.Q. (2009) APPL1: Role in Adiponectin Signaling and Beyond. *American Journal of Physiology, Endocrinology and Metabolism*, **296**, E22-E36. http://dx.doi.org/10.1152/ajpendo.90731.2008

[72] Prior, J.C. (2007) FSH and Bone—Important Physiology or Not? *Trends in Molecular Medicine*, **13**, 1-3. http://dx.doi.org/10.1016/j.molmed.2006.11.004

[73] Lee, R.C., Feinbaum, R.L. and Ambros, V. (1993) The C. Elegans Heterochronic Gene *Lin*-4 Encodes Small RNAs with Antisense Complementarity to *Lin*-14. *Cell*, **75**, 843-854. http://dx.doi.org/10.1016/0092-8674(93)90529-Y

[74] Guo, L., Zhao, R.C. and Wu, Y. (2011) The Role of MicroRNAs in Self-Renewal and Differentiation of Mesenchymal Stem Cells. *Experimental Hematology*, **39**, 608-616. http://dx.doi.org/10.1016/j.exphem.2011.01.011

[75] Lian, J.B., Stein, G.S., van Wijnen, A.J., Stein, J.L., Hassan, M.Q., Gaur, T., *et al.* (2012) MicroRNA Control of Bone Formation and Homeostasis. *Nature Reviews Endocrinology*, **8**, 212-227. http://dx.doi.org/10.1038/nrendo.2011.234

[76] Turner, R.T., Maran, A., Lotinun, S., Hefferan, T., Evans, G.L., Zhang, M., *et al.* (2001) Animal Models for Osteoporosis. *Reviews in Endocrine and Metabolic Disorders*, **2**, 117-127. http://dx.doi.org/10.1023/A:1010067326811

[77] Pietschmann, P., Skalicky, M., Kneissel, M., Rauner, M., Hofbauer, G., Stupphann, D., *et al.* (2007) Bone Structure and Metabolism in a Rodent Model of Male Senile Osteoporosis. *Experimental Gerontology*, **42**, 1099-1108. http://dx.doi.org/10.1016/j.exger.2007.08.008

Permissions

All chapters in this book were first published by Scientific Research Publishing; hereby published with permission under the Creative Commons Attribution License or equivalent. Every chapter published in this book has been scrutinized by our experts. Their significance has been extensively debated. The topics covered herein carry significant findings which will fuel the growth of the discipline. They may even be implemented as practical applications or may be referred to as a beginning point for another development.

The contributors of this book come from diverse backgrounds, making this book a truly international effort. This book will bring forth new frontiers with its revolutionizing research information and detailed analysis of the nascent developments around the world.

We would like to thank all the contributing authors for lending their expertise to make the book truly unique. They have played a crucial role in the development of this book. Without their invaluable contributions this book wouldn't have been possible. They have made vital efforts to compile up to date information on the varied aspects of this subject to make this book a valuable addition to the collection of many professionals and students.

This book was conceptualized with the vision of imparting up-to-date information and advanced data in this field. To ensure the same, a matchless editorial board was set up. Every individual on the board went through rigorous rounds of assessment to prove their worth. After which they invested a large part of their time researching and compiling the most relevant data for our readers.

The editorial board has been involved in producing this book since its inception. They have spent rigorous hours researching and exploring the diverse topics which have resulted in the successful publishing of this book. They have passed on their knowledge of decades through this book. To expedite this challenging task, the publisher supported the team at every step. A small team of assistant editors was also appointed to further simplify the editing procedure and attain best results for the readers.

Apart from the editorial board, the designing team has also invested a significant amount of their time in understanding the subject and creating the most relevant covers. They scrutinized every image to scout for the most suitable representation of the subject and create an appropriate cover for the book.

The publishing team has been an ardent support to the editorial, designing and production team. Their endless efforts to recruit the best for this project, has resulted in the accomplishment of this book. They are a veteran in the field of academics and their pool of knowledge is as vast as their experience in printing. Their expertise and guidance has proved useful at every step. Their uncompromising quality standards have made this book an exceptional effort. Their encouragement from time to time has been an inspiration for everyone.

The publisher and the editorial board hope that this book will prove to be a valuable piece of knowledge for researchers, students, practitioners and scholars across the globe.

List of Contributors

Xueyan Lin, Miaomiao Wu, Guimei Liu, Yun Wang, Qiuling Hou, Kerong Shi and Zhonghua Wang
College of Animal Science and Technology, Shandong Agricultural University, Tai'an, China

Caio Antonio Carbonari, Giovanna Larissa Gimenes Cotrick Gomes, Edivaldo Domingues Velini, Renato Fernandes Machado, Plinio Saulo Simões and Gabrielle de Castro Macedo
Department of Crop Science, College of Agricultural Sciences, São Paulo State University (UNESP), Botucatu, Brazil

Godson O. Osuji, Aruna Weerasooriya, Peter A. Y. Ampim, Laura Carson, Paul Johnson, Yoonsung Jung, Eustace Duffus, Sela Woldesenbet, Sanique South, Edna Idan, Dewisha Johnson, Diadrian Clarke, Billy Lawton, Alfred Parks, Ali Fares, Alton Johnson
Plant Systems Research Unit, College of Agriculture and Human Sciences, Prairie View A & M University, Prairie View, USA

Marco A. A. Souza, Osmário J. L. Araújo, Diego M. C. Brito, Rosane N. Castro and Sonia R. Souza
Department of Chemistry, Universidade Federal Rural do Rio de Janeiro, Seropédica, Brazil

Manlio S. Fernandes
Soil Department, Universidade Federal Rural do Rio de Janeiro, Seropédica, Brazil

Pierre Pandin, Marie Renard, Alessia Bianchini, Philippe Desjardin and Luc Van Obbergh
Department of Anesthesia & Critical Care, Erasmus Academic Hospital, Université Libre de Bruxelles, Brussels, Belgium

Luca Mattei, Antonietta Colatrella, Olimpia Bitterman, Paola Bianchi, Chiara Giuliani, Giona Roma, Camilla Festa, Gianluca Merola, Vincenzo Toscano and Angela Napoli
Faculty of Medicine and Psychology, Sapienza University of Rome, Rome, Italy

Bor Luen Tang
Department of Biochemistry, Yong Loo Lin School of Medicine, National University of Singapore, Singapore

Hala Safwat Mohamed El-Bassiouny, Amany Abd El-Monem Attia and Maha Mohamed Abd Allah
Botany Department, Agriculture and Biology Division, National Research Center, Cairo, Egypt

Bakry Ahmed Bakry
Agronomy Department, Agriculture and Biology Division, National Research Center, Cairo, Egypt

Mozhgan Afkhamizadeh, Reza Rajabian and Armaghan Moravej Aleali
Endocrine Research Center, Ghaem Hospital, Mashhad University of Medical Sciences, Mashhad, Iran

Seyed Bahman Ghaderian
Health Research Institute, Diabetes Research Center, Ahvaz Jundishapur University of Medical Science, Ahvaz, Iran

Arnold M. Mahesan
Jones Institute for Reproductive Medicine, Eastern Virginia Medical School, Norfolk, VA, USA

Dotun Ogunyemi and B. M. Paul
Department of Obstetrics and Gynecology, Oakland University William Beaumont School of Medicine; Royal Oak, MI, USA

Eric Kim, Anthea and Y.-D. Ida Chen
LA Biomedical Research Center, Harbor-UCLA Medical Center, Torrance, CA, USA

Manel Ayoub, Nedra Grira, Nejla Stambouli, Chakib Mazigh and Zied Aouni
Biochemistry Department, Research Unit, Military Hospital of Tunis, Tunis, Tunisia

Chedia Zouaoui and Borni Zidi
Endocrinology Department, Research Unit, Military Hospital of Tunis, Tunis, Tunisia

Radhia Kochkar and Ezzedine Ghazouani
Immunology Department, Military Hospital of Tunis, Tunis, Tunisia

Chaker Bouguerra
Epidemiology Department, Research Unit, Military Hospital of Tunis, Tunis, Tunisia

Andrey Kratnov and Elena Timganova
Department of Therapy, Yaroslavl State Medical University, Yaroslavl, Russia

Young-Sil Lee, Midori Asai, Sun-Sil Choi, Takayuki Yonezawa, Kazuo Nagai and Byung-Yoon Cha
Research Institute for Biological Functions, Chubu University, Kasugai, Japan

Toshiaki Teruya
Faculty of Education, University of the Ryukyus, Nishihara, Japan

Je-Tae Woo
Department of Biological Chemistry, Chubu University, Kasugai, Japan

Department of Research and Development, Erina Co., Inc., Tokyo, Japan

Jitender Sharma and Surendra K. Bansal
Department of Biochemistry, Vallabhbhai Patel Chest Institute, University of Delhi, Delhi, India

Bala K. Menon
Department of Respiratory Allergy and Applied Immunology, Vallabhbhai Patel Chest Institute, University of Delhi, Delhi, India

Vannan K. Vijayan
Department of Pulmonary Medicine, Vallabhbhai Patel Chest Institute, University of Delhi, Delhi, India
Bhopal Memorial Hospital and Research Centre, Bhopal, India

Valentina Bashkatova, Sergey Sudakov, Galina Nazarova and Elena Alexeeva
P.K. Anokhin Research Institute of Normal Physiology, Moscow, Russia

Carlos Fernandes Baptista and Maria de Nazareth Gamboa Ritto
Gynecology Department, Escola Paulista de Medicina/ Universidade Federal de São Paulo (EPM-UNIFESP), São Paulo, Brazil
Departmento de Cirurgia Geral e Especializada, Universidade Federal do Rio de Janeiro (UNIRIO), Rio de Janeiro, Brazil

Samuel Marcos Ribeiro de Noronha and Silvana Aparecida Alves Corrêa de Noronha
Surgery Department, Escola Paulista de Medicina/ Universidade Federal de São Paulo (EPM-UNIFESP), São Paulo, Brazil

Eduardo Henrique da Silva Freitas
Gynecology Department, Escola Paulista de Medicina/ Universidade Federal de São Paulo (EPM-UNIFESP), São Paulo, Brazil
Departmento de Medicina Geral, Universidade Federal do Rio de Janeiro (UNIRIO), Rio de Janeiro, Brazil

Melquíades Pereira Júnior, Mauro Abi Haidar, Ismael Dale Cotrim Guerreiro da Silva and Marisa Teresinha Patriarca
Gynecology Department, Escola Paulista de Medicina/ Universidade Federal de São Paulo (EPM-UNIFESP), São Paulo, Brazil

Paula Cerezini
Department of Agronomy, Universidade Estadual de Londrina, Londrina, Brazil

Antonio Eduardo Pípolo, Mariangela Hungria and Marco Antonio Nogueira
Embrapa Soybean, Londrina, Brazil

Yanbin Hua, Yuqin Song, Caifang Tian and Liulin Li
College of Horticulture, Shanxi Agricultural University, Taigu, Shanxi, China

Jie Li
College of Horticulture, Shanxi Agricultural University, Taigu, Shanxi, China
College of Forestry, Shanxi Agricultural University, Taigu, Shanxi, China

Xin-Gen Zhou
AgriLife Research and Extension Center, Texas A&M University System, Beaumont, TX, USA

Santiago Imperial and Josep J. Centelles
Departament de Bioquímica i Biologia Molecular (Biologia), Facultat de Biologia, Universitat de Barcelona, Barcelona, Spain

Dimitra A. Loka, Derrick M. Oosterhuis and Cristiane Pilon
Altheimer Laboratory, Department of Crop, Soil and Environmental Sciences, University of Arkansas, Fayetteville, AR, USA

Anna Gałęba
Department of Social Medicine, Poznan University of Medical Sciences, Poznan, Poland
Private Practice of Aesthetic Medicine and Anti-Aging, Warszawa and Poznan, Poland

Jerzy T. Marcinkowski
Department of Social Medicine, Poznan University of Medical Sciences, Poznan, Poland

Fábio Ferreira do Espírito Santo and Denise Rosso Tenório Wanderley Rocha
Division of Endocrinology, IPEMED Medical School, Salvador, Brazil

Alberto Krayyem Arbex
Division of Endocrinology, IPEMED Medical School, Salvador, Brazil
Visiting Scientist of the Harvard T. H. Chan School of Public Health, Harvard University, Boston, USA

Teruhiko Matsushima, Noriko Yoshimura and Yuumi Koseki
Department of Human Life Science, Jissen Women's University, Tokyo, Japan

Etienne Z. Gnimpieba and Abalo Chango
Department of Nutritional Sciences and Health, EGEAL UPSP: 2007.05.137-Institut Polytechnique Lasalle Beauvais, Beauvais, France

Souad Bousserouel
Laboratoire de Prévention Nutritionnelle du Cancer, Inserm U682-IRCAD, Strasbourg, France

Elizabeth Jeya Vardhini Samuel
Department of General Medicine, MM Hospital, Tanjore, India

Nagarajan Natarajan
Department of General Medicine, Pondicherry Institute of Medical Sciences, Pondicherry, India

Sri Kumar
Dhonavur Fellowship Hospital, Dhonavur, India

Márcio Shigueaki Mito, Cristiane Vizioli de Castro, Rosane Marina Peralta and Adelar Bracht
Laboratory of Liver Metabolism, Department of Biochemistry, University of Maringá, Maringá, Brazil

Yuan Yu Lin, Ching Yi Chen, Chih Chien Chen, Han Jen Lin, Harry John Mersmann and Shinn Chih Wu
Department of Animal Science and Technology, National Taiwan University, Taiwan

Shih Torng Ding
Department of Animal Science and Technology, National Taiwan University, Taiwan
Institute of Biotechnology, National Taiwan University, Taiwan

Stephan Pflugmacher
Technische Universität Berlin, Institute of Ecology, Chair Ecological Impact Research and Ecotoxicology, Berlin, Germany
Korea Institute of Science and Technology, Centre for Water Resource Cycle Research, Seoul, Republic of Korea

Sandra Kühn and Valeska Contardo-Jara
Technische Universität Berlin, Institute of Ecology, Chair Ecological Impact Research and Ecotoxicology, Berlin, Germany

Sang-Hyup Lee
Korea Institute of Science and Technology, Centre for Water Resource Cycle Research, Seoul, Republic of Korea
Graduate School of Convergence Green Technology and Policy, Korea University, Seoul, Republic of Korea

Jae-Woo Choi
Korea Institute of Science and Technology, Centre for Water Resource Cycle Research, Seoul, Republic of Korea
Department of Energy and Environmental Engineering, University of Science and Technology (UST), Daejeon, Republic of Korea

Seungyun Bai
KIST Europe Forschungsgesellschaft mbH, Campus E71, Environment and Bio Group, Saarbrücken, Germany

Kyu-Sang Kwon
Korea Institute of Science and Technology, Centre for Water Resource Cycle Research, Seoul, Republic of Korea

www.ingramcontent.com/pod-product-compliance
Lightning Source LLC
Chambersburg PA
CBHW081710240326
41458CB00156B/4840

* 9 7 8 1 6 3 2 4 2 4 6 7 9 *